RADIOLOGY 101
The Basics and Fundamentals of Imaging

FOURTH EDITION

RADIOLOGY 101
The Basics and Fundamentals of Imaging

FOURTH EDITION

EDITORS

Wilbur L. Smith, MD
Professor and Chair
Diagnostic Radiology
Wayne State University School of Medicine
Academic Radiology (3L8)
Detroit Receiving Hospital
Detroit, Michigan

Thomas A. Farrell, MB, FRCR, MBA
Section Head, Interventional Radiology
NorthShore University HealthSystem
Clinical Assistant Professor of Radiology
Department of Radiology
The University of Chicago Pritzker School of Medicine
Evanston, Illinois

 Wolters Kluwer | Lippincott Williams & Wilkins
Health

Philadelphia · Baltimore · New York · London
Buenos Aires · Hong Kong · Sydney · Tokyo

Senior Executive Editor: Jonathan W. Pine, Jr.
Product Manager: Amy G. Dinkel
Vendor Manager: Bridgett Dougherty
Senior Manufacturing Coordinator: Beth Welsh
Senior Marketing Manager: Kimberly Schonberger
Senior Designer: Joan Wendt
Production Service: Aptara, Inc.

Printed in China

Library of Congress Cataloging-in-Publication Data
Radiology 101 : basics and fundamentals of imaging / editors, Wilbur L.
Smith, Thomas A. Farrell. – Fourth edition.
    p. ; cm.
  Radiology one o one
  Radiology one hundred one
  Radiology one hundred and one
  Basics and fundamentals of imaging
  Includes bibliographical references and index.
  ISBN 978-1-4511-4457-4 (alk. paper)
  I. Smith, Wilbur L., editor of compilation. II. Farrell, Thomas A. (Clinical assistant professor of radiology), editor of compilation. III. Title: Radiology one o one. IV. Title: Radiology one hundred one. V. Title: Radiology one hundred and one. VI. Title: Basics and fundamentals of imaging.
  [DNLM: 1. Diagnostic Imaging. 2. Radiology. WN 180]
  RC78
  616.07'54–dc23
                                                                 2013025390

Care has been taken to confirm the accuracy of the information presented and to describe generally accepted practices. However, the authors, editors, and publisher are not responsible for errors or omissions or for any consequences from application of the information in this book and make no warranty, expressed or implied, with respect to the currency, completeness, or accuracy of the contents of the publication. Application of the information in a particular situation remains the professional responsibility of the practitioner.

The authors, editors, and publisher have exerted every effort to ensure that drug selection and dosage set forth in this text are in accordance with current recommendations and practice at the time of publication. However, in view of ongoing research, changes in government regulations, and the constant flow of information relating to drug therapy and drug reactions, the reader is urged to check the package insert for each drug for any change in indications and dosage and for added warnings and precautions. This is particularly important when the recommended agent is a new or infrequently employed drug.

Some drugs and medical devices presented in the publication have Food and Drug Administration (FDA) clearance for limited use in restricted research settings. It is the responsibility of the health care provider to ascertain the FDA status of each drug or device planned for use in their clinical practice.

To purchase additional copies of this book, call our customer service department at (800) 638-3030 or fax orders to (301) 223-2320. International customers should call (301) 223-2300.

Visit Lippincott Williams & Wilkins on the Internet: at LWW.com. Lippincott Williams & Wilkins customer service representatives are available from 8:30 am to 6 pm, EST.

10 9 8 7 6 5 4 3 2 1

A teacher affects eternity; he can never tell where his influence stops.

Henry Adams (American Philosopher)

Almost 25 years ago a jovial roguish man with a dry wit decided to devote the rest of his professional career to teaching students the art of radiology. Coming from a practice in the Midwest he decided to join the faculty at the University of Iowa to "have some fun." His "fun" resulted in innumerable publications, grants, and teaching awards both national and university wide. His recognition of the need to spread his lighthearted and practical philosophy of learning led to the first three editions of this book. At the outset, Bill Erkonen was a practical man and insisted the book be written to let the reader have fun. The book has always been published in soft cover intentionally aiming to keep the costs low, within the budget of students. Bill is now fully retired and age is taking its toll but his spirit lives on in those he teaches and inspires today. This book is dedicated to his ongoing joy in teaching.

—Wilbur Smith

Contributing Authors

Carol A. Boles, MD
Associate Professor of Radiology
Department of Diagnostic Radiology
Wake Forest Baptist Medical Center
Winston-Salem, North Carolina

William E. Erkonen, MD
Associate Professor Emeritus of radiology
Department of Radiology
The University of Iowa
Iowa City, Iowa

Laurie L. Fajardo, MD, MBA, FACR
Clinical Assistant Professor of Radiology
Department of Radiology
The University of Chicago
NorthShore University HealthSystem
Evanston, Illinois

Thomas A. Farrell, MB, FRCR, MBA
Section Head, Interventional Radiology
NorthShore University HealthSystem
Clinical Assistant Professor of Radiology
Department of Radiology
The University of Chicago Pritzker School of Medicine
Evanston, Illinois

David M. Kuehn, MD
Associate Professor
Department of Radiology
The University of Iowa
Iowa City, Iowa

Vincent A. Magnotta, PhD
Associate Professor
Department of Radiology
The University of Iowa
Iowa City, Iowa

T. Shawn Sato, MD
Senior Radiology Resident
The University of Iowa
Iowa City, Iowa

Yutaka Sato, MD, FACR
Professor
Department of Radiology
The University of Iowa
Iowa City, Iowa

Ethan A. Smith, MD
Clinical Assistant Professor
Section of Pediatric Radiology
Department of Radiology
C.S. Mott Children's Hospital
University of Michigan Health System
Ann Arbor, Michigan

Wilbur L. Smith, MD
Professor and Chair
Diagnostic Radiology
Wayne State University School of Medicine
Academic Radiology (3L8)
Detroit Receiving Hospital
Detroit, Michigan

Brad H. Thompson, MD
Associate Professor
Department of Radiology
Division of Thoracic Imaging
Carver College of Medicine
University of Iowa Hospitals and Clinics
Iowa City, Iowa

Limin Yang, MD, PhD
Clinical Assistant Professor
Department of Radiology
The University of Iowa
Iowa City, Iowa

Preface

The astute reader will notice that the following four paragraphs of this preface are identical to those penned by Dr. Erkonen in the last edition. The reason is, we could not think how to say it any better. Bill established a philosophy and legacy that we have attempted to carry through to the new edition. There is a truism in Radiology, "Human diseases don't change much, just the way we image them."

The specialty of radiology has been around for over 100 years and has played a critical role in patient diagnosis and care. During the last 30 years the role of radiology in patient diagnosis and care has soared on the wings of extraordinary technologic advances. As you read this work, remember that diseases have not changed a lot, but the way we look at them has due to these new and improved technologies.

All too often, educators incorrectly assume that the students know something about the subject that they are about to study. Therefore, the third edition of *Radiology 101* assumes that the reader's knowledge of radiology is at the most basic level.

The primary purpose of this book is to give the reader a "feel" for radiologic anatomy and the radiologic manifestations of some common disease processes. After reading this book, you will be better prepared for consultation with the radiologist, and this usually leads to an appropriate diagnostic workup. As one develops an understanding of what radiology has to offer, improved patient diagnosis and care are likely to follow. In addition, the reader will be able to approach an image without feeling intimidated. You might say, "it will prepare you for the wards and boards." The book is not intended to transform the reader into a radiologist look-alike. Rather, it is designed to be a primer or general field guide to the basics of radiology.

Anatomy is the language of radiology. A solid foundation in good old-fashioned normal radiologic anatomy is essential to understand the various manifestations of diseases on radiologic images. Thus, this book places heavy emphasis on images, stressing normal anatomy and commonly encountered radiologic pathology. We present clearly labeled images of normal anatomy from a variety of angles not only on radiographs but also on other commonly used imaging modalities such as computed tomography, magnetic resonance imaging, and ultrasonography.

The fourth edition contains several updates and one new feature. The text and illustrations are updated to reflect the increasing applications of molecular imaging, digital imaging, and magnetic resonance imaging. New chapter authors have been added, each an expert in their field yet writing in a style that is concise and readable. In doing this we have attempted to maintain emphasis on the core role of basic imaging techniques such as bone radiographs, chest radiographs and basic ultrasound which form the basis suggesting advanced diagnostic imaging may be needed.

A short new chapter has been added on the appropriate use of imaging. Included in that chapter is a brief section on radiation exposure, a factor of increasing concern when requesting imaging examinations. Indications for examinations are a dynamic concept therefore the chapter emphasizes more where to find updated information, then specific prescriptions for imaging usage.

Adult learning theory suggests that testing on material engages learners beyond the more passive role of a reader. We have therefore added questions at the end of each chapter which the reader can use to self-assess their learning.

Above all we hope that this text continues to serve as an introduction to the wonderful field of imaging. We aspired to write a text that is easy to read and comprehend rather than one that is encyclopedic. Please reader, have fun and enjoy while you learn.

Acknowledgments

The editors thank our many contributing authors all of whom bear some professional association with Dr. Erkonen and/or the Department of Radiology of the University of Iowa. No acknowledgment could be complete without the recognition of Edmund (Tony) Franken, MD who brought together the critical elements for this effort.

We also wish to recognize our many assistants who helped us master the new world of publishing and the dedicated editorial staff who pushed and prodded even some of the Luddites among the authors until everything came together.

Finally Dr. Farrell and I thank our families who put up with us for many long evenings of rewrites and modifications. Dr. Farrell thanks his wife Laurie and daughters Niamh and Ciara, whose patience and forbearance made this book possible. And to his first teachers – his parents. It is especially gratifying to see that some of the family members of the original authors are now practicing the same profession and even contributing to the heritage the book represents.

Contents

SECTION I
Basic Principles

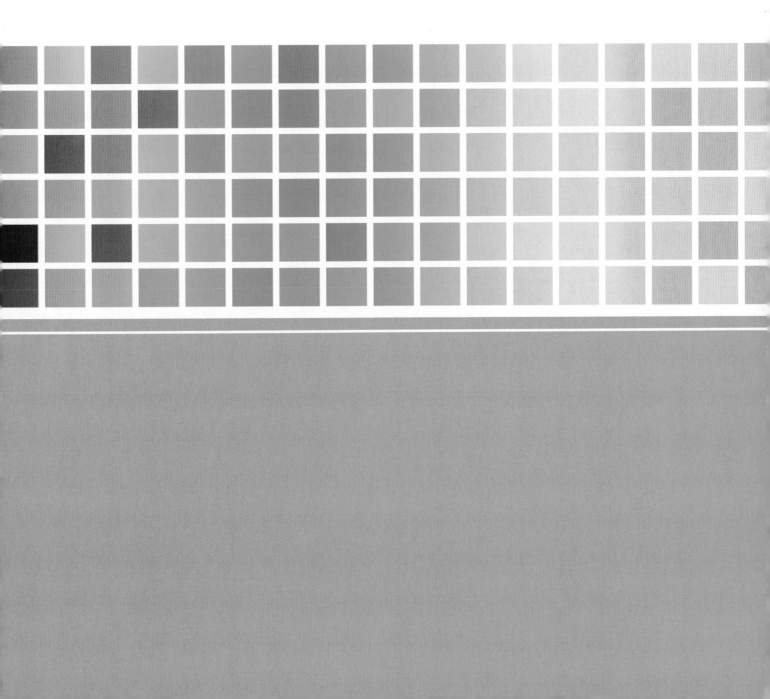

Radiography, Computed Tomography, Magnetic Resonance Imaging, and Ultrasonography: Principles and Indications

Vincent A. Magnotta • Wilbur L. Smith • William E. Erkonen

Few of us take the time to study, let alone enjoy, the physics of the technology that we use in our everyday lives. Almost everybody drives an automobile, for instance, but only a few of us have working knowledge about what goes on under our car hoods. The medical technology that produces imaging studies is often met with a similar reception: We all want to drive the car, so to speak, but we do not necessarily want to understand the principles underlying the computed tomograms or magnetic resonance (MR) images that we study. Yet, a basic understanding of imaging modalities is extremely important, because you will most likely be reviewing images throughout your professional career and the results of these consultations will affect your making a clinical decision. The interpretation of imaging studies is to a considerable degree dependent on understanding how the images are produced. One does not necessarily have to be a mechanic to be a skilled driver, but you do need to know when to put fuel in the car. Similarly, reaching a basic understanding of how imaging studies are produced is a necessary first step to critically viewing the images themselves. This chapter is designed to demonstrate the elementary physics of radiologic diagnostic imaging.

RADIOGRAPHY

Radiographs are the most common imaging consultations requested by clinicians. So let us set off on the right foot by referring to radiologic images as *radiographs, images,* or *films,* but not *x-rays.* After all, x-rays are electromagnetic waves produced in an x-ray tube. It is acceptable for a layperson to refer to a radiograph as an x-ray, but the knowledgeable clinician and healthcare worker should avoid the term. Your usage of appropriate terminology demonstrates your *savoir-faire* (the ability to say and do the right thing) to your colleagues and patients.

    Whenever possible, radiographs are accomplished in the radiology department. The number of views obtained during a standard or routine study depends on the anatomic site being imaged. The common radiographic views are named according to the direction of the x-ray beam and referred to as posteroanterior (PA), anteroposterior (AP), oblique, and lateral views.

    The chest will be used to illustrate these basic radiographic terms, but this terminology applies to almost all anatomic sites. PA indicates that the central x-ray beam

3

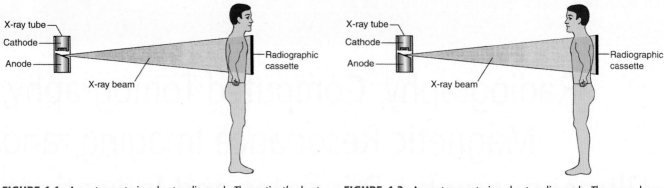

FIGURE 1.1. A posteroanterior chest radiograph. The patient's chest is pressed against the cassette with hands on the hips. The x-ray beam emanating from the x-ray tube passes through the patient's chest in a posterior-to-anterior or back-to-front direction. The x-rays that pass completely through the patient eventually strike the radiographic film and screens inside the radiographic cassette.

FIGURE 1.3. An anteroposterior chest radiograph. The x-ray beam passes through the patient's chest in an anterior-to-posterior or front-to-back direction. Note that the patient's hands are on the hips.

travels from posterior to anterior or back to front as it traverses the chest or any other anatomic site (Fig. 1.1). Lateral indicates that the x-ray beam travels through the patient from side to side (Fig. 1.2). When the patient is unable to cooperate for these routine views, a single AP upright or supine view is obtained. AP means that the x-ray beam passes through the chest or other anatomic site from anterior to posterior or front to back (Fig. 1.3). PA and AP radiographs have similar appearances but subtle difference in magnification of structures, particularly the heart. When the patient cannot tolerate a transfer to the radiology facility, a portable study is obtained, which means that a portable x-ray machine is brought to the patient wherever he or she is located. AP is the standard portable technique with the patient sitting or supine (Fig. 1.4). Portable radiographic equipment generates less powerful x-ray beams than fixed units and therefore, the prevalence of suboptimal images is greater.

Radiographs have traditionally been described in terms of shades of black, white, and gray. What causes a structure to appear black, white, or gray on a radiograph? Actually, it is the density of the object being imaged that determines how much of the x-ray beam will be absorbed or attenuated (Fig. 1.5). In other words, as the density of an object increases, fewer x-rays pass through it. It is the variable density of structures that results in the four basic radiographic classifications: Air (black), fat (black), water

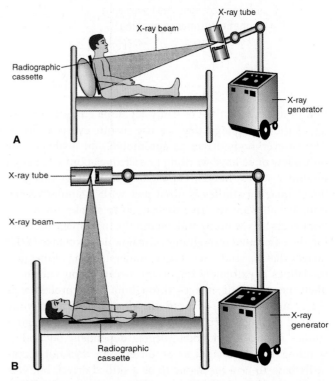

FIGURE 1.4. An anteroposterior portable chest radiograph with the patient either sitting **(A)** or supine **(B)**. The x-ray beam passes through the patient's chest in an anterior-to-posterior direction. The x-ray machine has wheels and this allows it to be used wherever needed throughout the hospital.

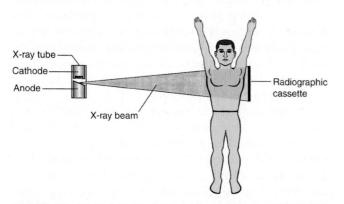

FIGURE 1.2. A lateral chest radiograph. The x-ray beam passes through the patient's chest from side to side. The x-rays that pass completely through the patient eventually strike the radiographic film and screens. Note that the patient's arms are positioned as not to project over the chest.

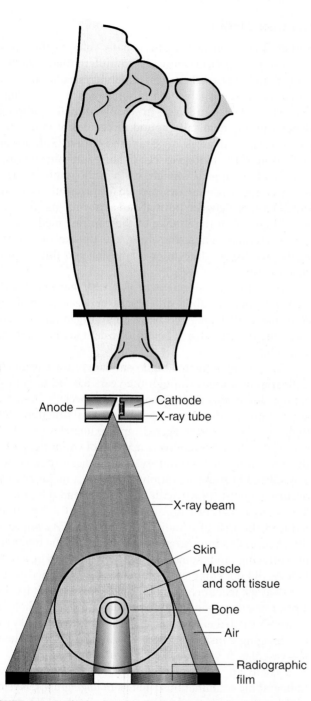

FIGURE 1.5. A: The level in the distal thigh through which the x-ray beam is passing in **(B)**. **B:** Cross-section of the distal thigh at the level indicated in **(A)**. Notice that when the x-ray beam passes through air, the result is a black area on the radiograph. When the x-ray beam strikes bone, the result is a white area on the radiograph. If the x-ray beam passes through soft tissues, the result is a gray appearance on the film.

Table 1.1	
Basic Radiograph Film Densities or Appearances	
Object	**Film Density**
Air	Black
Fat	Black
Bone	White
Metal	White
Calcium	White
Organs, muscles, soft tissues	Shades of gray

its density is slightly greater than that of air. Fat will appear black on a radiograph but slightly less black than air. High-density objects such as bones, teeth, calcium deposits in tumors, metallic foreign bodies, right and left lead film markers, and intravascularly injected contrast media absorb all or nearly all of the x-ray beam. As a result, the radiographic film receives little or no x-ray exposure, and these dense structures appear white. Muscles, organs (heart, liver, spleen), and other soft tissues appear as shades of gray, and the shades of gray range somewhere between white and black depending on the structure's density. These shades of gray are referred to as *water density*.

In the "old days" when films were widely employed as an image storage/display medium, radiographic screens are positioned on both sides of a sheet of film inside the lighttight cassette or film holder (Fig. 1.6A). The chemical structure of the screens causes them to emit light flashes or to fluoresce when struck by x-rays (Fig. 1.6B). Actually, it is the fluoresced light from the screens on both sides of the film that accounts for the major exposure of the radiographic film. The direct incident x-rays striking the radiographic film account for only a small proportion of the film exposure. The use of screens decreases the amount of radiation required to produce a radiograph, and this in turn decreases the patient's exposure to radiation. *It is important to remember that radiographic films, photographic films, and the currently used phosphor plates for digital radiography (DR) all respond in a similar manner to light and x-rays. While film recording is going the way of the dodo, this principal remains valid.*

Computed Radiography (Digital Radiography)

In conventional radiography, the radiographic image is recorded on film that goes through chemical processing for development. Computed radiography (CR) or digital radiography (DR) is the process of producing a digital radiographic image. Instead of film, a special phosphor plate is exposed to the x-ray beam. The image information is obtained by scanning the phosphor plate with a laser beam that causes light to be released from the phosphor plate. The intensity of the emitted light depends on the local radiation exposure. This emitted light is intensified by a

(gray), and metal or bone (white; Table 1.1). For example, the lungs primarily consist of low-density air, which absorbs very little of the x-ray beam. Thus, air allows a large amount of the x-ray beam to strike or expose the radiographic film. As a result, air in the lungs will appear black on a radiograph. Similarly, fat has a low density, but

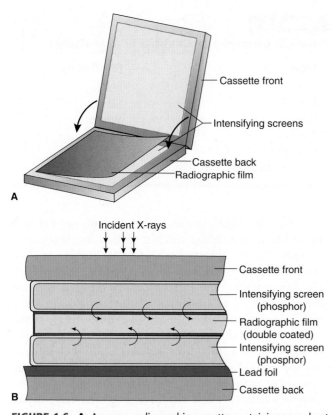

A

B

FIGURE 1.6. A: An open radiographic cassette containing one sheet of radiographic film and two intensifying screens. A radiographic screen is positioned on each side of the film, and the screens emit a light flash (fluoresce) when struck by an x-ray. Also, some x-rays directly strike the radiographic film. This combination of light flashes from the screens and x-rays directly striking the film causes the radiographic film to be exposed. This is similar to photographic film. **B:** Cross-sectional illustration of a radiographic cassette. Note the lead foil in the back of the cassette that is designed to stop any x-rays that have penetrated the full thickness of the cassette. The *curved arrows* represent light flashes that are created when x-rays strike the screens.

photomultiplier tube and is subsequently converted into an electron stream. The electron stream is digitized, and the digital data are converted into an image by computer. The resulting image can be viewed on a monitor or transferred to a radiographic film. The beauty of this system is that the digital image can be transferred via networks to multiple sites in or out of the hospital, and the digital images are easily stored in a computer or on a server. For example, a digital chest radiograph obtained in an intensive care unit can be transmitted to the radiology department for consultation and interpretation in a matter of seconds. Then the radiologist can send this image via a network back to the intensive care unit or to the referring physician's office and this digital information would be stored in a computer (server) for future recall. This technology is used routinely in the practice of medicine to share images between the radiologist and referring physicians.

Contrast Media

Radiographic contrast media usually refer to the use of intravascular pharmaceuticals to differentiate between normal and abnormal tissues, to define vascular anatomy, and to improve visualization of some organs. These high-density pharmaceuticals in conventional radiology depend upon chemically bound molecules of iodine that cause varying degrees of x-ray absorption. Soft tissues such as muscles, blood vessels, organs, and some diseased tissues often appear similar on a radiograph. Usually, when contrast agents are injected intravascularly to tell the difference between normal and abnormal tissues there is a difference in the uptake of the contrast media in the various tissues. Thus, the more the uptake of contrast media in a tissue, the whiter it appears, and this is called *enhancement*.

It is this enhancement or contrast that enables the viewer to detect subtle differences between normal and abnormal soft tissues and between an organ and the surrounding tissues. Also, it beautifully demonstrates arteries and veins.

The use of iodinated high-osmolar contrast agents for radiographic studies through the years has led to complications due to this high-osmolar load especially in infants and in individuals with compromised renal function. With high-osmolar contrast agents, approximately 7% of the people developed reactions consisting of vomiting, pain at the injection site, respiratory symptoms, urticaria, and generalized burning sensation. However, a major advance occurred in the 1990s with the widespread adoption of low-osmolar contrast agents (LOCAs) that substantially reduced the risk of osmolar reactions. LOCAs improved the comfort of administration and decreased the frequency of annoying and sometimes life-threatening reactions. LOCAs did not completely eliminate the incidence of serious contrast reaction and nephropathy. If a patient has had a prior reaction, one should consult with one's radiologist to weigh the benefit versus the risk and possible alternative imaging considered especially in patients with diabetes, vascular disease, or renal dysfunction.

There are many uses for iodinated compounds in radiographic examinations such as in *angiography, myelography, arthrography,* and *computed tomography (CT)*. *Angiography* is merely the injection of an iodinated contrast media directly into a vein or artery via a needle and/or catheter (see Chapter 11). *Arthrography* is the injection of contrast media and/or air into a joint. Air may be used alone or in combination with these compounds to improve contrast. It has been used to image multiple joints such as rotator cuff injuries of the shoulder and to assess meniscus injuries in the knee. Since the advent of CT and magnetic resonance imaging (MRI), the arthrogram has become less important. *Myelography* is the placement of contrast media in the spinal subarachnoid space, usually via a lumbar puncture. This procedure is useful for diagnosing diseases in and around the spinal canal and cord. Because of the advent of the less invasive CT and MRI modalities, the use of myelogram studies has been decreasing.

Another type of contrast media is used for the gastro-intestinal (GI) tract. A heavy metal-based compound (usually barium) defines the mucosal pattern very well. To accomplish a GI contrast examination, the barium sulfate suspension is introduced into the GI tract by oral ingestion (upper GI series) or through an intestinal tube (small bowel series) or as an enema (barium enema). When air along with the barium is introduced into the GI tract, the result is called a double-contrast study. Barium studies are safer, better tolerated by patients, and relatively inexpensive compared with the more invasive GI endoscopic studies. Barium studies can be effective in diagnosing a wide variety of GI pathology, as they are quite sensitive and specific. With the widespread use of CT to study GI pathology, both barium- and iodine-based contrast agents have been utilized. Owing to the contrast sensitivity of CT, a much lower concentration (not volume) of barium or iodine is employed for bowel visualization.

When the integrity of the GI tract is in question, there exists a potential for catastrophic extravasation of the barium into the mediastinum and peritoneum. In these situations, barium studies are contraindicated and a water-soluble iodinated compound should be used. As a general rule, images produced with water-soluble contrast agents are less informative than barium studies, because the water-soluble agents are less dense than barium, do not adhere as well to mucosa, and result in poorer contrast.

In MRI, standard iodinated contrast agents are of no use. Instead, we use magnetically active compounds such as gadolinium or other metals such as iron oxide with unpaired electrons (paramagnetic effects) to enhance imaging certain disease processes. Gadolinium does not produce an MR signal but does cause changes in local magnetic fields by inducing T1 shortening in tissues where it has localized. It is useful for imaging tumors, infections, and acute cerebral vascular accidents. Although the principles of MRI and CT differ, the practical outcomes are similar. They both cause lesion enhancing or in other words a lesion is whiter than the surrounding tissues (Fig. 1.7).

Gadolinium generally has a low risk for reactions and/or nephropathy, but it can cause a severe connective tissue disorder, *nephrogenic sclerosing fibrosis (NSF)*. NSF virtually only occurs in patients who are on dialysis or have a creatinine clearance less than 30 mg/dL. This disease is a very serious complication and is similar to scleroderma. The takeaway lesson on gadolinium is *to consult with your radiologist* on any patient with known renal failure or a history of NSF before requesting a contrast-enhanced MRI examination.

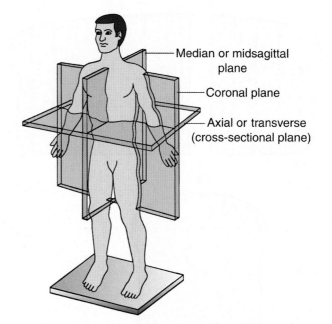

FIGURE 1.7. Sagittal, coronal, and axial anatomic planes.

COMPUTED TOMOGRAPHY

CT involves sectional anatomy imaging or anatomy in the sagittal, coronal, and axial (cross-sectional, transverse) planes. These terms, which can be confusing, are clearly illustrated in Figure 1.7. Sectional anatomy has always been important to physicians and other healthcare workers, but the newer imaging modalities of CT, MRI, and ultrasonography (US) demand an in-depth understanding of anatomy displayed in this manner.

CT, sometimes referred to as computerized axial tomography (CAT) scan technology, was developed in the 1970s. The rock group, The Beatles gave a big boost to CT development when it invested a significant amount of money in a business called Electric Musical Instruments Limited (EMI). It was EMI engineers who subsequently developed CT technology. Initially, EMI scanners were used exclusively for brain imaging, but this technology was rapidly extended to the abdomen, thorax, spine, and extremities.

CT imaging is best understood if the anatomic site to be examined is thought of as a loaf of sliced bread; an image of each slice of bread is created without imaging the other slices (Fig. 1.8). This is in contradistinction to a radiograph, which captures the whole loaf of bread as in a photograph.

The external appearance of a typical CT unit or machine is illustrated in Figure 1.9. CT images are produced by a combination of x-rays, computers, and detectors. A computer-controlled couch transfers the patient in short increments through the opening in the scanner housing. In the original, now near-extinct standard CT unit, the x-ray tube located in the housing (gantry) rotates around the patient, and each anatomic slice to be imaged

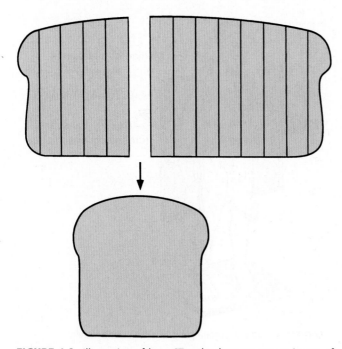

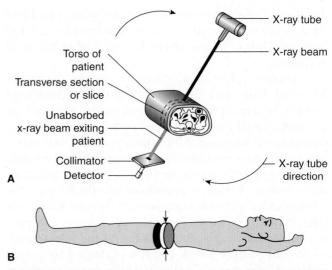

FIGURE 1.10. A: Illustration of how the x-ray tube circles the patient's abdomen to produce an image (slice) as shown in **(B)**. **B:** Demonstration of how a CT scan creates a thin-slice axial image of the abdomen (*arrows*) without imaging the remainder of the abdomen.

FIGURE 1.8. Illustration of how CT technology creates an image of a single slice of bread from a loaf of sliced bread without imaging the other slices.

is exposed to a pencil-thin x-ray beam (Fig. 1.10). Each image or slice requires only a few seconds; therefore, breath-holding is usually not an issue. The thickness of these axial images or slices can be varied from 1 to 10 mm depending on the indications for the study. For example, in the abdomen and lungs we commonly use a 10-mm slice thickness because the structures are large. A slice thickness of only a few millimeters is used to image small structures like those found in the middle and inner ear. An average CT study takes approximately 10 to 20 minutes depending on the circumstances.

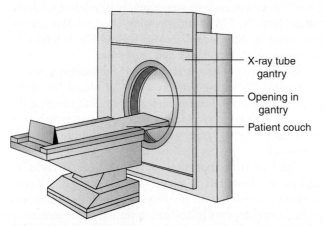

FIGURE 1.9. A standard CT scanner or machine. The patient couch or cradle is fed through the opening in the x-ray tube gantry or housing, and the anatomic part to be imaged is centered in this opening. The x-ray tube is located inside the gantry and moves around the patient to create an image.

As in a radiograph, the amount of the x-ray beam that passes through each slice or section of the patient will be inversely proportional to the density of the traversed tissues. The x-rays that pass completely through the patient eventually strike detectors (not film), and the detectors subsequently convert these incident x-rays to an electron stream. This electron stream is digitized or converted to numbers referred to as CT units or Hounsfield units; then computer software converts these numbers to corresponding shades of black, white, and gray. A dense structure, such as bone, will absorb most of the x-ray beam and allow only a small amount of x-rays to strike the detectors. The result is a white density on the image. On the other hand, air will absorb little of the x-ray beam, allowing a large number of x-rays to strike the detectors. The result is a black density on the image. Soft tissue structures appear gray on the image.

This CT digital information can be displayed on a video monitor, stored on magnetic tape, transmitted across computer networks, or printed on radiographic film via a format camera.

Because CT technology uses x-rays, the image densities of the anatomic structures being examined are the same on both CT images and radiographs. In other words, air appears black on both a CT image and a radiograph and bone appears white on both modalities. One major difference between a radiograph and a CT image is that a radiograph displays the entire anatomic structure, whereas a CT image allows us to visualize slices of a structure; using CT the x-rays are recorded by devices called detectors and converted to digital data.

CT imaging is accomplished with and/or without intravenously injected contrast media. The intravenous contrast media enhance or increase the density of blood

Table 1.2

Some Common Indications for CT Imaging

Trauma
Intracranial hemorrhage (suspected or known)
Abdominal injury, especially to organs
Fracture detection and evaluation
Spine alignment
Detection of foreign bodies (especially in joints)
Diagnosis of primary and secondary neoplasms
    (liver, renal, brain, lung, and bone)
Tumor staging

vessels, vascular soft tissues, organs, and tumors as in a radiograph. This enhancement assists in distinguishing between normal tissue and a pathologic process. Contrast media are not needed when searching for intracerebral hemorrhage or a suspected fracture or for evaluating a fracture fragment within a joint. However, contrast is used when evaluating the liver, kidney, and brain for primary and secondary neoplasms. A few of the common indications for CT imaging are listed in Table 1.2. Oral GI contrast agents may be administered prior to an abdominal CT to delineate the contrast-filled GI tract from other abdominal structures.

Helical or spiral CT technology is similar to standard CT but with a few new twists. In helical or spiral CT, the patient continuously moves through the gantry while the x-ray tube continuously encircles the patient (Fig. 1.11). This combination of the patient and the x-ray tube continuously moving, results in a spiral configuration. This technology can produce slices which may vary in thickness from 1 to 10 mm. The resolution and contrast of these images are

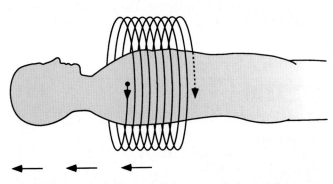

FIGURE 1.11. A helical or spiral CT scanner. The x-ray tube continuously circles the patient while the patient couch moves continuously through the opening in the x-ray tube gantry. The combination of continuous patient and x-ray tube movement results in a spiral configuration, hence the name "helical." In a standard CT or nonhelical scanner, the patient couch moves in short increments toward the gantry opening and stops intermittently to allow the x-ray tube to move around the patient. Thus, the x-ray tube moves around the patient only when the couch is stationary.

better than on standard CT images, resulting in improved images in areas such as the thorax and the abdomen.

Multislice/Dynamic Computed Tomography

The early conventional CT scanners had only a single row of detectors, thus only one tomographic slice or image was generated with each rotation of the x-ray tube around the patient. The current state of the art is multislice CT. This equipment has multiple contiguous rows of detectors that yield multiple tomographic slices with only one rotation of the x-ray tube around the patient. There can be many detector rings in one CT unit, thus resulting in multiple image slices of a 15-cm segment of anatomy. Hence, large volumes can be scanned in short periods of time, and the slice thickness varies depending on the structure being imaged. For example, one rotation around the cervical spine encompassing the base of the skull to T3 would take 11 seconds. Subsequently, with software this data can immediately create a three-dimensional (3D) reconstruction and even a cine. The resulting 3D image can be rotated and examined visually in multiple orientations. The data is digital and affords the opportunity to electronically edited out structures such as the ribs from the images.

This increased speed of volume coverage by the multislice CT is especially beneficial in CT angiography or dynamic CT. For example, in CT angiography or dynamic CT the multislice scanner can cover the entire abdominal aorta in 15 seconds. Following a bolus injection of contrast media, serial angiographic images of the aorta or any area of interest can be made to observe the movement of contrast media through the area of interest during the arterial and venous phases. Some advantages and disadvantages of the multidetector CT are listed in Table 1.3.

Dual-Source Computed Tomography

Dual-source CT scanners utilize two different x-ray energies that originate from a single tube that is rapidly switched between energies or from two separate x-ray tubes. Dual-energy scanners also utilize multiple detectors and helical scanning. The gray value in CT images is dependent not only on the density and thickness of the object being measured, but also the energy of the x-rays.

Table 1.3

Advantages and Disadvantages of Multislice CT

Advantages
Static and cine or movie images
Noninvasive
Rapid filming results in decreased motion artifact
Good spatial resolution

Disadvantages
Expensive

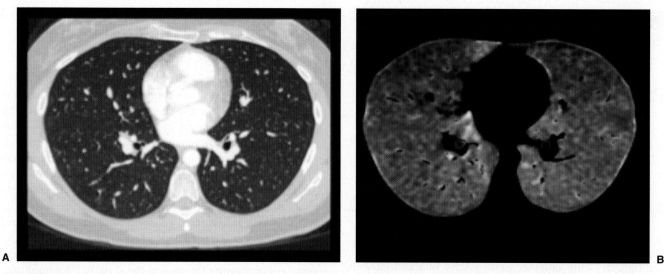

FIGURE 1.12. Dual-energy dynamic contrast-enhanced lung perfusion blood volume study obtained from a normal subject. **A:** Cross-sectional CT image generated with a 140-kV x-ray. **B:** The resulting blood volume. This demonstrates the ability of dual-energy imaging to determine tissue composition. (Image courtesy of Drs. Eric A. Hoffman, PhD and John D. Newell Jr, MD, Iowa Comprehensive Lung Imaging Center, University of Iowa Carver College of Medicine.)

That is, an image generated with low- and high-energy x-rays will have different gray values for the same object. The two images resulting from the low- and high-energy x-rays can be combined using a weighted subtraction. Dual-energy imaging has a number of applications including direct removal of bone for angiographic imaging, plaque characterization, lung perfusion (Fig. 1.12), identification of ligaments and tendons, and assessment of tissue composition. Radiation dose is a potential concern using dual-source scanners. Low tube currents can be used to acquire images with doses similar to convention CT images; however, image noise will be higher. The dose can be further reduced using dual-source imaging by creating virtual unenhanced images from the dual-energy images, thus eliminating the need for precontrast scans.

MAGNETIC RESONANCE IMAGING

MRI or MR is another method for displaying anatomy in the axial, sagittal, and coronal planes, and the slice thicknesses of the images vary between 1 and 10 mm. MRI is especially good for coronal and sagittal imaging, whereas axial imaging is the forte of CT. One of the main strengths of MRI is its ability to detect small changes (contrast) within soft tissues, and MRI soft-tissue contrast is considerably better than that found on CT images and radiographs.

CT and MR imaging modalities are digital-based technologies that require computers to convert digital information to shades of black, white, and gray. The major difference in the two technologies is that in MRI, the patient is exposed to external magnetic fields and radiofrequency waves, whereas during a CT study the patient is exposed to x-rays. The magnetic fields used in MRI are believed to be harmless. While most studies have shown that MRI is safe for the fetus, several animal studies have suggested that there is the potential for teratogenic effects during early fetal development. The safety concerns to the fetus are primarily related to teratogenesis and acoustic damage. Therefore, MRI should be used cautiously, especially during the first trimester. However, maternal safety is the same as that for imaging a nonpregnant patient.

MR scanning can be a problem for people who are prone to develop claustrophobia, because they are surrounded by a tunnel-like structure for approximately 30 to 45 minutes. Some of the advantages and disadvantages of MRI are summarized in Table 1.4. There are a few contraindications for an MRI study, and these are listed in Table 1.5.

Table 1.4
Advantages and Disadvantages of MRI
Advantages
Static and cine or movie images
Multiple plane images
Good contrast
No known health hazards
Good for soft-tissue injuries of the knee, ankle, and shoulder joints
Disadvantages
More expensive than CT
Long scan times may result in claustrophobia and motion artifacts

Table 1.5
Contraindications for MRI Studies
Cerebral aneurysms clipped by ferromagnetic clips
Cardiac pacemakers
Inner ear implants
Metallic foreign bodies in and around the eyes

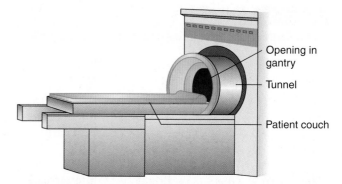

FIGURE 1.13. Illustration of an MRI scanner. Notice that its external appearance is similar to that of a CT scanner. The main difference, of course, is that there is a magnetic field rather than an x-ray tube around the gantry opening.

The external appearance of an MRI scanner or machine is similar to that of a CT scanner with the exception that the opening in the MRI gantry is more tunnel-like (Fig. 1.13). As in CT, the patient is comfortably positioned supine, prone, or decubitus on a couch. The couch moves only when examining the extremities or areas of interest longer than 40 cm. The patient hears and feels a jackhammer-like thumping while the study is in progress.

The underlying physics of MRI is complicated and strange sounding terms proliferate. Let us keep it simple: Human *MRI is essentially the imaging of protons.* The most commonly imaged proton is hydrogen, as it is abundant in the human body and is easily manipulated by a magnetic field; however, other nuclei can also be imaged. Because the hydrogen proton has a positive charge and is constantly spinning at a fixed frequency (*spin frequency*), a small magnetic field with a north pole and a south pole surrounds the proton, a moving charged particle creates a surrounding magnetic field. Thus, these hydrogen protons act like magnets and align themselves within an external magnetic field much like nails in a magnetic field or the needle of a compass.

While in the MRI scanner, or magnet, short bursts of radio-frequency waves are broadcast into the patient from radio transmitters. The broadcast radio wave frequency is the same as the spin frequency of the proton being imaged (hydrogen in this case). The hydrogen protons absorb the broadcast radio wave energy and become energized or *resonate*, hence the term MR. Once the radio-frequency wave broadcast is discontinued, the protons revert or decay back to their normal or steady state that existed prior to the radio wave broadcast. As the hydrogen protons decay back

to their normal state or relax, they continue to resonate and broadcast radio waves that can be detected by a radio wave receiver set to the same frequency as the broadcast radio waves and the hydrogen proton spin frequency (Fig. 1.14). The intensity of the radio wave signal detected by the receiver coil indicates the numbers and locations of the resonating hydrogen protons. These analog (wave) data received by the receiver coil are subsequently converted to numbers (digitized), and the numbers are converted to shades of black, white, and gray by computers.

For example, there are many hydrogen atoms and protons present in fat, and the received radio wave signal will be intense or very bright. However, there is much less hydrogen in bone cortex, and the received radio wave signal is of low intensity or black. The overall result is a 3D proton density plot or map of the anatomic slice being examined. Now comes the complicated part. The received radio wave signal intensity from the patient is determined not only by the number of hydrogen atoms but also by the T1 and T2 relaxation times. If the radio receivers listen early during the decay following the discontinuance of the radio wave broadcast, it is called a T1-weighted sequence. In a T1 image, the fat is white and the gray soft tissue detail is excellent. If the radio receivers listen late during the decay, it is called a T2-weighted sequence wherein the water in soft tissues is now a lighter gray and fat appears

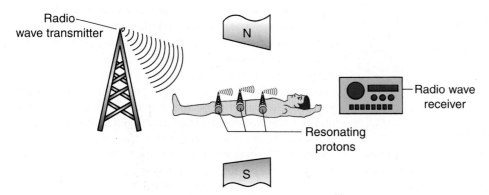

FIGURE 1.14. The general principles of MRI physics. The frequencies of the radio wave transmitter, the radio wave receiver, and the spin frequency of hydrogen atom protons are the same.

Table 1.6

A Comparison of Structure Appearances on Images[a]

Object	CT and Radiographs	MRI T1	T2
Air	Black	Dark	Dark
Fat	Black	Very bright	Intermediate to dark
Muscles	Gray	Dark	Dark
Bone cortex	White	Dark	Dark
Bone marrow	Gray	Bright	Intermediate to dark
Gadolinium		Very bright	Bright

[a]On MR images, the words dark, low-intensity signal, and black are synonymous; bright, high-intensity signal, and white are synonymous; and intermediate-intensity-signal and gray are synonymous.

gray. The simplest way to think of T1 and T2 is as two different technical ways to look at the same structure. This is analogous to the PA and lateral radiographs being two different ways to view a bone or the chest. We tend to use T1 imaging when seeking anatomic information. T2 imaging is helpful when searching for pathology, because most pathology tends to contain considerable amounts of water or hydrogen and T2 causes water to light up like a light bulb. In general, T1 images have good resolution and T2 images have better contrast than T1 images.

Although human anatomy is always the same no matter what the imaging modality, the appearances of anatomic structures are very different on MR and CT images. Sometimes it is difficult for the beginner to differentiate between a CT image and an MR image. The secret is to *look to the fat*. If the subcutaneous fat is black, it is a CT image as fat appears black on studies that use x-rays. If the subcutaneous fat is white (high-intensity signal), then it has to be an MRI. Next, *look to the bones*. Bones should have a gray medullary canal and a white cortex on radiographs and CT images. The medullary canal contains bone marrow, and the gray is due to the large amount of fat in bone marrow. On a T1 MR image nearly all of the bone medullary cavities appear homogeneously white, as the bone marrow is fat that emits a high-intensity signal and appears white. Also, on MRI the cortex of the bone will appear black (dark or low-intensity signal), whereas on CT images the cortex is white. Soft tissues and organs appear as shades of gray on both CT and MR. Air appears black on CT and has a low-intensity signal (black or dark) on MR. Table 1.6 compares the appearances of various structures on MR and CT images.

Magnetic Resonance Angiography

Magnetic resonance angiography (MRA) is a special non-interventional study that can image vessels without using needles, catheters, or iodinated contrast media. As a general rule, flowing blood appears black on most MR images, but by using a special imaging technique (gradient-echo pulse sequence) the arterial and venous blood appears as a high-intensity signal, or bright (Fig. 1.15). This procedure allows reconstruction of 3D images of the vasculature that can be reconstructed with the digital information. MRA has been effective for imaging arteries and veins in the head and neck, abdomen, chest, and extremities. Gadolinium is the contrast media utilized when imaging smaller vessels, as in the distal extremities. However, as a general rule, contrast media is not needed for imaging larger blood vessels.

Functional Magnetic Resonance Imaging

This procedure gives us a good way to assess brain and cardiac function as oxygenated and deoxygenated blood cause magnetic signal variations that can be detected by MRI scanning. This makes it possible to identify areas that are active or inactive such as in the brain as working areas of the brain consume more oxygen. Functional magnetic resonance imaging (fMRI) is good for cognitive tests. fMRI is used in normal controls to study how the brain functions and has been used extensively for presurgical planning.

fMRI is a technique that sensitizes the acquired signal intensity to changes in regional blood flow that occur while performing a cognitive task. The primary method for collecting fMRI data is the blood oxygenation level dependence (BOLD) method. A change in the relative hemoglobin oxygenation generates the underlying signal that is acquired during a rapid dynamic acquisition using a $T2^*$-weighted echo-planar imaging sequence. The signal intensity–time series acquired during the dynamic acquisition is correlated with a description of the task being performed.

With the limited coverage required to study the brain during fMRI studies, the couch remains in a static position and the patient remains immobile.

Functional Cardiac Magnetic Resonance Imaging

Several methods have been employed to assess cardiac function using MRI. Cine studies acquire the MRI signal and reconstruct images across several phases of the cardiac cycle. From these images, it is possible to measure left ventricle volume and ejection fraction. Tagging sequences place a series of lines or grid across the image using selective spatial presaturation pulses (spatial modulation of magnetization). This is performed prior to a cine-imaging sequence. The change in the grid positions can be used to extract information regarding myocardial contraction and strain. Other techniques such as delayed contrast enhancement can be used to distinguish infarct from viable myocardium. Normal myocardial tissue will appear dark on this sequence while areas of bright signal within the myocardium are regions of infarct/scar.

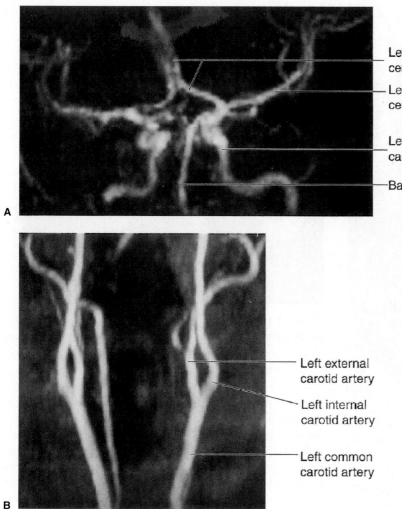

A

B

FIGURE 1.15. **A:** MRA axial image of the circle of Willis arteries (normal). **B:** MRA coronal image of the carotid arteries (normal).

Left anterior cerebral artery

Left middle cerebral artery

Left internal carotid artery

Basilar artery

Left external carotid artery

Left internal carotid artery

Left common carotid artery

Diffusion-Weighted Imaging Magnetic Resonance

Because free diffusion of protons is inhibited by cell membranes, diffusion-weighted imaging magnetic resonance (DWIMR) is particularly sensitive to cellular injuries of multiple etiologies. In DWIMR, the abnormal motion of water molecules in the brain is detected from the additional loss in the dephasing signal as the water molecules diffuse through the tissues. As a result, DWIMR is routinely used in the diagnosis of ischemic stroke and can reliably detect hypoxic ischemia within minutes of symptom onset (Fig. 1.16).

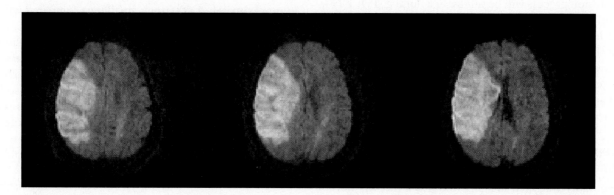

FIGURE 1.16. Three slices from a diffusion-weighted MRI scan in a patient with an acute stroke. The bright area shows the region of infarct and ischemia.

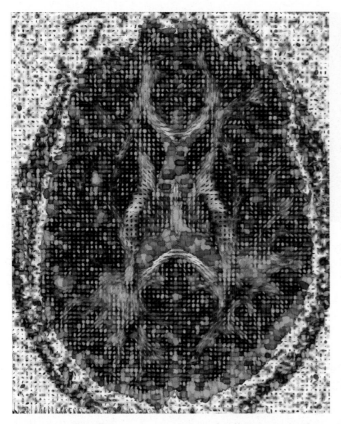

FIGURE 1.17. Diffusion tensor analysis of diffusion-weighted images. Glyphs of the diffusion orientation are displayed over a fractional anisotropy image. The glyphs are color-coded, based on the primary direction of water motion: Red (right–left), green (anterior–posterior), and blue (superior–inferior). The glyphs show uniform and large water mobility in the ventricles representing by the large spherical glyphs. The splenium and the genu of the corpus callosum show the well defined right–left fiber orientation in this region.

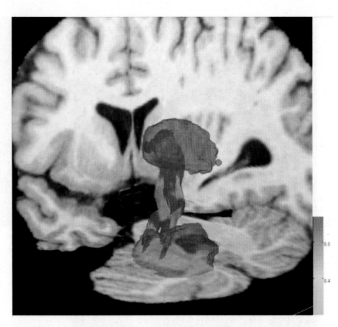

FIGURE 1.18. Fiber tracts generated from diffusion-weighted images between the cerebellum and the thalamus. The fiber tracts are overlaid on a volumetric T1-weighted image. The cerebellum and the thalamic regions used to define the fiber tracts are shown in red.

The water diffusion process can be mathematically modeled as a tensor, which can be used to define the orientation of the underlying tissue. Gray matter and CSF do not have any underlying structure and the diffusion process can be modeled as a sphere. However, white matter and muscle fibers have a defined orientation and the shape of the diffusion process will be similar to a hotdog (Fig. 1.17). This orientation information can be combined across voxels in the image to form a representation of white matter fiber tracks (Fig. 1.18). The generation of fiber tracks from DWIMR is known as tractography. Analysis of the tensor also provides scalar measures of the diffusion process that describe the shape, fractional anisotropy (FA), amount of diffusion, and mean diffusivity (MD).

Susceptibility-Weighted Magnetic Resonance Imaging

Susceptibility-weighted imaging (SWI) is a recently developed MR imaging technique that utilizes susceptibility differences between tissues to form its contrast. For example, deoxygenated hemoglobin is paramagnetic. High-resolution 3D imaging is used to generate a static image of the local field variations that result from paramagnetic particles. Dephasing of the MR signal due to local susceptibility changes are measured and used to weigh the resulting image. SWI is very sensitive to venous blood, hemorrhage, and iron storage. This imaging technique has shown great potential for assessing traumatic brain injury, stroke/hemorrhage, multiple sclerosis, and tumors (Fig. 1.19).

Magnetic Resonance Spectroscopy

Magnetic resonance spectroscopy (MRS) is a method that evaluates the metabolite concentrations in the body. In this technique, the signal from protons contained within water is suppressed, and the protons in various metabolites such as N-acetyl aspartate (NAA), choline, creatine, and lactate are detected. The signal from these metabolites is approximately 1,000 times smaller as compared with the signal from water. Therefore, voxels on order of 1 cc are used. This technique is often used to evaluate lesions to determine whether they are cancerous, since tumors have been shown to have an elevated concentration of choline with a reduction in NAA (Fig. 1.20). MRS has also been used to diagnose acute stroke by showing an increase in lactate. MRS is also useful for looking at disorders of metabolism and inflammatory diseases.

ULTRASONOGRAPHY

US is a useful diagnostic imaging tool that is noninvasive and does not use x-rays or radiation. US has significantly

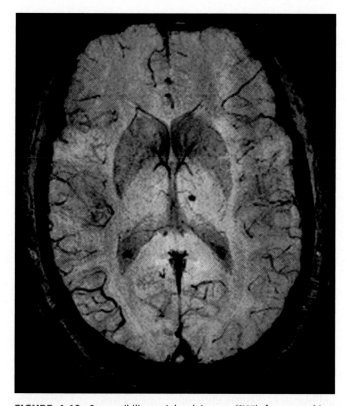

FIGURE 1.19. Susceptibility-weighted image (SWI) from a subject with traumatic brain injury. The venous vasculature appears dark on the images due to deoxygenated hemoglobin. A dark microbleed lesion appears in the left thalamus resulting from the traumatic brain injury.

Table 1.7
Some Common Imaging Applications for Diagnostic US
Obstetrics Pediatric brain Testicle and prostate Female pelvis Chest for pleural fluid drainage Abdomen (kidney, pancreas, liver, and gallbladder) Vascular disease Rotator cuff of the shoulder

improved the diagnosis, treatment, and management of a number of diseases. Some common areas where US imaging is used are listed in Table 1.7. US has achieved excellent patient acceptance because it is safe (no ionizing radiation), fast, painless, and relatively inexpensive when compared with the other imaging modalities. The advantages and disadvantages of US are listed in Table 1.8.

Ultrasound technology produces sectional anatomy images or slices in multiple planes much like CT and MRI. A US machine consists of an ultrasound wave source, a computer, and a transducer (Fig. 1.21). The US machine emits high-frequency sound waves, ranging from 1 to 10 MHz, whose frequencies are considerably above the human ear's audible range of 20 to 20,000 Hz. Short bursts of these high-frequency sound waves are alternately broadcast into the patient via the transducer, and some of the

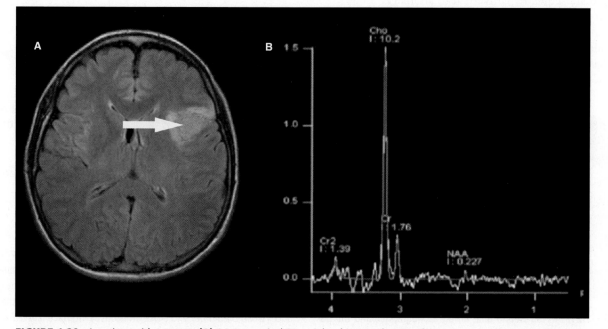

FIGURE 1.20. A patient with a tumor. **(A)** An anatomical T1-weighted image showing the tumor mass. The *arrow* shows the region where the MRS data were collected. **(B)** Graph of metabolite concentrations. The graph shows increased choline (Cho) and reduced *N*-acetyl aspartate. These are typical findings for MRS studies in tumors.

Table 1.8

Advantages and Disadvantages of US Diagnostic Imaging

Advantages

Multiple plane imaging including obliques
Safe—no known biologic harm at diagnostic sound frequency levels
Painless (noninvasive)
Less expensive than CT and MRI
Equipment cost is less than that of CT and MRI
Real time or cine is possible
Very portable

Disadvantages

Requires technical skill or is operator dependent
Not good for bone and lung imaging

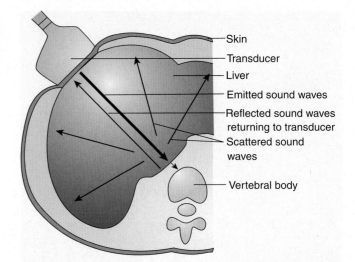

FIGURE 1.22. A transducer placed on the skin overlying the liver. The transducer broadcasts short bursts of high-frequency sound waves into the liver and deeper structures. Reflected sound waves are intermittently received by the transducer when it is not broadcasting sound waves. Note that some of the sound waves are deflected away from the transducer and are of no use for imaging.

reflected sound waves from the body tissues are intermittently received by the transducer (Fig. 1.22). The acoustic impedance (Z) of a structure determines the amount of sound energy transmitted and reflected at its boundary (Z = tissue density × sound velocity). When a sound wave encounters an acoustic interface or the boundary between two media of different acoustic impedance, the sound waves may be absorbed, deflected, or reflected (Fig. 1.23).

The analog sound waves that are reflected directly back to the transducer are subsequently digitized. Next, a computer converts this digital information to an image with shades of black, white, and gray. US, like MRI and CT, depends on computer technology to store digital information and subsequently converts it to an image.

Normal organs and tissues have their own characteristic echo pattern, whereas diseased organs and tissues have altered echo patterns. Solid organs usually have a homogeneous echo pattern, whereas fluid-filled organs and masses such as the urinary bladder, cysts, some tumors,

gallbladder, pleural effusions, and ascites have relatively fewer internal echoes.

The terminology used to describe an US image plane is slightly different from that used to describe CT and MR image planes. In US, an axial view may be referred to as a transverse scan, and a sagittal view may be called a longitudinal scan or view (Fig. 1.24). As previously noted, a significant part of medicine is just learning the lingo.

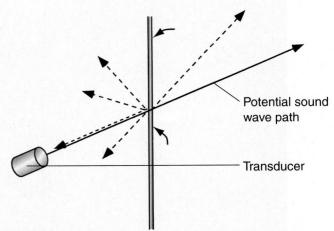

FIGURE 1.23. Illustration of what can happen to sound waves when they encounter an acoustic interface. An acoustic interface represents the intersection of two structures that possess different acoustic impedances or densities. When the sound waves are broadcast from the transducer (*solid black line*) and strike an acoustic interface (*curved arrows*), a number of things can happen to them such as the following: They can be reflected back to the transducer, be deflected away from the transducer, pass through the interface, or be absorbed at the interface.

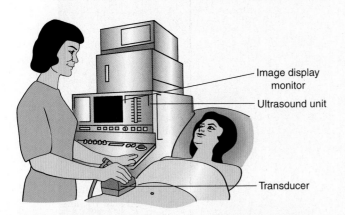

FIGURE 1.21. An ultrasound unit, an ultrasonographer, and the patient. The transducer is centered over the abdomen. The ultrasonographer moves the transducer with the right hand while making technical adjustments on the US unit with the left hand.

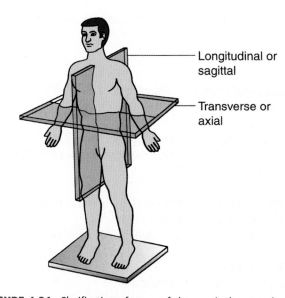

Longitudinal or sagittal

Transverse or axial

FIGURE 1.24. Clarification of some of the terminology used to describe sectional anatomy planes on US images.

While an US study is in progress, the images are viewed on a monitor. The monitor is analogous to a movie screen or television, and this viewing mode is called real time. This allows onlookers to observe a beating heart or the anatomy and movements of an intrauterine fetus. Also, static images may be reproduced on film by a format camera.

A small portable unit is now available for use in emergency situations. The laptop-sized computer is placed on a nearby flat surface. The transducer is approximately the size of one's hand and can be easily held over the area of interest to obtain urgently needed information such as when looking for abdominal fluid in trauma cases. This is called *FAST* or Focused Assessment with Sonography for Trauma.

PICTURE ARCHIVING SYSTEMS

The picture archive and computer system (PACS) is a comprehensive computer-based system designed to easily store and rapidly retrieve medical images. As one might expect, this is a challenging task as the size and number of images continue to grow rapidly. In recent years, the development of a standardized image format called Digital Imaging and Communications in Medicine (DICOM) has made the handling of medical images from a wide variety of modalities and manufacturers possible.

Key Points

- There are four basic densities or appearances to observe on radiographs and CT images: *Air,* which appears black; *fat,* which also appears black; *soft tissues and organs,* which appear gray; *and metal, calcium, and bone,* which appear white.
- Plain radiography images are produced by x-rays and radiographic film. CR or digital radiographs are produced by phosphor plates, x-rays, laser scanning, and computers. CT images are produced by x-rays, detectors, and computers. MR images are produced by magnetic fields, radio-frequency waves, and computers. US images are produced by high-frequency sound waves, transducers, and computers.
- Sectional anatomy is the imaging of anatomy in multiple planes, including the axial plane (transverse or cross-sectional), the sagittal plane, and the coronal plane.
- A key to distinguishing an MRI image from a CT image is that the fat on an MRI appears white, whereas fat on a CT appears black. Look to the fat.
- T1 MR images tend to have excellent resolution and are, therefore, used to procure anatomic information. T2 MR images have better contrast than T1 images. T2 images cause water to light up; therefore, T2 imaging is frequently used when searching for pathology, as most pathology tends to contain a lot of water.
- The high resolution of CT makes it effective for imaging anatomy. MRI has high soft-tissue contrast that makes it especially useful for soft tissue imaging.
- Commonly used contrast agents include barium sulfate, high- and low-osmolar iodinated compounds, ionic iodinated and nonionic (low-osmolar) contrast media, air, and gadolinium. Images produced with water-soluble iodinated agents are generally less informative than barium studies, because they are less dense and result in poorer contrast.

SUGGESTED READING

1. Bushberg JT, Seibert JA, Leidholdt EM Jr, et al. *Essential physics of medical imaging.* Philadelphia, PA: Lippincott Williams & Wilkins, 2002.
2. Cherry SR, Sorenson JA, Phelps ME. *Physics in nuclear medicine,* 3rd ed. Philadelphia, PA: WB Saunders, 1993.
3. Hashemi RH, Bradley WG. *MRI: the basics.* Baltimore, MD: Williams & Wilkins, 1997.

▪▪▪▪▪▪▪ QUESTIONS

1. X-rays are
   a. images on film
   b. images on a PACS unit
   c. electromagnetic waves
   d. all of the above

2. The basic densities discriminated on a radiograph are
   a. bone
   b. water
   c. air
   d. all of the above

3. CR (computed radiography) and DR (direct radiography) are imaging systems that
   a. do away with the need for film
   b. facilitate portable techniques
   c. use a recording phosphor
   d. record analog images

4. Regarding radiographic contrast, which is/are correct?
   a. It contains bound iodine molecules
   b. Low-osmolar compounds (LOCA) are more toxic than high-osmolar compounds (HOCA)
   c. It should not be used intravascularly
   d. All of the above

5. Gadolinium, used for MRI contrast, acts by
   a. inducing local T1 shortening in magnetic fields
   b. absorbing magnetic energy
   c. balanced outer ring electrons alter precession in a magnetic field
   d. showing lesions distinctly on T2W images

6. Computed tomography
   a. was invented by the Beatles
   b. measures absorbed energy on Hounsfield units
   c. is an x-ray technique
   d. a and c only
   e. b and c only

7. Magnetic resonance imaging does not
   a. produce images in multiple planes
   b. use x-ray energy
   c. produce studies more cheaply than CT
   d. produce good spatial contrast but poorer tissue contrast than CT

8. Special MRI sequences to demonstrate specific molecules or activities include
   a. diffusion-weighted imaging for cytotoxic edema
   b. functional MRI to demonstrate changes in oxygenation of hemoglobin
   c. susceptibility MRI to demonstrate tissue iron
   d. all of the above

9. Indications for ultrasound include all but which of the following?
   a. Testicular torsion
   b. Ovarian cysts
   c. Pneumonia
   d. Abdominal aortic aneurysm

10. A picture archiving and communications system (PACS) is
   a. a sophisticated analog device to show high-resolution reconstructions
   b. a billing system for radiology
   c. a device using Digital Imaging and Communication in Medicine (DICOM) protocols
   d. an audio dictation device

Correctly Using Imaging for Your Patients

Wilbur L. Smith

■■■■■ **Chapter Outline**

Imaging Appropriately
Radiation Protection
Key Points

IMAGING APPROPRIATELY

Modern medicine is confusing both for patients and physicians. Imaging tests are essential to make or confirm many diagnoses but the plethora of possibilities and the heightened patient diagnostic expectations confound everyone. Just look at media where you can see actors posing as "doctors" performing and reading their own MRI studies to make a rare diagnosis and administer the unique curative drug that they just happen to have in their desk drawer. We all know it is either fiction or advertising, but it is what the public has come to expect. The complexity of imaging examination's technical performance, sequencing, and selection is the subject of reams of studies and the object of years of training. Have you ever looked at the control panel for a modern CT or MRI scanner? Could you turn it on without fear of blowing the whole place up, let alone assure the proper examination sequences and time the contrast administration? Enough said, the message is getting the right imaging examination for your patient performed in a competent and diagnostic manner requires teamwork and consultation, so let us consider the process.

First, there has to be recognition of your patient's need for a study. Sometimes this is easy and straightforward; a patient comes to you with cough and fever and you hear rales in his chest. A simple chest x-ray is likely the imaging of choice as there is a high clinical probability that the patient has pneumonia. Great so far, no need for elaborate consultation, get the test and when it is interpreted as positive, treat. But let us say that after a couple of days of improvement on antibiotics the patient comes back a week later clinically worse with the return of the initial symp-

toms. What now, should you change antibiotics, put on a TB skin test, and/or consider more imaging? Perhaps now it is time to consult but with whom: Infectious disease expert or the radiologist? Each offers a valuable perspective and, most importantly, can help you do the "right thing" for your patient. The radiologist upon review may see a hilar mass which he/she originally thought a lymph node but now thinks may be an endobronchial lesion causing a postobstructive pneumonia. In that case, the antibiotic change suggested by infectious disease consultation is unlikely to be of much value and a definitive CT would be best. On the other hand, if the mass was a lymph node the TB skin test that the infectious disease expert suggested is a great idea. The point is that there is no shame in seeking help; we are not all the great TV doctors who are wise and omniscient. Our patients are also not TV patients who have rare and exotic diseases where the more tests the better regardless of whether they or society can afford them.

The critical assessment of using the correct imaging modality for the correct patient for the correct reason is everyone's concern. Imaging is expensive, carries some risk, and if inappropriately applied may lead to either false-positive or falsely reassuring results. An unnecessary test, particularly in the older population often results in findings called "Incidentalomas." An "Incidentaloma" is defined as a finding of questionable significance which is not related to the reason for performing the test in the first place. One retrospective study showed that individuals over the age of 70 years will almost invariably have an "Incidentaloma" finding on an abdomen and pelvis CT scan and that the older the patient the greater the number of "Incidentalomas" per patient will be discovered. "Incidentalomas" often result in a plethora of further unnecessary tests or treatments. Fortunately, the harm done is usually economic and perhaps societal owing to increased radiation dose but occasionally a false-positive finding results in surgery or a diagnostic disaster such as a serious contrast reaction. Always question results unrelated to the reason an examination was performed in the first place. Sometimes incidental findings are critical or may affect future care but more often they are "Incidentalomas."

The next rule of appropriate imaging is using your radiologist as a consultant. You would not think of spending $2,000 without knowing what you were getting for it but when you request an MRI without careful consideration that is exactly what you are doing. Radiologists spend a lot of time learning the strengths and limitations of their tools; not taking advantage of that experience is unwise. One of the functions that you should demand of your radiology service is the ability to provide a prospective consultation on the proper sequencing of examinations, utility of examinations, and risks of examinations. How else can you provide your patients with the highest levels of care? Radiologists who spend years of their lives learning to recommend the appropriate imaging are happy to talk to you for free. What a bargain in today's healthcare. It seems an oxymoron that radiologists by consulting often serve counter to their direct economic interests by discouraging performance of unnecessary tests. Consider an example; you obtain a chest radiograph on a 28-year-old man who was otherwise healthy but had chest wall trauma. The radiograph is negative for fractures but shows a 3-mm diameter nodule in the right upper lobe. What does that mean? Unless you are familiar with the literature on pulmonary nodules your first call should be to the radiologist before you order a chest CT or other expensive imaging. Hopefully, the radiologist would ask you if the patient is high or low risk for malignancy (read heavy smoker) and if low risk tell you not to do any more imaging. If high risk, a follow-up chest x-ray in 12 months is a good recommendation and may well suffice to deal with the issue. In either case your patient and the healthcare system are better served than had you immediately requested a chest CT. I know it seems an economic paradox but most radiologists would prefer not to perform a nonindicated examination.

Not all questions are as easily dealt with as the simple chest nodule and the American College of Radiology (ACR) has responded to the need for appropriate imaging by forming multidisciplinary committees to assess the value of imaging for multiple clinical scenarios and conditions. These recommendations are developed by expert panels using literature review, clinician experts and subspecialty expert radiologists to rate the appropriateness of imaging for many clinical situations. The recommendations are free, online, and open to all, including your patients, on the ACR.org website. The recommendations include a numerical assessment of appropriateness of various types of imaging as well as a relative scale of radiation dose from the study. There is now a movement to build these criteria into the decision-making algorithms of the electronic medical record. This means that before ordering an examination you would automatically be presented with queries as to whether or not the examination you requested was appropriate for the clinical situation. Of course no appropriateness criteria can be encyclopedic and these may be good reasons to deviate from the ACR criteria, but at least knowing about them and consulting the radiologist will give you a solid basis for decision making.

One of the other key adverse effects of an unnecessary test is ionizing radiation. The cancer scare has probably been overdone on an individual basis but there is a real risk of increased ionizing radiation exposure to the population gene pool as opposed to the individual. The next section of this chapter deals with a simple and practical approach to understanding the risks of diagnostic test radiation exposure.

RADIATION PROTECTION

Radiation exposure owing to diagnostic imaging is everyone's concern, the challenge is to keep this concern in the proper perspective; hysteria often trumps reason. If a patient has a potentially serious condition that cannot be diagnosed without radiation-based imaging, then there should be no hesitation, do the imaging! On the other hand, if the diagnosis is highly unlikely after reviewing the whole clinical picture, or if an equally efficacious means of making the diagnosis exists without using ionizing radiation (MRI, ultrasound, or nonimaging test), then avoid x-ray–based testing. Several factors must be assessed but remember an un-indicated test is likely to lead to a false-positive finding! False-positive findings never do anyone any good and can cost a lot of money or pain to disprove. Remember the most effective patient radiation protection is not to do an unnecessary test!

Now let us assume that you have analyzed the situation and the test is really needed; what is next? You need to know enough of the language of radiation protection to explain the need for the test and the risks. Remember your patient has been on the internet and seen all the stories about radiation overexposure. In fact the Environmental Protection Agency website has a fancy do it yourself radiation calculator where you plug in such factors as airplane trips and geographic area of your domicile as well as your medical exposure to calculate your annual radiation exposure. With all this data it is almost certain your patient will have questions regarding the procedure and the level of radiation exposure for a study. All x-ray studies do not involve equal radiation doses and a sense of proportion is important. Table 2.2 demonstrates the doses from several common imaging examinations.

Table 2.1

Average Radiation Exposures

Living in the Midwest for a day	0.03 mSv
Chest radiograph	0.1 mSv
Dental radiograph	0.005 mSv
Head CT	2 mSv
Chest CT (conventional dose)	7 mSv
Abdominal and pelvic CT	10 mSv

Comparing these doses to the background radiation from just existing on earth is often helpful in explaining radiation safety for your patients. As you can readily see CT is the major medical source of radiation exposure for the United States' population.

In order to respond effectively to your patient's questions, knowing indications for CT imaging as well as the advantages of CT as compared to other imaging modalities (Table 2.1) is helpful. Your local radiologist is always a valuable resource to help answer these questions. Remember, it is not your job to be all knowing, just how to find the right information at the right time for the patient. That said it always helps to understand the language and to answer questions as to the safety of procedure when your patients ask.

If the radiation-based test is necessary you need to understand the concept of ALARA (as little as reasonably acceptable). This concept, based on the old axiom of do no harm, is useful in other areas as well as radiation safety, but is particularly apt in the radiology protection arena. For any examination using ionizing radiation the technique is adjustable and will affect the total radiation dose. Here you need to know two terms, the milligray (mGy) and the millisievert (mSv). These terms are related but very different. Milligray is a measure of ionization and strictly speaking is an ion chamber value of how much ionizing radiation is applied while mSv is a measure corrected for the biologic effect on tissues in the course of the beam. Think of it this way, the same amount of ionizing radiation (mGy) applied to a radiosensitive tissue such as the lens of the eye will cause more damage than the same mGy hitting an insensitive tissue such as the bones of the orbit. The Sievert is the more critical measure but the Gray is the most frequently reported. The reason for that is simple, most radiation-producing diagnostic machines report Gray directly at the end of the examination. That said using high-dose techniques in the diagnostic radiology ranges will almost certainly guarantee prettier pictures, but how "pretty" do the images need to be in order to make the diagnosis? The recent interest in monitoring CT doses and the mandatory accreditation of CT facilities is a step in the right direction although it is not as simple as it

sounds. The radiologist and radiology professionals must constantly monitor the facility and equipment to ensure optimal performance. This is where ALARA comes in; using only the minimum radiation dose technique needed to make the diagnosis is optimally the ALARA principle. How do we achieve that, by adjusting techniques so that we give lower dose, by scanning only the tissues in question, and by using the best radiation protection of all . . . NOT DOING UNNECESSARY EXAMINATIONS.

After you protect your patient, you need to protect yourself. A single view chest x-ray, even if it is aimed right at you, is only slightly more than a day's exposure from natural background and about equal to the radiation from a 4-hour airplane ride. While the dose from a single radiograph is small, the cumulative dose especially for someone working with x-rays on a daily basis can be significant. Fluoroscopy, which continuously generates x-rays, can have substantially more radiation exposure resulting in skin damaging doses to both the patient and unshielded personnel. Whenever you work in a radiation area be sure you wear your protective garb and you put on your radiation monitoring badge.

Pediatric patients and pregnant patients are a special concern. Kids have longer anticipated lives, exposing them to potential cancer induction and germ cell genetic mutations induced by radiation will likely carry throughout their reproductive lives. The Society for Pediatric Radiology recognized this and initiated an "Image Gently" program which has had measurable success in applying the ALARA principles to pediatric imaging. Clearly there is a risk benefit analysis which is needed for any use of ionizing radiation but in kids, there is extra need for consideration of alternative to imaging with ionizing radiation. In pregnancy the greatest concern is in the period of organogenesis during the first and early second trimesters. Third trimester fetuses are pretty radiation resistant. If you should get into a question of radiation protection in pregnancy be sure to consult your radiologist, preferably before exposing the patient.

Key Points

- If the simple first test does not solve the issue, consult someone else.
- Radiologists and specialist clinicians each bring a different and valuable approach to a diagnostic dilemma; having both benefits your patient.
- Unnecessary imaging examinations often result in false-positive findings. These can be dangerous!
- ALARA is the key to decisions on using ionizing radiation wisely.
- Children and early pregnancy fetuses are at far greater risk from diagnostic radiation's long-term ill effects than adults.

FURTHER READINGS

1. Patient safety. RadiologyInfo.org Web site. http://www.radiology info.org/en/safety/index.cfm. Accessed March 4, 2013.
2. Radiation: Non-ionizing and ionizing. United States Environmental Protection Agency Web site. http://www.epa. gov/radiation/understand. Updated August 7, 2012. Accessed March 4, 2013.
3. Stabin MG. Doses from medical radiation sources. Health Physics Society Web site. http://hps.org/hpspublications/ articles/dosesfrommedicalradiation.html. Updated March 4, 2013. Accessed March 4, 2013.

■■■■■■■ QUESTIONS

1. True or false: Consultation and interpretation are expected services of a Radiology department.

2. True or false: Federal guidelines requiring certification of CT facilities assure compliance with ALARA principles.

3. True or false: Radiation exposure from a chest radiograph is about quadruple the exposure from living a day on earth.

4. True or false: Most humans over the age of 70 years will have at least one incidental finding on an abdomen and pelvis CT.

5. True or false: Diagnostic radiation exposure in adults over the age of 70 years is likely to cause an excessive incidence of cancer.

6. True or false: If you only occasionally perform fluoroscopy in the OR radiation protection equipment is uncomfortable and unnecessary.

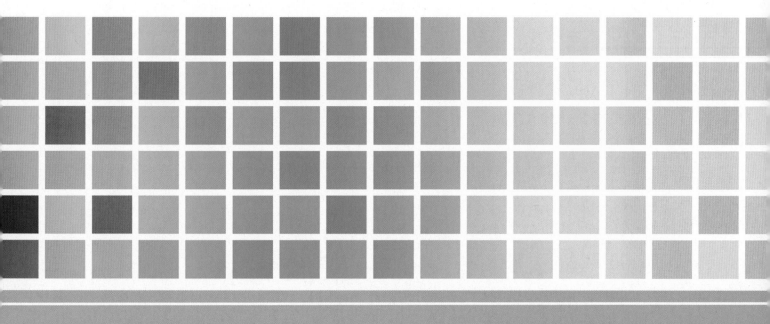

SECTION II
Imaging

Chest

Brad H. Thompson • William E. Erkonen

The chest radiograph is the most commonly performed radiographic examination accounting for 45% of all radiographic examinations in the United States. Since all clinicians should be adept and comfortable reviewing chest films, it is our goal through this chapter to provide a primer on how to logically interpret chest radiographs and discuss those disease processes which are commonly encountered.

RADIOGRAPHIC TECHNIQUE

The chest radiographic examination consists of two projections, namely *posteroanterior (PA) and lateral views*. When the patient's condition precludes these standard views, a single portable anteroposterior (AP) view can be obtained with the realization that portable AP films of the chest (which do not include a lateral projection) are generally less sensitive for detecting disease, and are subject to technical limitations such as magnification and suboptimal patient positioning. Every effort should be made to get the patient to make a maximum inspiration for the portable examination as a suboptimal inspiration contributes to a nondiagnostic examination. For these reasons,

obtaining PA and lateral radiographs is preferable. What constitutes a good quality chest image? First, examination of the image should reveal that the spine is barely visible behind the heart. Secondly, the lungs should not be black, and thirdly the blood vessels in the lung should be easily seen and crisp. The diaphragm should be seen at the level of the eighth to tenth posterior ribs as evidence of a good inspiratory effort. A standard PA chest film exposes the patient to 0.1 milliSieverts (mSv) of radiation, which is similar to 10 days' exposure to environmental background radiation. In comparison, the dose of a standard chest CT is approximately 8 mSv, which is comparable to 3 years' exposure to natural background radiation. According to the American College Radiology Appropriateness Criteria, routine admission and preoperative chest radiography is not appropriate in an asymptomatic whose history and physical are unremarkable (1).

The radiographic techniques and positioning are optimized for evaluation of the lungs primarily, and do not generally provide for a sufficient diagnostic evaluation of extrapulmonary structures such as the ribs or spine. Dedicated rib or spine views provide better radiographic detail of these structures.

HOW TO REVIEW THE CHEST RADIOGRAPHS

Frontal

Correct patient identification may seem elementary, but errors do occur, especially in a busy work environment resulting in inappropriate management decisions. Fortunately, with the advent of digital imaging and picture archive and communication systems (PACS), these errors are rare.

The next step is verifying optimal patient positioning and correct left–right annotation. All images must be routinely annotated with left or right side markers by the technologist. For all frontal projection chest radiographs (either AP or PA), the right (R) and left (L) markers indicate the patient's right and left side, respectively (Fig. 3.1).

One ground rule worth remembering is that "you only see what you know" and lack of knowledge about chest anatomy and normal radiographic findings will only limit your success in film interpretation. Also the more images you see, the greater your data bank (and expertise) becomes. Anatomically there are three lobes (upper, lower,

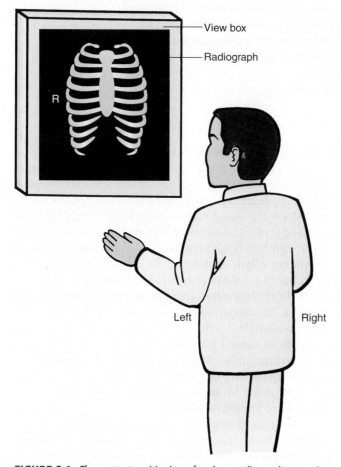

FIGURE 3.1. The correct positioning of a chest radiograph on an image display. The patient's right side on the film should always be opposite the viewer's left side.

Table 3.1
Checklist for Frontal Chest Film Review

Patient ID, time of examination
Side marker
Trachea central?
Heart size and shape
Aortic arch (side and width)
AP window
Location of hilae
Pulmonary vessel size
Lungs for symmetry and lucency
Diaphragm location
Ribs, spine, and soft tissues
Do not forget the four corners (shoulders and under the diaphragm)

and mid) and two fissures (major and minor) on the right and two lobes separated by one fissure on the left. Each lobe in turn is divided into segments, each with its own bronchus and blood supply.

When first reviewing a chest film, we suggest the observer render an initial *Gestalt* impression by examining the entire image for any obvious abnormality such as an enlarged heart or a lung mass. Then, we suggest reviewing the film in a logical and methodical approach. Checklists reduce human error and they are a feature of everyday life. The use of a mental checklist is essential to avoid overlooking radiographic abnormalities. The following checklist or system is suggested in Table 3.1. We find it useful to start at the top of the film and identify the tracheal air column. This accomplishes two goals: Firstly, the trachea on a correctly centered PA film should be midline and should be superimposed over the spinous processes of the upper thoracic spine, and the scapulae should be clear of the lungs. This ensures that the patient is not rotated (Fig. 3.2). Secondly, any deviation of the trachea off midline on a correctly centered film indicates a potential mediastinal or thyroid mass.

Next, follow the trachea inferiorly to arrive at the cardiac outline, for an evaluation of the heart size. The transverse diameter of the heart should not exceed 50% of the transverse diameter of the thoracic cage measured at the same level. This is called the *cardiothoracic ratio* (Fig. 3.3). This measurement, however, is only accurate on PA films as there is considerable magnification of the cardiac silhouette on AP projections which makes an accurate determination of heart size on portable films generally unreliable. To illustrate the nature of this magnification, consider the analogy of the shadow cast of your hand by a flashlight; the closer your hand is to the surface/shadow, the more accurate the size of the silhouette. For this reason, PA films are performed with the anterior chest wall closest to the film cassette with the term PA denoting the direction of the x-rays

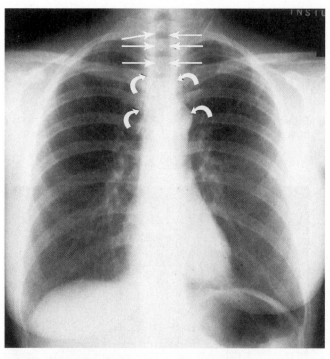

FIGURE 3.2. *Normal chest PA radiograph.* The vertical trachea (*straight arrows*) should always be midline. The narrow mediastinum is water density (*curved arrows*).

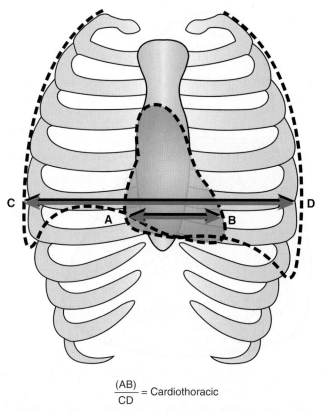

$$\frac{(AB)}{CD} = \text{Cardiothoracic}$$

FIGURE 3.3. *The cardiothoracic ratio.* The CTR is calculated by measuring the transverse diameter of the heart (*A–B*) and dividing by the transverse thoracic measurement (*C–D*).

(posterior to anterior). Poor inspiratory effort and recumbency can further exaggerate the cardiac size.

Next, evaluate the shape of the cardiac silhouette which has multiple components. The convex right cardiac border is formed by the right atrial shadow, which resides just below the vertical straight border rendered by the superior vena cava (SVC) (Fig. 3.4). The left ventricle constitutes the left heart border and the cardiac apex. The superior left cardiac border should be concave in most cases (Fig. 3.4). The right ventricle is directly superimposed

on the cardiac silhouette and is not a border-forming structure on frontal radiographs. Similarly, a normal sized left atrium is also not visible on PA or AP radiographs (Fig. 3.5). In cases of left atrial enlargement, the superior left heart border becomes convex, and in severe cases, the right lateral border of the left atrium may become

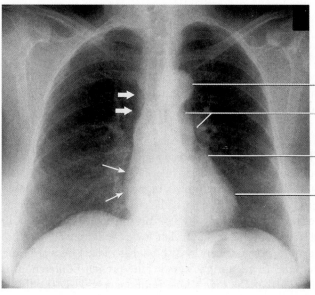

Aortic arch (knob)

Main and left pulmonary arteries

Left atrial appendage

Left ventricle

FIGURE 3.4. *Normal chest posteroanterior (PA) radiograph.* The convex right cardiac border is formed by the right atrium (*straight thin arrows*), and the *heavy arrows* indicate the location of the superior vena cava. The left cardiac and great vessels border might be considered as four skiing moguls. From cephalad to caudad the moguls are the aortic arch, the main and left pulmonary arteries, the left atrial appendage, and the left ventricle.

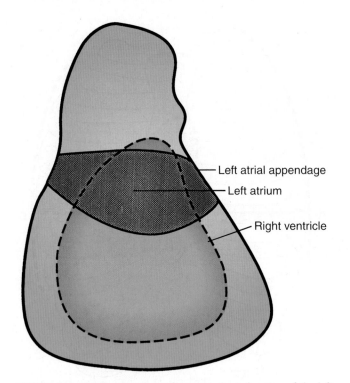

FIGURE 3.5. *Cardiac chambers.* The approximate location of the left atrium and right ventricle on a normal PA or AP chest radiograph. These cardiac chambers cannot be delineated on normal studies. However, the left atrial appendage can occasionally be seen in normal patients, especially younger females.

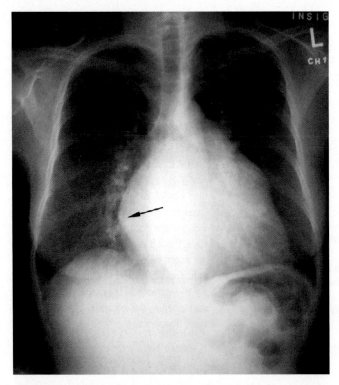

FIGURE 3.6. *Left atrial enlargement.* PA radiograph. This film shows the double density sign (*arrow*) produced by the overlapping of the left atrium with the right heart border (right atrium). Also, note the outward convexity of the upper left heart border typically seen with left atrial enlargement.

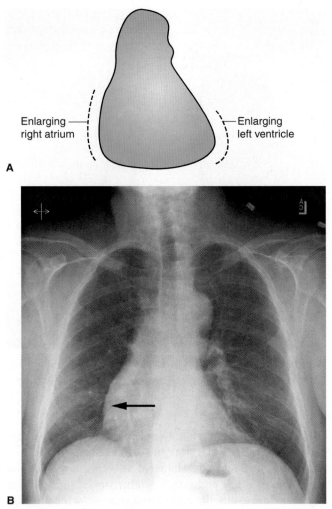

FIGURE 3.7. *Right atrial and left ventricular enlargement.* Cardiac silhouette changes during right atrium and left ventricle enlargement. **A:** As the right atrium enlarges, the convex right heart border enlarges to the patient's right. As the left ventricle enlarges, the cardiac apex moves to the patient's left and downward. **B:** PA chest radiograph showing right atrial enlargement (*arrow*).

superimposed over the right atrial shadow, producing what is known as the *double-density sign* (Fig. 3.6). As the left ventricle enlarges, the cardiac apex moves down and out. As the right atrium enlarges, the right heart border becomes protuberant (Fig. 3.7).

Next, your review should take you superiorly to the aortic arch, pulmonary arteries, and the main stem bronchi. The left and right pulmonary arteries and the main stem bronchi form the primary hilar shadows. On normal chest radiographs, the left hilum is higher than the right hilum in approximately 70% of normal chest films and is at the same level in the remaining 30% of cases. A lower left than right hilum should alert one to left lower collapse. The pulmonary arteries and their lobar branches radiate outward from the hila. In an upright person, the pressure differential is enough that the lower lobe pulmonary vessels should be

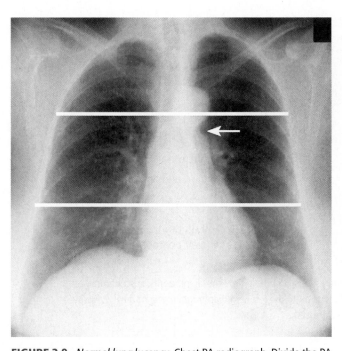

FIGURE 3.8. *Normal lung lucency.* Chest PA radiograph. Divide the PA or AP chest radiograph into horizontal thirds and compare the right and left lung fields moving in a head to foot direction. Note the aortopulmonary window (*arrow*).

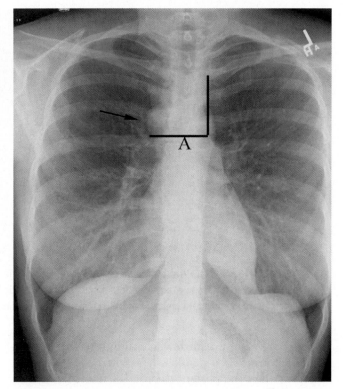

FIGURE 3.9. *Normal vascular pedicle.* The vascular pedicle is determined by drawing a horizontal line (*A*) from the junction of the azygos vein (*arrow*) and SVC over to a perpendicular line drawn from the left subclavian artery inferiorly along the transverse portion of the thoracic aorta (aortic arch).

larger than the upper lobe vessels because of greater blood flow. The main pulmonary artery can be prominent in the young and athletic, especially in females. The *aortopulmonary window* is the concavity or space immediately below the aortic arch and above the left pulmonary artery (Fig. 3.8). Convexity of the aortopulmonary window raises the suspicion of either a mass or adenopathy occupying this space. It is important to remember that in the elderly the thoracic aorta commonly becomes tortuous or ectatic, and this should not be interpreted as abnormal. Now divide the lungs into horizontal thirds and compare the right and left lung fields for symmetry and lucency (Fig. 3.8).

Next, your attention should be directed to the *mediastinum* which is the extrapleural space between the lungs, specifically its contour and width. The vascular pedicle extends from the thoracic inlet to the base of the heart caudally. The right border of the pedicle is the SVC, and the left border is the aortic arch near the origin of the left subclavian artery (Figs. 3.2 and 3.9). Next, review both diaphragms; the right hemidiaphragm should normally be about 1 to 2 cm higher than the left due to the liver. The lateral recesses of the diaphragms form the lateral costophrenic gutters, which should be sharp and form an acute angle where the diaphragms insert laterally to the chest wall. Finally, determine the location of the gastric air bubble (if present), which should be underneath the left hemidiaphragm (Fig. 3.10).

The lower cervical spine, thoracic spine, shoulders, and ribs complete a routine review of a chest film (Figs. 3.10 and 3.11). On a PA radiograph, the horizontal portions of each rib are the posterior arcs and the anterior ribs are usually angled downward (Fig. 3.11). Rib abnormalities may be easier to detect by rotating the image 90 degrees (clock- or counterclockwise). Although the bony structures are not very well delineated on chest radiographs, significant abnormalities can be seen, emphasizing the need for review of the four corners of the radiograph (Fig. 3.12).

Three areas where lung lesions are commonly missed are behind the anterior first ribs, behind the heart, and behind the diaphragm.

Lateral

For lateral radiographs, it is customary to have the film oriented such that the patient is facing toward your left (Fig. 3.13). Once again, begin by reviewing the entire image looking for any obvious abnormalities. Following this, evaluate the size and shape of the cardiac silhouette, which lies anteriorly. On lateral projections, the right ventricle forms the anterior border of the cardiac silhouette. The left ventricle forms the major portion of the inferior–posterior cardiac border, and the left atrium forms the superior–posterior cardiac border. On most lateral chest radiographs, the posterior wall of the inferior vena cava can be seen as it enters from the abdomen into the right atrium (Fig. 3.13, *straight arrows*). The identification of

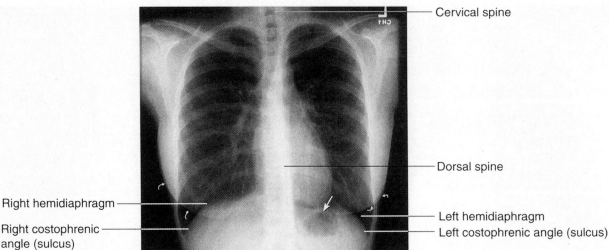

FIGURE 3.10. *Normal PA chest radiograph.* After comparing the lung fields, you next view the diaphragms, costophrenic angles, and lower dorsal spine. Note the close proximity of the gastric fundus air to the left hemidiaphragm (*straight arrow*). Always remember to identify both breast shadows in female patients (*curved arrows*).

the inferior vena cava shadow is useful in the determination of left ventricular size. The left ventricle is considered enlarged when the posterior border of the left ventricle resides 2 cm or more posterior to the inferior vena cava. Since the right atrium is a superimposed cardiac chamber, it is not visualized on the lateral projection.

The lateral film is the best view to evaluate the *hilar* structures. By drawing a vertical line down the tracheal air column, both hila can be distinguished (Fig. 3.14). The dominant shadow ventral to your line is largely composed of the right main pulmonary artery, which should be about

the size of the distal phalanx of your thumb. The left hilum, composed primarily of the left pulmonary artery, resides posterior to this line and should be about one-third the size of the right. Next, locate the sternum and search the retrosternal and pre-cardiac spaces for abnormal or pathologic soft tissue or air shadows (Fig. 3.15A). On the lateral view, the retrosternal lucency is due to the superimposition of the aerated upper lobes, whereas the right middle lobe and the lingular segment are projected over the cardiac silhouette. The lower lobes are located in the retrocardiac space overlying the spine extending inferiorly to

FIGURE 3.11. *Normal PA chest radiograph.* The posterior ribs (*straight arrows*) are horizontal and anterior ribs (*curved arrows*) are angled caudad or inferiorly. All of these structures must be included in your checklist as well as the shoulder girdles and cervical and dorsal spine areas.

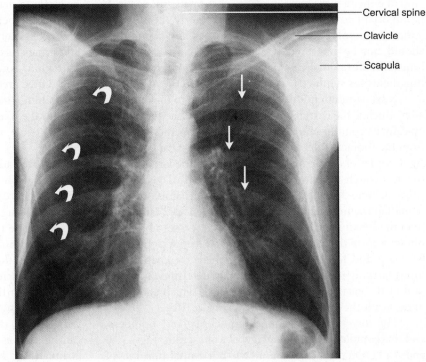

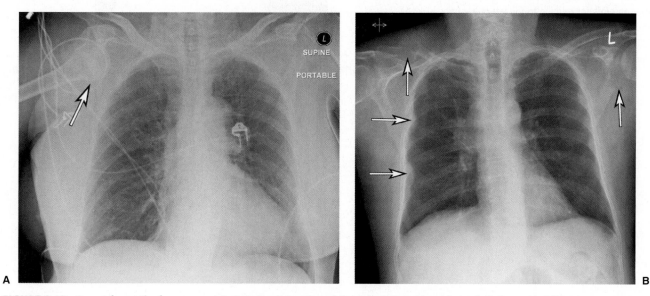

A

B

FIGURE 3.12. *Do not forget the four corners!* **A:** Anterior dislocation of the right humeral head (*arrow*). **B:** Several lytic bony lesions reflecting metastatic disease including the left scapula, right clavicle, and several ribs on the right side (*arrows*).

the diaphragms (Fig. 3.15B). It is important to understand the pulmonary lobar spatial relationships in locating pathologic pulmonary processes. The apical segments of the lower lobes extend as high as the fourth thoracic vertebra and the costophrenic recesses of the lower lobes may extend down to the second lumbar vertebra.

Finally, observe the contours of the diaphragms and the posterior costophrenic angles (or gutters). The right hemidiaphragm should be slightly lower in location and more magnified than the left on the lateral view. This is important in identifying and determining the location of a small pleural effusion, which may not be apparent on the frontal film. Note that the right hemidiaphragm can be seen in its entirety, because air in the right lower lobe abuts the soft tissue density hemidiaphragm allowing a sharp interface to be formed. On the left, only the cardiac apex and posterior hemidiaphragm are generally demonstrated, so the anterior aspect of the left diaphragm is usually obscured by its continuity with the heart and pericardial fat (Fig. 3.16).

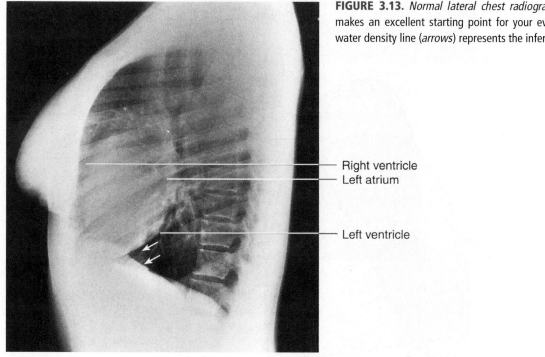

Right ventricle
Left atrium

Left ventricle

FIGURE 3.13. *Normal lateral chest radiograph.* The cardiac silhouette makes an excellent starting point for your evaluation. The faint vertical water density line (*arrows*) represents the inferior vena cava.

FIGURE 3.14. *Normal lateral chest radiograph.* The oval-shaped right pulmonary artery lies anterior and inferior relative to the left pulmonary artery. The left pulmonary artery crosses cephalad over the left main stem bronchus and it lies inferior to the aortic arch.

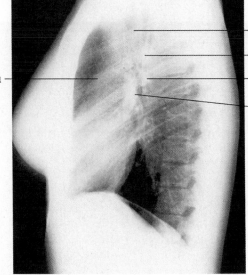

— Trachea

— Aortic arch

— Left pulmonary artery

— Right pulmonary artery

Ascending aorta —

FIGURE 3.15. A: *Normal lateral chest radiograph.* The anterior and posterior bony structures should always be routinely viewed. The spine appears *less* dense as you proceed caudally due to attenuation by the shoulders. **B:** Illustration of the spatial relationships of the pulmonary lobes on the lateral view. Note that the right middle lobe and the lingular segments of the left upper lobe (*curved arrows*) project over the heart (*straight arrow*). The lower lobes are primarily posterior structures. The major fissures extend obliquely up to approximately the T4 level.

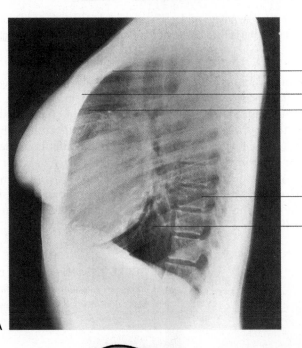

— Sternum manubrium

— Sternum body

— Retrosternal space (upper lobes)

— Dorsal vertebral body

— Retrocardiac space (lower lobes)

A

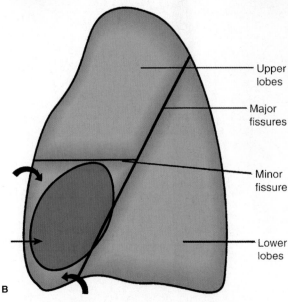

Upper lobes

Major fissures

Minor fissure

Lower lobes

B

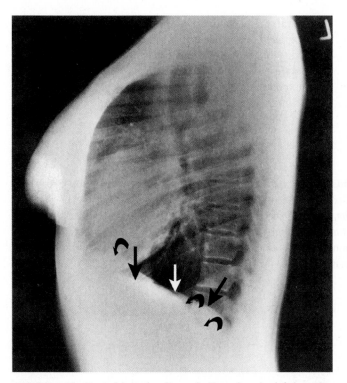

FIGURE 3.16. *Normal lateral radiograph.* Note that the left hemidiaphragm (*straight arrows*) is not visible anteriorly where it abuts the heart (water density). This is an excellent example of the silhouette sign. On the other hand, the entire right hemidiaphragm (*curved arrows*) is visible.

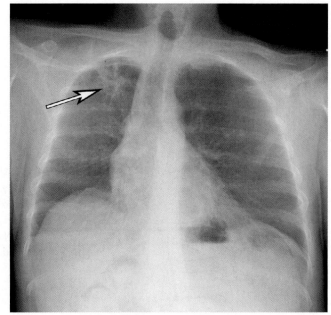

FIGURE 3.17. *Apicolordotic view.* This view is obtained with the patient leaning backward. Note how the clavicles project above the lung apices allowing better visualization of the upper lobes. This film shows a cavitary lesion in the right upper lobe (*arrow*) due to an atypical mycobacterial infection.

Additional Views

The *AP lordotic view,* which is an AP film taken with the patient leaning back is useful for visualization of upper lobe or apical pathology (Fig. 3.17). This projection displaces the clavicles above the thoracic inlet and enables better visualization of the lung apices.

Placing a patient on their side (decubitus position) and obtaining a film across the chest in the AP direction is described as a *decubitus* view. This view is helpful for detecting small amounts of pleural air or fluid, which may not be seen on the standard views described above (Fig. 3.18).

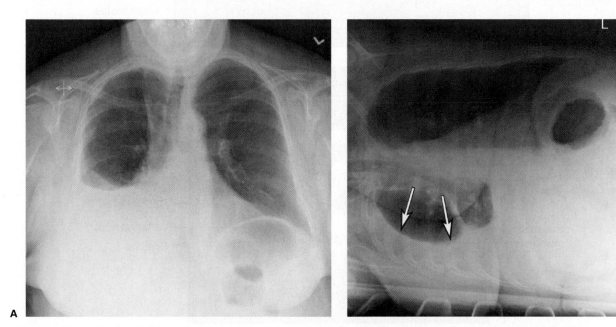

FIGURE 3.18. *Right pleural effusion.* **A:** PA chest film shows a moderate right pleural effusion. **B:** Right lateral decubitus film confirms that the right pleural effusion (*arrows*) is free flowing and not loculated.

NORMAL THORACIC CROSS-SECTIONAL ANATOMY

Multidetector (or spiral) CT (MDCT) allows imaging of the chest within one breath hold (~15 seconds or less). Figures 3.19 to 3.27 demonstrate normal cadaveric cross-sectional anatomy correlated with CT and magnetic resonance (MR).

In general, CT is preferred to MR for chest and pulmonary imaging because of faster examination times and less susceptibility to motion and respiratory artifacts. Some MDCT scanners are capable of scanning the heart in a heartbeat, with excellent spatial and temporal resolution allowing three-dimensional (3D) visualization of the coronary arteries (Fig. 3.28).

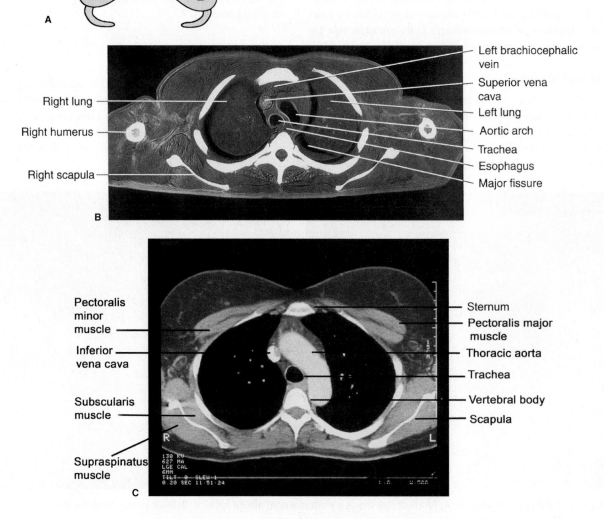

FIGURE 3.19. *Normal axial cross-sectional anatomy.* **A:** Approximate axial anatomic level through the aortic arch for **(B)** and **(C)**. **B:** Axial cadaver radiograph of the sectioned chest at the aortic arch level. Normal. A frozen cadaver was sectioned and then radiographed. **C:** Normal chest CT image at the aortic arch level with mediastinal windows.

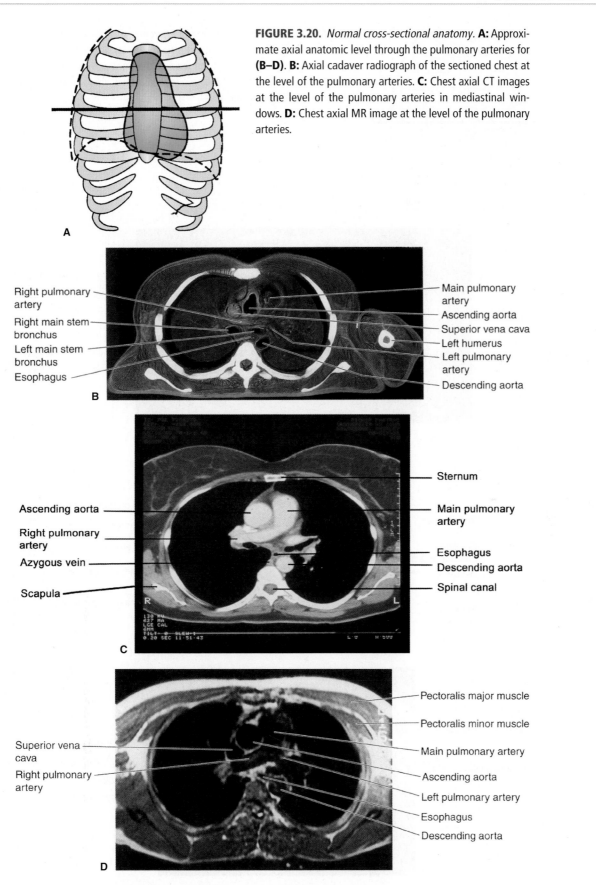

FIGURE 3.20. *Normal cross-sectional anatomy.* **A:** Approximate axial anatomic level through the pulmonary arteries for **(B–D)**. **B:** Axial cadaver radiograph of the sectioned chest at the level of the pulmonary arteries. **C:** Chest axial CT images at the level of the pulmonary arteries in mediastinal windows. **D:** Chest axial MR image at the level of the pulmonary arteries.

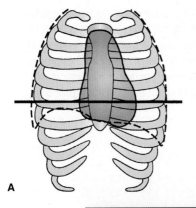

FIGURE 3.21. *Normal cross-sectional anatomy.* **A:** Approximate axial anatomic level through the right and left atria for **(B–D)**. **B:** Axial cadaver radiograph of the sectioned chest at the level of the right and left atria. **C:** Chest axial CT images at the level of the atria in mediastinal windows. **D:** Chest axial MR image at the level of the atria.

A

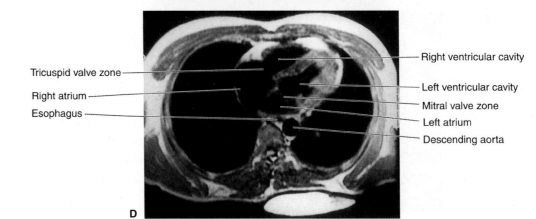

Left ventricular outflow tract

Esophagus

Right ventricular cavity
Interventricular septum
Right atrium
Left ventricular cavity
Left atrium
Pulmonary vein
Descending aorta

B

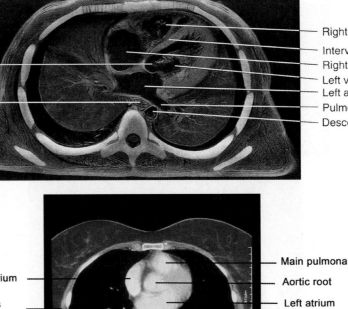

Right atrium

Serratus anterior muscle

Azygous vein

Spinous process

Main pulmonary artery

Aortic root

Left atrium

Descending aorta

Transverse process

C

Tricuspid valve zone

Right atrium

Esophagus

Right ventricular cavity

Left ventricular cavity

Mitral valve zone

Left atrium

Descending aorta

D

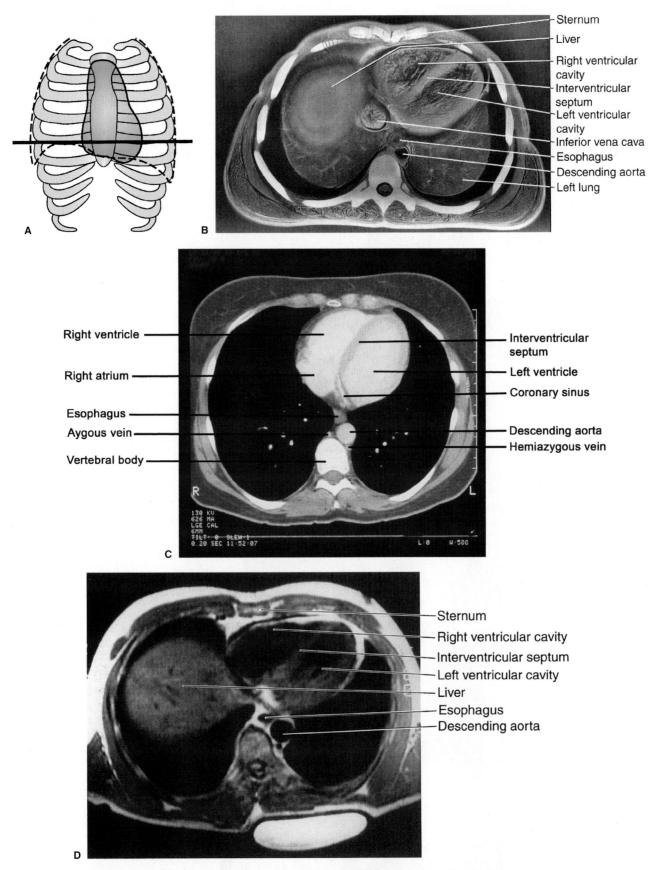

Sternum
Liver
Right ventricular cavity
Interventricular septum
Left ventricular cavity
Inferior vena cava
Esophagus
Descending aorta
Left lung

Right ventricle
Right atrium
Esophagus
Aygous vein
Vertebral body

Interventricular septum
Left ventricle
Coronary sinus
Descending aorta
Hemiazygous vein

Sternum
Right ventricular cavity
Interventricular septum
Left ventricular cavity
Liver
Esophagus
Descending aorta

FIGURE 3.22. *Normal cross-sectional anatomy.* **A:** Approximate axial anatomic level through the right and left ventricles for **(B–D)**. **B:** Axial cadaver radiograph of the sectioned chest at the level of the ventricles. **C:** Chest axial CT image through using a mediastinal window. Normal. **D:** Chest axial MR image at the level of the ventricles.

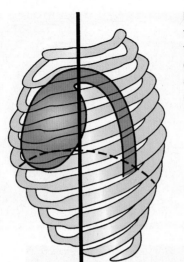

FIGURE 3.23. *Normal coronal sectional anatomy.* **A:** Illustration of the approximate coronal anatomic level through the left atrium for **(B)** and **(C)**. **B:** Coronal cadaver radiograph of the sectioned chest through the level of the left atrium. Normal. **C:** Chest coronal MR image through the right and left atria.

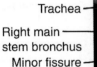

Trachea

Right main stem bronchus

Minor fissure

Liver

Hepatic vein

Aortic arch

Main pulmonary artery

Left main stem bronchus

Left atrium

Right and left hemidiaphragms

Gastric fundus

Spleen

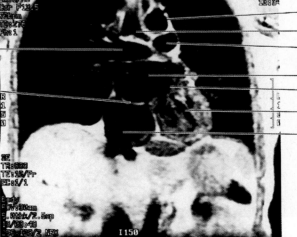

Right pulmonary artery

Interatrial septum

Aortic arch

Left main stem bronchus

Main pulmonary artery

Left atrium

Mitral valve zone

Left ventricular cavity

Right atrium

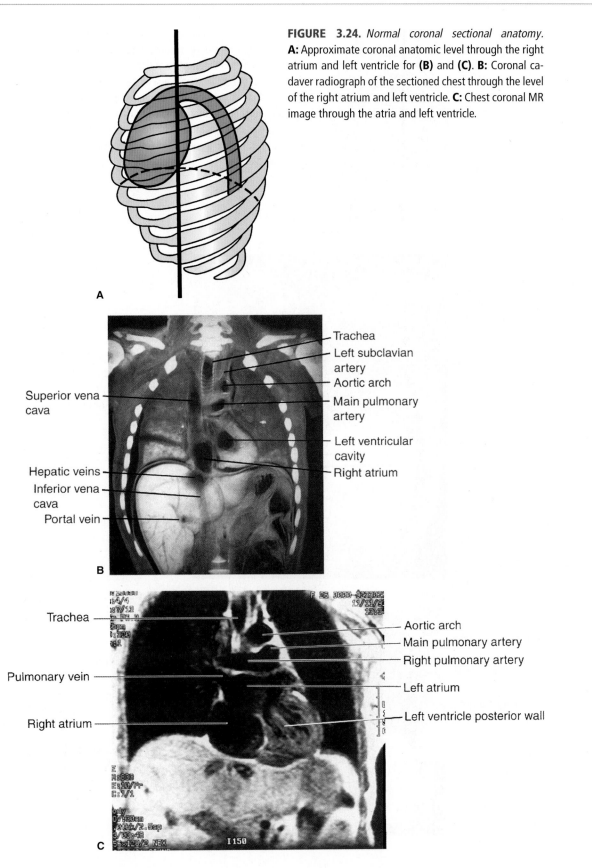

FIGURE 3.24. *Normal coronal sectional anatomy.* **A:** Approximate coronal anatomic level through the right atrium and left ventricle for **(B)** and **(C)**. **B:** Coronal cadaver radiograph of the sectioned chest through the level of the right atrium and left ventricle. **C:** Chest coronal MR image through the atria and left ventricle.

A

Superior vena cava

Hepatic veins

Inferior vena cava

Portal vein

Trachea
Left subclavian artery
Aortic arch
Main pulmonary artery

Left ventricular cavity

Right atrium

B

Trachea

Pulmonary vein

Right atrium

Aortic arch
Main pulmonary artery
Right pulmonary artery

Left atrium

Left ventricle posterior wall

C

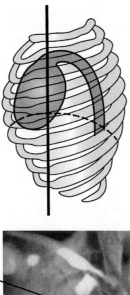

A

FIGURE 3.25. *Normal coronal sectional anatomy.* **A:** Illustration of the approximate coronal anatomic level through the left ventricle and the ascending aorta for **(B)** and **(C)**. **B:** Coronal cadaver radiograph of the sectioned chest through the left ventricle and the ascending aorta. Note that the convex right cardiac border is due to the right atrium (*straight arrows*). **C:** Chest coronal MR image through the left ventricle and the ascending aorta.

Ascending aorta

Minor fissure

Aortic arch
Main pulmonary artery
Left atrial appendage
Right atrial appendage
Left ventricular cavity

Right atrium

Hepatic vein
Liver
Portal vein

B

Ascending aorta

Right lung

Right atrium

Main pulmonary artery

Left atrial appendage

Left lung

Left ventricular cavity

Liver

C

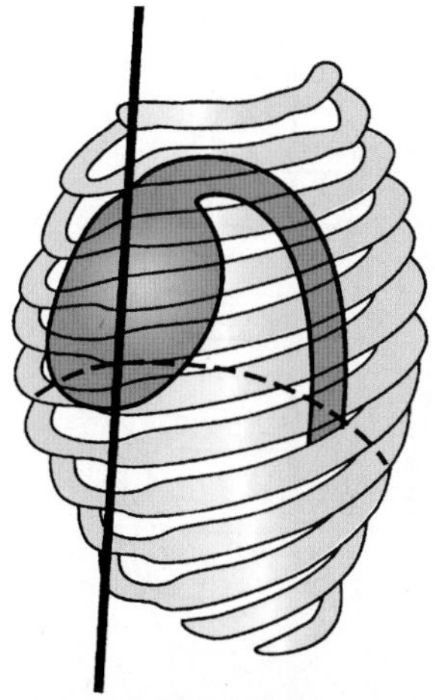

FIGURE 3.26. *Normal coronal sectional anatomy.* **A:** Illustration of the approximate coronal anatomic level through the ventricles for **(B)** and **(C)**. **B:** Coronal cadaver radiograph of the sectioned chest through the ventricles. Normal. **C:** Chest coronal MR image through the ventricles.

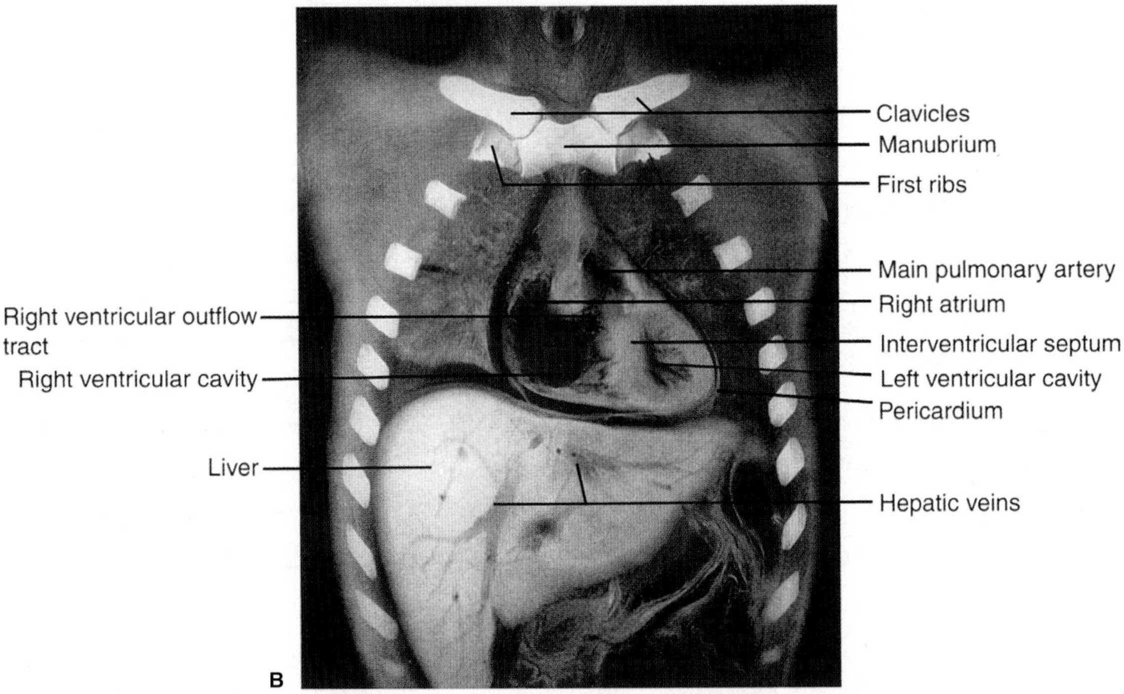

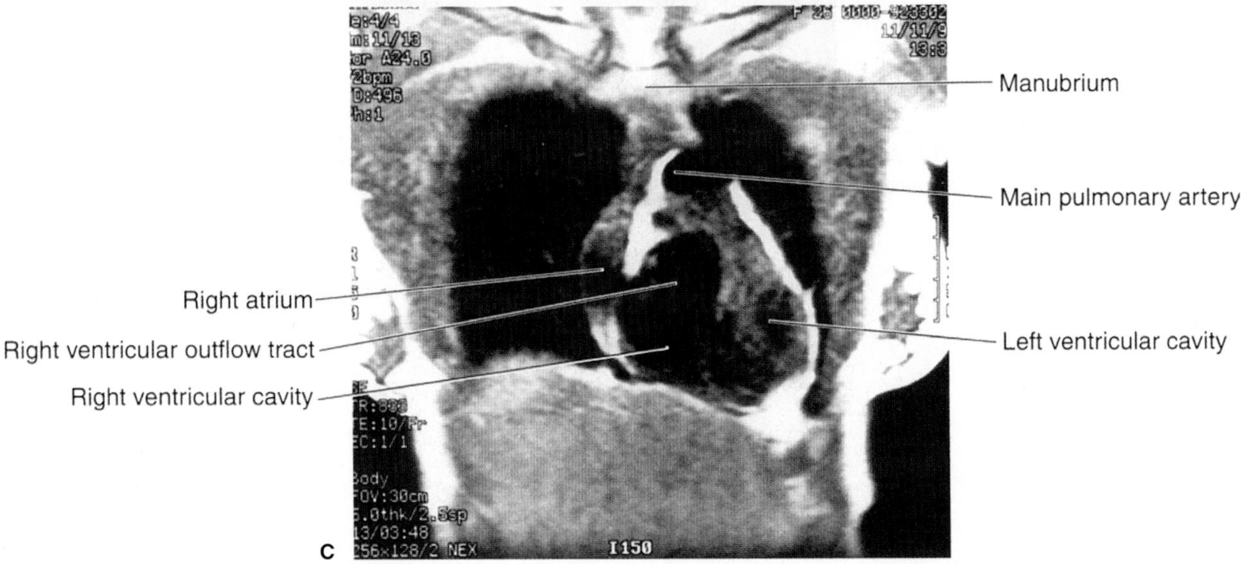

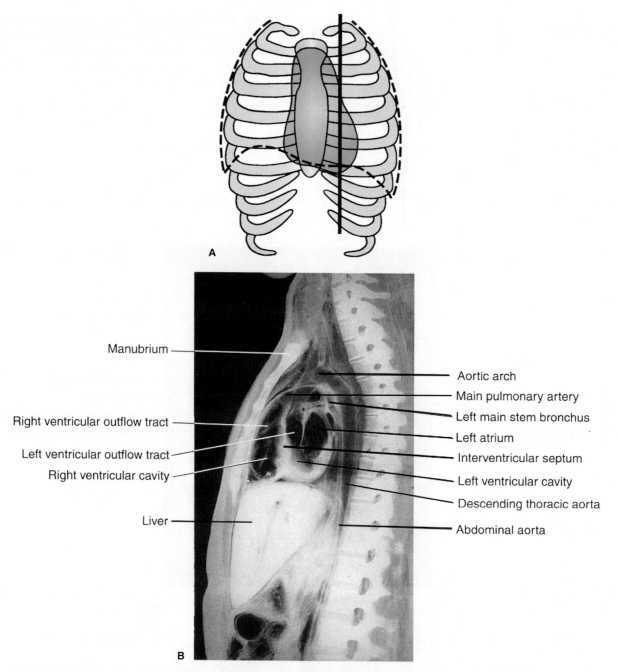

FIGURE 3.27. *Normal sagittal anatomy.* **A:** An illustration of the approximate sagittal anatomic level for **(B)**. **B:** Sagittal cadaver radiograph of the sectioned chest through the right ventricular outflow tract and the right ventricle.

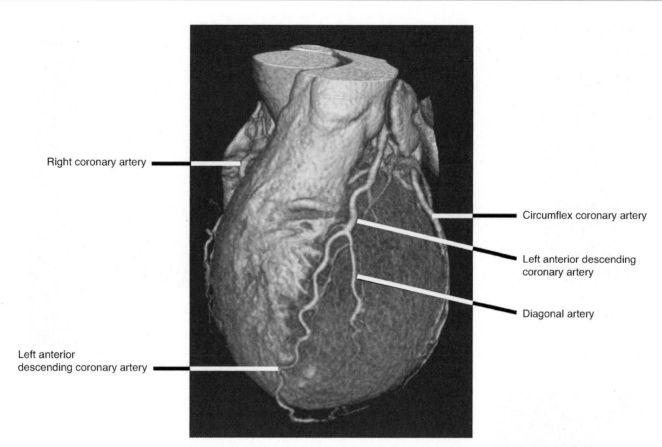

Right coronary artery

Circumflex coronary artery

Left anterior descending coronary artery

Diagonal artery

Left anterior descending coronary artery

FIGURE 3.28. *CTA surface rendered volumetric image of the left coronary circulation* provides a 3D perspective and demonstrate the left coronary arteries relative to underlying cardiac structures. The left anterior descending coronary artery supplies most of the left ventricle while the circumflex artery runs in the left atrio-ventricular groove. A portion of the right coronary artery is visible along the left side of the image.

CONGENITAL VASCULAR ANOMALIES

Embryonic migration of the azygos vein up over the superior recess of the right upper lobe creates a mock vertical fissure-like opacity (Fig. 3.29) which is created by indentation of both visceral and parietal pleural surfaces along the arc-like course of the azygos vein as it courses inferiorly to insert normally into the SVC. This azygos fissure, which is only visualized on PA radiographs as a thin curvilinear line and outlines an *azygos lobe* is a common normal variant and is of no clinical significance.

The most common thoracic aortic anomaly is a *right-sided aortic arch* (Fig. 3.30). On the PA radiograph, the right-sided arch often appears more cephalad than a normal left-sided arch. The most common types are right-sided aortic arch with aberrant left subclavian artery and the mirror-image type. The variant with aberrant left subclavian artery is rarely associated with congenital heart disease whereas the mirror-image type of right aortic arch is very strongly associated with congenital heart disease, most commonly tetralogy of Fallot.

Coarctation of the aorta is a focal stenosis at the junction of the aortic arch and the descending thoracic aorta. The

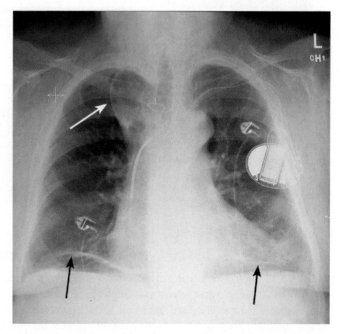

FIGURE 3.29. *Azygos lobe.* Chest PA radiograph. The azygos lobe is outlined with a *white arrow*. Also note the areas of discoid atelectasis in the lower lobes (*black arrows*) in the basilar regions of both lungs.

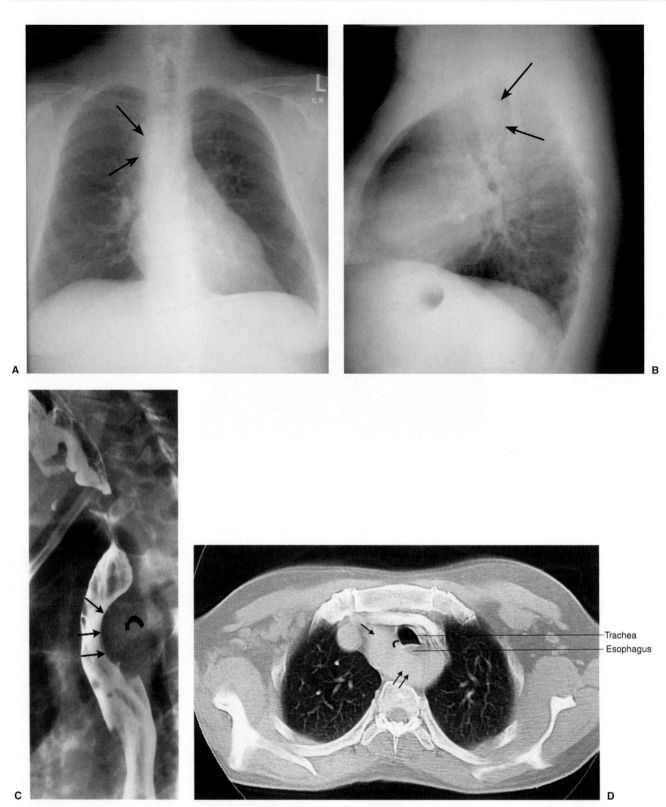

FIGURE 3.30. *Right-sided aortic arch and left descending thoracic aorta.* Chest PA **(A)** and lateral **(B)** radiographs, barium swallow **(C),** and chest CT **(D).** This 42-year-old male smoker was suspected of having cancer of the lung. **A:** A neoplastic mass was suspected on the PA radiograph, but this proved to be an ill-defined aortic knob to the right of the midline (*arrows*). The right aortic arch is indenting the right side of the trachea. **B:** The right-sided aortic arch indents the posterior aspect of the trachea (*arrows*) on the lateral radiograph. **C:** Barium swallow confirms a significant indentation on the posterior aspect of the barium-filled esophagus (*straight arrows*) secondary to the crossing aortic arch (*curved arrow*). **D:** The diagnosis is confirmed by chest CT that shows the right-sided aorta (*single straight arrow*) passing posterior to the esophagus and trachea (*double straight arrows*) to reach the left side of the thorax. Again, note the indentation on the right side of the trachea (*curved arrow*) secondary to the right-sided aortic arch.

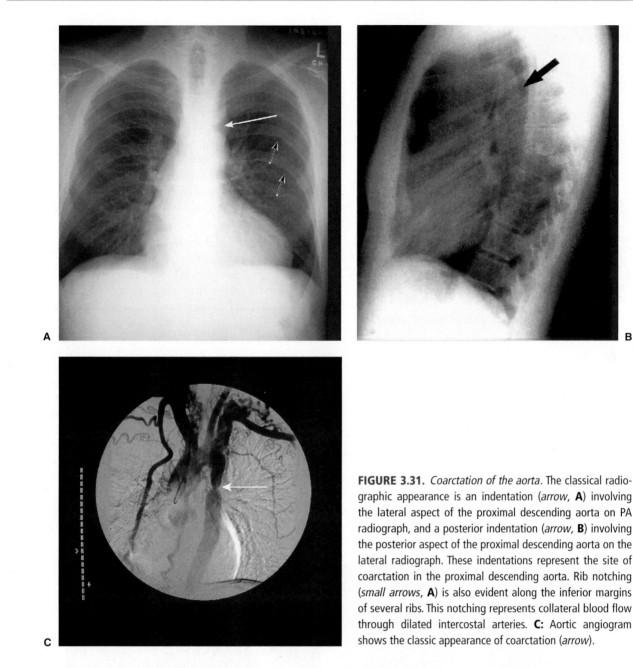

FIGURE 3.31. *Coarctation of the aorta.* The classical radiographic appearance is an indentation (*arrow,* **A**) involving the lateral aspect of the proximal descending aorta on PA radiograph, and a posterior indentation (*arrow,* **B**) involving the posterior aspect of the proximal descending aorta on the lateral radiograph. These indentations represent the site of coarctation in the proximal descending aorta. Rib notching (*small arrows,* **A**) is also evident along the inferior margins of several ribs. This notching represents collateral blood flow through dilated intercostal arteries. **C:** Aortic angiogram shows the classic appearance of coarctation (*arrow*).

degree of coarctation is variable, and the clinical features vary with the location and degree of stenosis. Patients may have a systolic murmur, cardiac enlargement, and pre- and poststenotic aortic dilatation depending on the location and severity of the stenosis (Fig. 3.31). Rib notching can occur along the inferior aspect of the ribs reflecting collateral blood flow through dilated intercostal arteries (Fig. 3.31B).

FOREIGN BODIES, LINES, AND TUBES

Occasionally objects on the skin may be mistaken for chest pathology. Examples included are hair braids and skin nodules (Figs. 3.32–3.35). Characteristically these are very well defined on the chest radiograph. An innocuous skin fold which appears as a well-defined line traversing the lung may be mistaken for the visceral pleural edge of a pneumothorax. Some foreign bodies such as central venous lines and endotracheal and nasogastric tubes are intentionally placed (Fig. 3.36) and it is important to recognize and document the course and location of these when caring for acutely ill patients. The optimal location of central venous lines is between the mid SVC and the mid right atrium. The optimal location for the tip of an endotracheal tube is 5 cm above the carina.

Air in the Wrong Places

A *pneumothorax* is an accumulation of air within the pleural space. It is most often spontaneous or may be due to trauma or iatrogenic causes such as lung biopsy (Table 3.2).The definitive radiographic diagnosis of pneumothorax is made

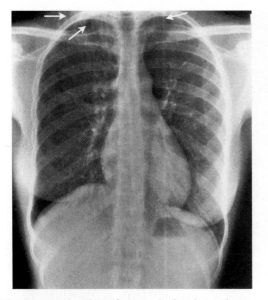

FIGURE 3.32. *Hair braid.* A soft tissue shadow (*arrows*) projects over the right supraclavicular region.

Table 3.2
Causes of Pneumothorax

Traumatic
1. Trauma: Rib fractures or penetrating chest wounds
2. Iatrogenic
    a. Thoracoscopy
    b. Thoracentesis
    c. Placement of central line
    d. Artificial ventilation (barotrauma)
    e. Post-thoracic surgery
    f. Transthoracic or bronchoscopic lung biopsy

Spontaneous
1. Rupture of a bleb or bullae
2. Secondary to underlying pulmonary disease (fibrosis, emphysema)
3. Secondary to pneumomediastinum

by identifying the *visceral pleura edge* of the collapsed lung (Fig. 3.37). Additional findings include an abnormally hyperlucent hemithorax and loss of peripheral lung markings on the affected side. Upright or decubitus films are useful ways to document the presence of pleural air. Expiratory films accentuate air trapping in the pleural space and may make small and subtle pneumothoraces more visible. Recumbent portable films on the other hand are unreliable for demonstrating even large pneumothoraces, because the air resides immediately ventral to the lung and is not visualized on a frontal view. A *tension pneumothorax* occurs when the air within the pleural space is sufficiently large to produce mass effect upon the mediastinal structures and ipsilateral diaphragm. If sufficiently great enough, the mass effect on the heart and great vessels can produce acute cardiovascular collapse due to diminished cardiac output (Fig. 3.38). A tension pneumothorax represents an emergency requiring immediate placement of chest tube to decompress the pleural space. For most pneumothoraces, the optimal location for chest tube placement

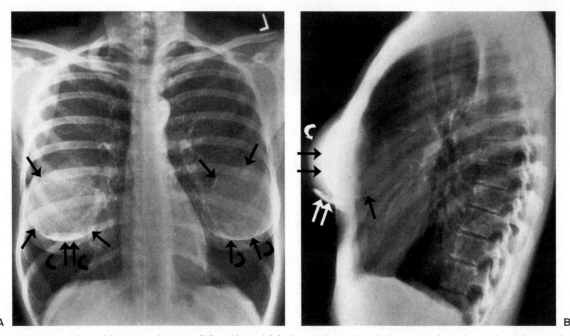

A   B

FIGURE 3.33. *Bilateral breast implants.* PA **(A)** and lateral **(B)** chest radiographs. The breast implants (*arrows*) exhibit peripheral calcifications along the capsules of each prosthesis.

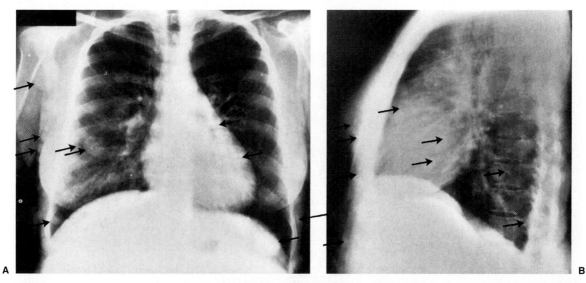

FIGURE 3.34. *Neurofibromatosis.* Chest PA **(A)** and lateral **(B)** radiographs. Multiple well-defined subcutaneous soft tissue nodules (*arrows*) project over the thorax which should not be mistaken for pulmonary nodules.

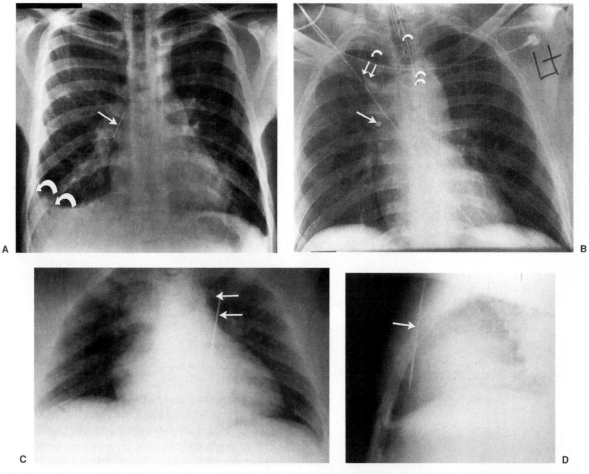

FIGURE 3.35. *Foreign bodies.* **A:** PA chest radiograph shows a metallic density (*straight arrow*) identified as an aspirated *straight pin* in the right bronchus intermedius. Note the right pleural effusion (*curved arrows*). It has been estimated that there must be at least 125 cc of pleural fluid before it is recognized on PA and AP views. **B:** Chest portable AP radiograph reveals a *tooth fragment* (*straight arrow*) in the right bronchial tree. The patient was involved in a motor vehicle accident, and a portion of a tooth was missing. The chest radiograph shows the tooth fragment projecting over the right upper bronchial tree. Note that the endotracheal tube (*single curved arrow at top*) lies to the patient's right of the nasogastric tube (*double curved arrows*). An azygos lobe is present, and the position of the azygos vein is more lateral and cephalad than normal (*double straight arrows*). The azygos lobe (*single curved arrow at left*) is visible. **C,D:** Chest AP **(C)** and lateral **(D)** radiographs reveal a *darning needle lodged in the right ventricle.* The child of this young mother accidentally stabbed her with a darning needle. The needle (*arrows*) projects over the right ventricle region in both views. It was successfully removed at thoracotomy.

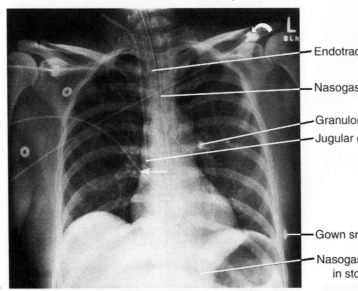

— Endotracheal tube tip

— Nasogastric tube in esophagus

— Granuloma
— Jugular central line tip

— Gown snap
— Nasogastric tube
   in stomach

A

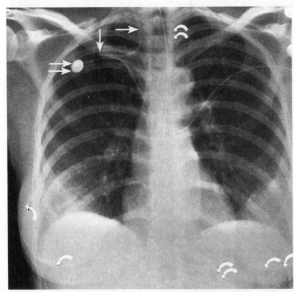

B

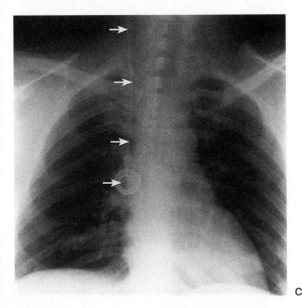

C

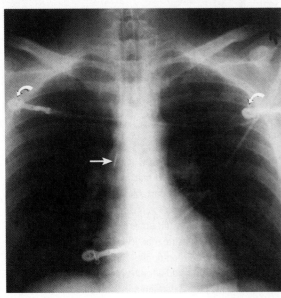

D

FIGURE 3.36. *Normal tube and line positions* **A:** Chest AP radiograph. The ET tip is 5 cm above the carina. The tip of the central line via a right jugular vein approach projects over the superior vena cava. The *curved arrow* points to a monitoring electrode that lies on the skin on the patient's left shoulder. **B:** Chest AP radiograph. Right jugular central line inadvertently passed into the right subclavian vein (*single straight arrow*). Bilateral breast implants are present (*single curved arrows*). A monitoring electrode (*double straight arrows*) and a nasogastric tube (*double curved arrows*) are also present. **C:** Chest AP radiograph. The Hickman line (*arrows*) with a chest port catheter is directed cephalad up into the right jugular vein rather than caudad toward the superior vena cava. The tip of the line is beyond the edge of the radiograph. **D:** Chest AP radiograph. Endotracheal tube (*straight arrow*) inadvertently placed in right intermediate bronchus. External monitoring electrodes are present (*curved arrows*).

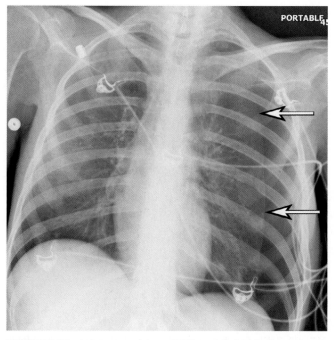

FIGURE 3.37. *Left pneumothorax.* AP chest radiograph shows a moderate left pneumothorax (*arrows*). Note the clear demarcation of the visceral pleural surface of the left lung.

Table 3.3

Causes of Pneumomediastinum

Traumatic
1. Closed chest trauma
2. Associated with pneumothorax
3. Esophageal or tracheobronchial perforation
4. Asthma
5. Ventilator induced (barotrauma)

Spontaneous
1. Bleb or bullae rupture
2. Idiopathic

Iatrogenic
1. Postsurgical (thoracotomy)
2. Esophageal resection or dilatation
3. Bronchoscopy

is the second intercostal space in the mid clavicular line. Most pleural effusions are percutaneously drained (thoracentesis) posteriorly below the seventh intercostal space.

Pneumomediastinum is a collection of air within the mediastinum, the causes of which are listed in Table 3.3. The presence of air within the mediastinum is usually an ominous sign in patients with a history of trauma or vomiting suggesting rupture of either the esophagus or trachea (Fig. 3.39). Spontaneous self-limiting pneumomediastinum may occur in young adults with asthma.

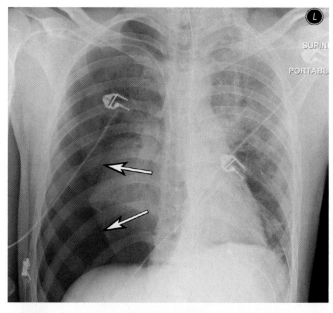

FIGURE 3.38. *Right tension pneumothorax.* Portable AP radiograph shows a large right pneumothorax with near complete collapse of the right lung (*arrows*). Note the depression of the right diaphragm and the deep right lateral costophrenic sulcus or angle (deep sulcus sign). Also, note the slight deviation of the cardiac silhouette to the left side.

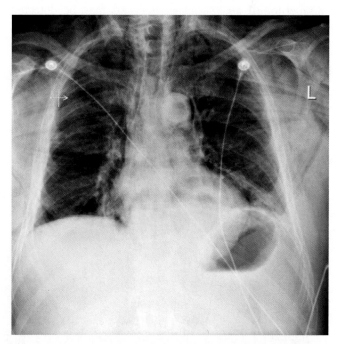

FIGURE 3.39. *Pneumomediastinum due to esophageal perforation.* PA chest radiograph shows extensive air within the mediastinum, as well as lucencies around the aortic arch and along the tracheal air column and associated subcutaneous air.

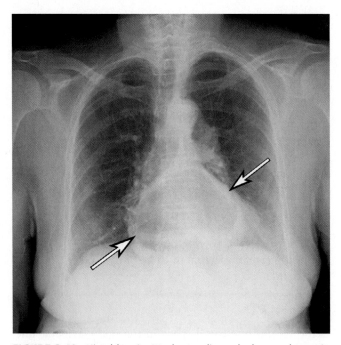

FIGURE 3.40. *Hiatal hernia.* PA chest radiograph shows a large air-filled bubble overlying the cardiac silhouette reflecting a herniation of the stomach up into the chest.

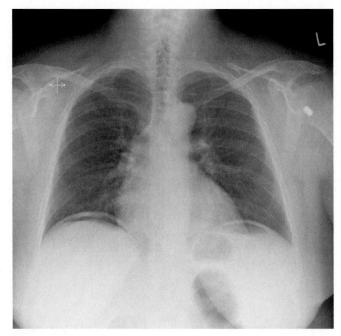

FIGURE 3.42. *Free intraperitoneal air.* PA chest radiograph showing crescentic air under both diaphragms due to a perforated gastric ulcer.

Hiatal hernias may be seen as an incidental retrocardiac lucency or density depending on the amount of air within (Fig. 3.40).

Abscess formation within the chest wall or back is seen as an air–fluid level is identified in the subcutaneous tissues (Fig. 3.41). Finally, as little as a few milliliters of free intraperitoneal air (*pneumoperitoneum*) may be detected just under the diaphragm on upright radiographs of the lower chest and upper abdomen (Fig. 3.42). This represents a significant finding and is due to visceral perforation.

Too Much Air in the Lungs

Chronic obstructive pulmonary disease (COPD) is a condition most often due to cigarette smoking, in which the

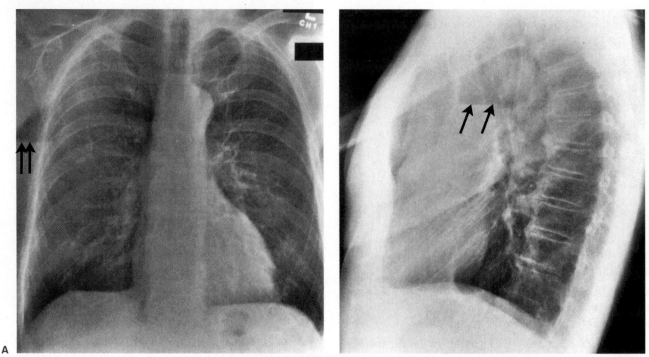

FIGURE 3.41. *Right axillary abscess.* PA **(A)** and lateral **(B)** chest radiographs. This patient developed an abscess after a right axillary node dissection. An air–fluid level (*arrows*) is seen on both views.

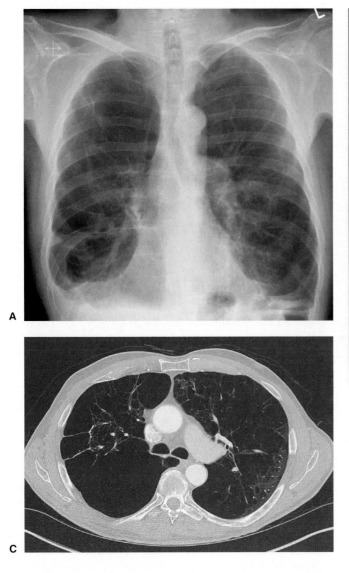

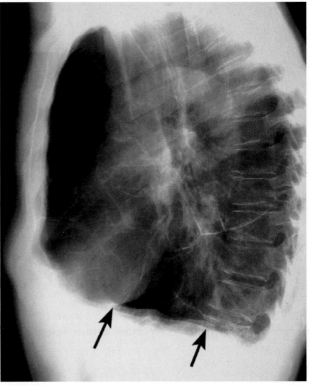

FIGURE 3.43. *Chronic obstructive pulmonary disease (COPD).* PA **(A)** and lateral **(B)** chest radiographs. The lungs are hyperlucent and hyperinflated. The diaphragms are flattened on both projections reflecting the increase in lung volumes. The retrosternal airspace is expanded and the AP dimension of the chest is greater than normal. **C:** Both lungs are lucid and void of normal lung markings reflecting both emphysema and bullous changes, which is better demonstrated on the corresponding chest CT.

lungs have become permanently damaged and the airways narrowed. Emphysema is enlargement/destruction of the alveoli distal to the terminal bronchioles without associated fibrosis. Radiographically, this is manifested as an increase in lung volumes and lucency. Due to air trapping and lung destruction, the lungs typically look hyperinflated and abnormally dark on a chest radiograph. Pulmonary cysts or bullae may also contribute to the findings of hyperinflation and translucency (Fig. 3.43A,B). Chest radiography is an insensitive screening method for diagnosing mild and moderate emphysema. High resolution CT (HRCT) on the other hand offers superior information about lung morphology and is the best modality for detecting and quantifying emphysema and/or bullous lung disease (Fig. 3.43C).

In contrast, chronic interstitial lung disease is a spectrum of disorders of various etiologies (many unknown) characterized by the presence of lung fibrosis. Radiologically, pulmonary fibrosis is characterized by the development of linear or reticular changes in the lungs in association with *diminished* lung volumes (Fig. 3.44). Usually a progressive disease, HRCT, and open lung biopsy aid in the diagnosis.

Two Signs and Two Patterns

The reason we see a border of a structure on an image is because it is contiguous with another structure of different radiographic density. This phenomenon is known as the *silhouette sign* which is the blurring or obscuration of a normal radiographic border when two contiguous structures are of similar density. Because most pathologic processes within the chest are fluid or soft tissue in density, the silhouette sign facilitates the detection and localization of these abnormalities. For example, left lower lobe pneumonia or atelectasis will obscure the border of the left hemidiaphragm. Similarly, since the right middle lobe is adjacent to the right cardiac border, any right middle lobe collapse or consolidation obscures the right cardiac border

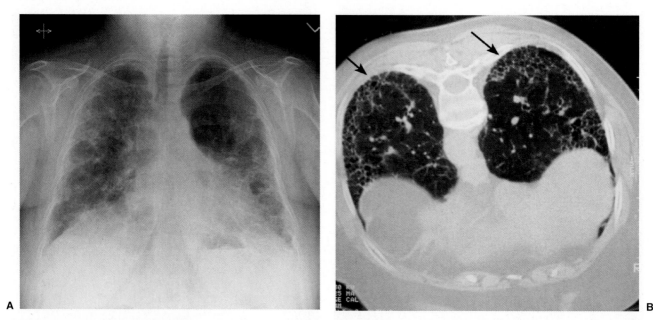

A   B

FIGURE 3.44. *Pulmonary fibrosis.* **A:** PA chest film shows extensive bilateral symmetric interstitial or reticular changes through-out both lungs reflecting pulmonary fibrosis. **B:** These interstitial changes are better demonstrated on the corresponding prone chest CT, which shows the fine interstitial markings of pulmonary fibrosis (*arrows*).

on the frontal radiograph (Fig. 3.45). The same observation also holds true for disease processes within the lingular segment of the left upper lobe, which will obscure the left heart border.

Bronchi are usually not seen on a chest film because they contain and are surrounded by air. However, when the alveoli fill with fluid such as occurs in pneumonia, pulmonary edema, and hemorrhage, the bronchi may

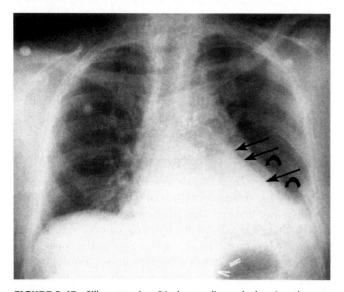

FIGURE 3.45. *Silhouette sign.* PA chest radiograph showing obscuration of the left hemidiaphragm due to left lower lobe collapse, because the density of the collapsed lung and left hemidiaphragm are juxtaposed. The *straight arrows* indicate the left lower lobe and the *curved arrows* indicate the heart.

become more conspicuous producing a sign called an *air bronchogram.*

Turning our attention to the lung parenchyma, the *pattern of airspace (alveolar) disease* is typically one of fluffy and confluent opacification. The appearance and the finding of an air bronchogram are hallmarks of *airspace disease.* In contrast, an *interstitial pattern* is due to thickening of the lung interstitium (the supporting structures) and may be subclassified as nodular (metastases, sarcoidosis, silicosis) or reticular (lines) (pulmonary interstitial edema, idiopathic pulmonary fibrosis) or a combination of both (reticulonodular). The appearance is inhomogeneous and does not respect lobar boundaries. An advanced interstitial pattern is seen in honeycombing due to pulmonary fibrosis. The two patterns, airspace and interstitial, may overlap and coexist and one may transition into the other but it is worthwhile trying to classify parenchymal lung into these two main categories.

ATELECTASIS, PLEURAL DISEASE, AND PULMONARY EMBOLI

Atelectasis

Atelectasis (or collapse) represents the loss of aeration of lung tissue. Atelectasis varies in extent from being subsegmental and appearing as linear shadows within the lungs (discoid atelectasis) (Fig. 3.46) to a complete collapse of an entire lobe or lung (Fig. 3.47). The appearance of each of the collapsed individual lobes is shown in Figure 3.48. In addition to the unique appearances of the various lobar abnormalities, five types of atelectasis are described: *Passive*

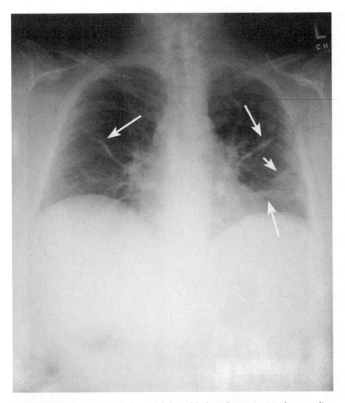

FIGURE 3.46. *Bilateral discoid (plate-like) atelectasis.* PA chest radiograph. The *arrows* indicate the typical appearance of regions of discoid atelectasis, which are commonly found in postoperative, post-trauma, severely ill, or debilitated patients.

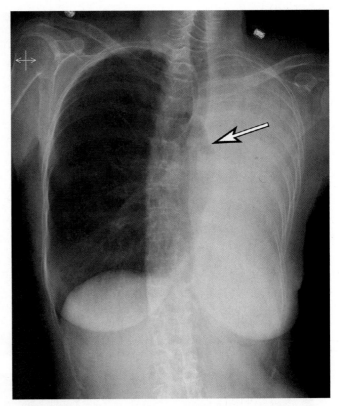

FIGURE 3.47. *Complete left lung collapse.* AP chest film shows complete collapse of the left lung which is due to mucous plugging in the left mainstem bronchus. Note how there is an abrupt loss of the normal pneumatization of the left mainstem bronchus (*arrow*) at the site of the mucous plug. This is known as the bronchial cut-off sign.

atelectasis refers to atelectatic lung usually arising from prolonged recumbency or shallow tidal volumes. *Compressive* atelectasis refers to areas of atelectasis which is compressed by an adjacent abnormality, such as a large pleural effusion. *Adhesive* atelectasis occurs when alveoli collapse due to insufficient surfactant such as occurring in hyaline membrane disease in neonates. *Postobstructive* atelectasis occurs when there is complete airway occlusion (tumor, foreign body, or mucous plugging) (Fig. 3.47). *Cicatricial* or rounded atelectasis occurs when lung tissue curls into a spherical opacity residing adjacent to a pre-existing pleural abnormality such as pleural thickening or calcification (Fig. 3.49). It is important to understand that atelectasis is not by itself a primary disease process but rather an indicator of underlying lung disease or airway abnormality. The causes of atelectasis and radiographic signs of atelectasis are listed in Tables 3.4 and 3.5, respectively.

Pleural Disease

A *pleural effusion* is an abnormal collection of fluid in the pleural space due either to an increased production or a reduced absorption. Less than 5 mL of pleural fluid is normally present to lubricate movement of the pleural surfaces during respiration. Pleural effusions are generally classified as *transudates or exudates,* based on the mechanism of fluid

formation and pleural fluid chemistry. Transudates result from an imbalance in oncotic and hydrostatic pressures and have a serum albumin and LDH level less than exudates which are usually the result of inflammation or reduced lymphatic drainage. On a PA chest film the first 175 mL is not seen as the fluid accumulates in the

Table 3.4
Causes of Atelectasis

1. Postobstructive
   a. Tumor in airway
   b. Foreign body or mucous plug in airway
   c. Infection
   d. Mainstem intubation
2. Postoperative
3. Extrinsic compression
   a. Pleural disorders: Fluid/blood/pus/tumors
   b. Pneumothorax
4. Restrictive motion
   a. Trauma
   b. Neuromuscular diseases
   c. Infections

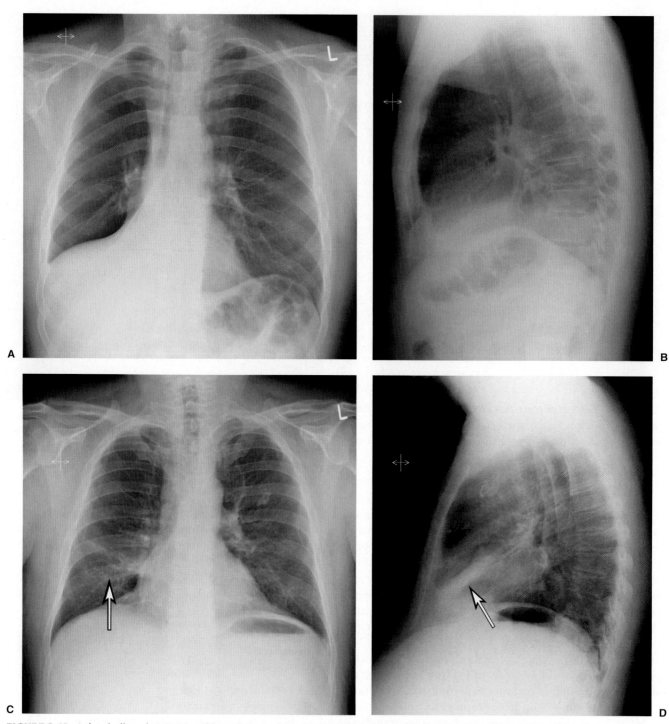

FIGURE 3.48. *Lobar (collapse).* **A,B:** PA and lateral views of the chest showing combined *right lower and middle* lobe collapse. The frontal projection shows obscuration of both the right diaphragm and right heart border (silhouette sign) and the lateral projection shows opacity overlying the lower thoracic spine due to the collapsed lower lobe (spine sign). **C,D:** *Right middle lobe* collapse. Note the partial obscuration of the right heart border on the frontal film due to atelectasis (*arrow*, **C**) and the band of atelectasis overlying the heart shadow on the lateral film (*arrow*, **D**).

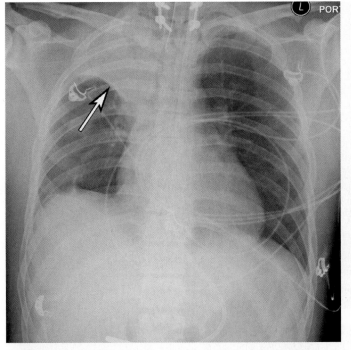

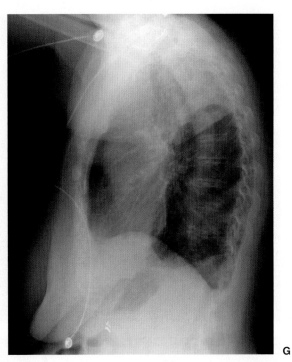

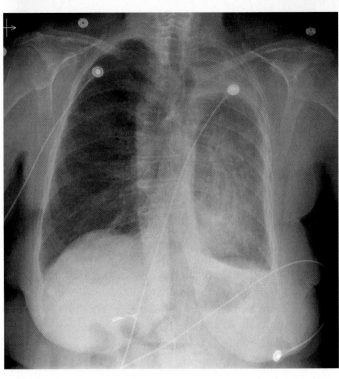

FIGURE 3.48. (*Continued*) **E:** *Right upper lobe* collapse. AP chest radiograph showing the typical wedge shaped appearance of right upper lobe collapse (*arrow*). Note the elevation of the right diaphragm reflecting the associated volume loss. **F,G:** *Left upper lobe* collapse. PA and lateral chest films show veil-like volume loss of the left lung due to complete left upper lobe collapse with associated deviation of the trachea and the heart to the left side. On the lateral film, the collapsed left upper lobe which resides anteriorly produces the generalized ground-glass changes of the left lung which are apparent on the frontal projection.

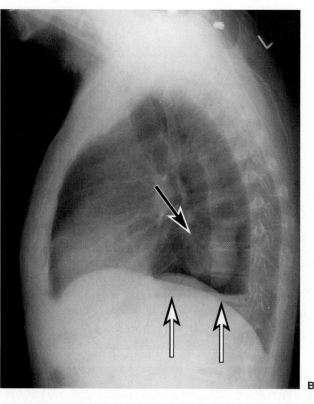

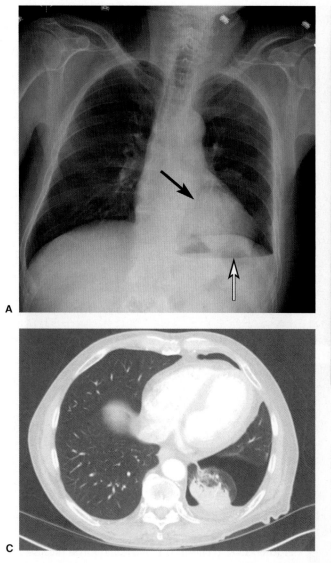

FIGURE 3.49. *Round(ed) atelectasis.* PA **(A)** and lateral films **(B)** of the chest show a spherical opacity in the left lower lobe postero-medially (*black arrows*), which, on the corresponding chest CT **(C)**, reflects an area of round atelectasis. Note the conspicuous volume loss of the left lower lobe. Also, note on the CT the presence of both air and fluid in the left pleural space (*white arrows*). This hydropneumothorax occurred after transbronchial biopsies of the left lower lobe.

subpulmonic and costophrenic regions first. With further accumulation, the hemidiaphragm and costophrenic sinus are obscured leading to the characteristic meniscus sign with the highest point in the midaxillary line. Massive pleural effusion may be seen as complete opacification of

the hemithorax with displacement of the mediastinum and hemidiaphragm away from the effusion. A pleural effusion associated with pneumonia is called *parapneumonic* effusions, which if secondarily infected will result in the accumulation of pus within the pleural space and it is then termed *empyema. Hydropneumothorax* occurs when there is both air and fluid in the pleural space, with loss of the meniscus sign.

Other examples of pleural pathology include masses and calcification. Solid pleural masses include lung carcinoma abutting the pleura and malignant mesothelioma. Pleural calcification may be due to healed empyema, tuberculosis, and asbestos exposure.

Pulmonary Embolism

Pulmonary embolism (PE) is a common cause of cardiovascular morbidity and mortality. Typically, a thrombus originating in lower extremity and/or pelvic veins migrates to the pulmonary arteries causing acute chest pain, dyspnea, and reduced cardiac output.

Table 3.5

Radiographic Signs of Atelectasis

Primary
1. Loss of volume of involved segment, lobe, or lung
2. Consolidated lung tissue
3. Air bronchograms (absent in postobstructive atelectasis)
4. Coaptation of bronchi and vessels

Secondary
1. Upward elevation of the ipsilateral hemidiaphragm
2. Mediastinal shift toward side of collapse
3. Closer spacing of ribs

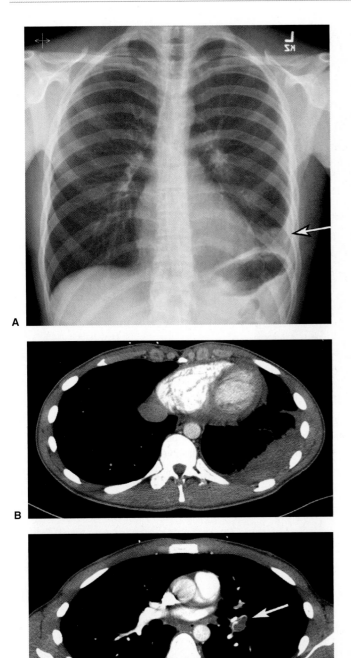

A

B

C

FIGURE 3.50. *Pulmonary embolism.* Patient presented with acute shortness of breath and chest pain. The PA film **(A)** shows a subtle peripheral pleural-based opacity in the left lower lobe (*arrow*), which on corresponding chest CT **(B)** relates to a large area of peripheral left lower lobe consolidation/infarction (Hampton hump). **C:** CT angiography revealed a large occlusive left lower lobe acute pulmonary embolus (*arrow*).

The chest film findings in patients with acute PE are variable and may be normal in up to 20% of patients. Abnormal findings include atelectasis, effusion, and pulmonary infarction (Fig. 3.50). A CT Chest is the current gold standard for making the diagnosis (Fig. 3.50C) and

this test has replaced ventilation/perfusion (V/Q) scanning and pulmonary angiography (Fig. 3.51). However, ventilation/perfusion scans are still useful in patients who cannot receive IV contrast due to impaired renal function or those with a history of prior contrast allergy. See Chapter 10 for more on V/Q scanning. Rarely, thrombus may originate from central venous lines, which when infected can cause septic pulmonary emboli which result in cavitary lung abscesses (Fig. 3.52).

PULMONARY INFECTIONS

Because of the myriad of potential pathogens, it is difficult to determine the microbiologic cause of pneumonia based on the radiographic appearances alone. In general, pneumonias appear as airspace infiltrate or consolidation. The findings range from a segmental infiltrate to complete opacification of both lungs (Figs. 3.53–3.57). Lung abscess, a complication of pneumonia especially with *Staphylococcus aureus, Streptococcus pyogenes,* and gram-negative organisms, appears as a cavity associated with lung consolidation (Figs. 3.58–3.59).

Atypical pneumonias are characterized by a lack of exudate into alveoli. Instead, the interstitium of the lung becomes inflamed with the result that airspace consolidation is minimal or lacking and chest film is opacified disproportionately to the severity of clinical features. Table 3.6 lists common causes of atypical pneumonia and examples are shown in Figures 3.60 and 3.61. *Immunosuppressed* patients are particularly susceptible to fungal and mycobacterial infections. Despite new therapies and improved public health measures, *pulmonary tuberculosis* continues to be a persistent and problematic disease. As much as one-third of the world's population has been infected with *Mycobacterium tuberculosis* which typically involves the lungs, but can also affect other organs. Most tuberculous infections are asymptomatic and *latent (primary),* but about one in ten latent infections progresses to *active disease (post primary)* which, if untreated has a 50% mortality rate. In active pulmonary TB, infiltrates or consolidations and/or cavities are often seen in the upper lungs with or without mediastinal or hilar lymphadenopathy. As many as 25% of people with active TB may be asymptomatic and it may become a chronic illness causing bronchiectasis and

Table 3.6
Causes of Atypical Pneumonia
Cytomegalovirus
Legionnaires' disease
Measles
Mycoplasma
Pneumocystis
Tuberculosis
Varicella

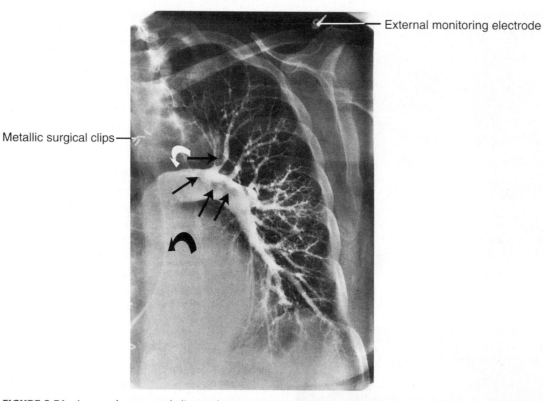

External monitoring electrode

Metallic surgical clips

FIGURE 3.51. *Acute pulmonary embolism: Pulmonary angiogram.* This 72-year-old woman had 72-hour status post coronary artery bypass grafting and developed acute shortness of breath and hypoxia. There are multiple pulmonary emboli (*straight arrows*) within the left main pulmonary artery and its branches secondary to lower extremity deep vein thrombosis. The angiographic catheter (*curved arrows*) is visible in the left pulmonary artery.

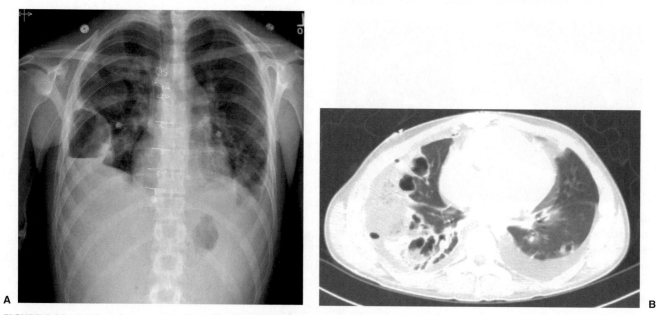

A   B

FIGURE 3.52. *Septic pulmonary emboli.* **A:** PA chest film shows numerous cystic lung lesions (abscesses) on the right side along with a right pleural effusion. **B:** Corresponding chest CT image shows to better advantage these scattered pulmonary abscesses, which are bilateral and which have the peripheral distribution typical of septic embolic disease.

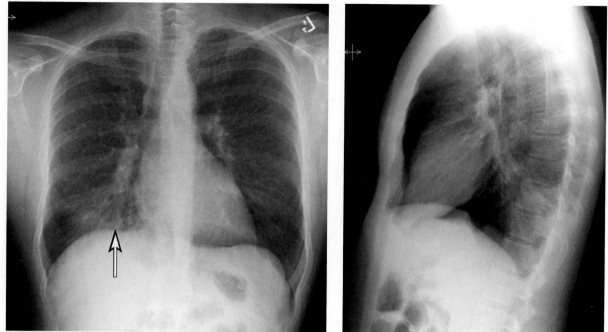

FIGURE 3.53. *Right lower lobe pneumonia.* PA **(A)** and lateral **(B)** views of the chest show airspace disease in the right lower lobe (*arrow,* **A**). Note on the lateral projection the corresponding "spine sign" produced by the infiltrate which overlies the lower thoracic spine. The spine sign refers to additional density overlying the spine by a superimposed opacity which in this case was due to the right lower lobe infiltrate.

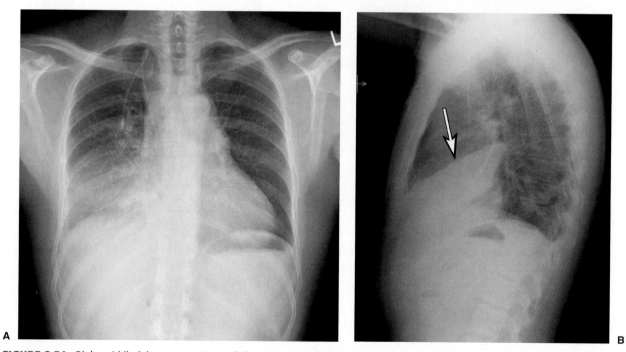

FIGURE 3.54. *Right middle lobe pneumonia.* PA **(A)** and lateral **(B)** films show a confluent opacity in the right middle lobe (*arrows*).

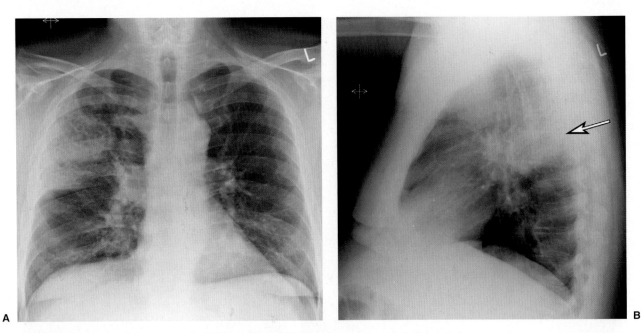

A   B

FIGURE 3.55. *Right upper lobe pneumonia.* PA **(A)** and lateral **(B)** films show pneumonia in the posterior segment of the right upper lobe (*arrow*, **B**).

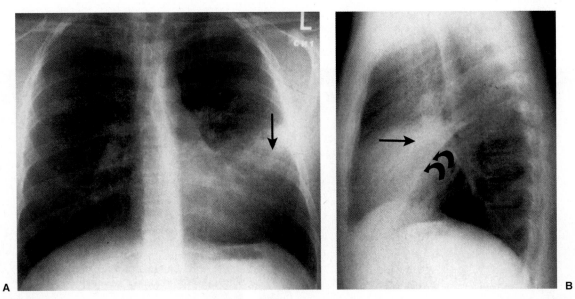

A   B

FIGURE 3.56. *Lingular pneumonia.* PA **(A)** and lateral **(B)** films show an infiltrate in the lingula (*arrows*). Note the obscuration of the left heart border on the PA projection (silhouette sign).

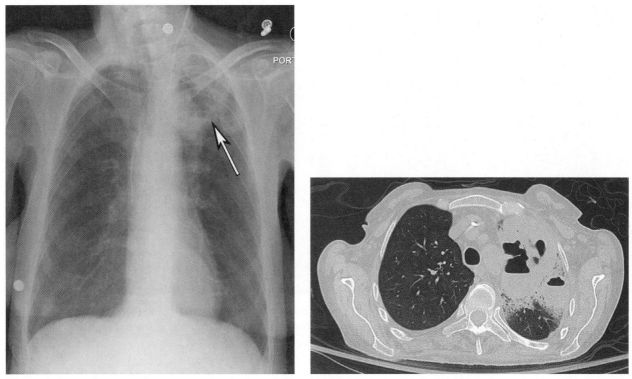

FIGURE 3.57. *Pulmonary abscess.* PA chest radiograph **(A)** and chest CT image **(B)** show a large left upper lobe consolidation with cavitation (*arrow*, **A**) typical of a pulmonary abscess which in this case was due to *Staphylococcus aureus.*

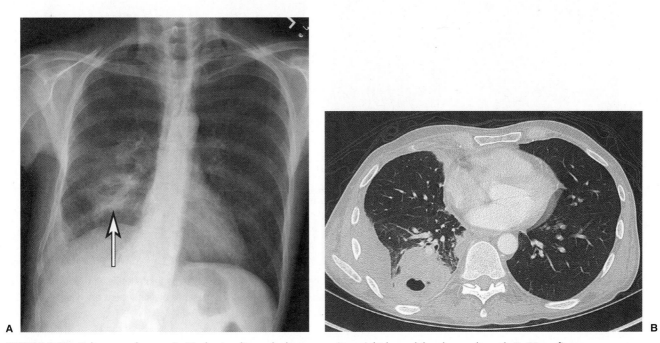

FIGURE 3.58. *Pulmonary abscess.* **A:** PA chest radiograph shows a cavitary right lower lobe abscess (*arrow*). **B:** CT confirms the cavitation.

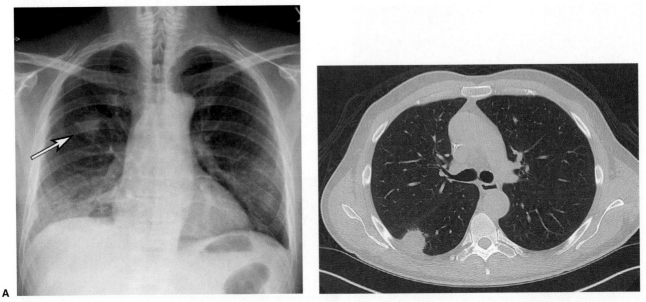

A   B

FIGURE 3.59. *Acute pulmonary aspergillosis.* PA chest radiograph **(A)** and chest CT image **(B)** both show a conspicuous nodule (*arrow,* **A**) in a patient with profound neutropenia after bone marrow transplant for leukemia. The nodules in *aspergillosis* have a solid and slight spiculated morphology mimicking a bronchogenic carcinoma.

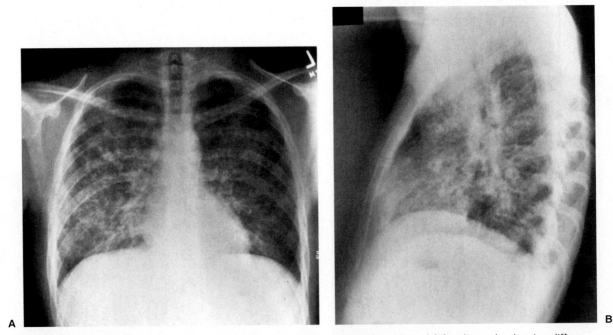

A   B

FIGURE 3.60. *Atypical pneumonia due to varicella (chicken pox).* Chest PA **(A)** and lateral **(B)** radiographs showing diffuse reticulonodular infiltrates throughout both lung fields. These patients are acutely ill, and the presence of skin lesions are diagnostically helpful.

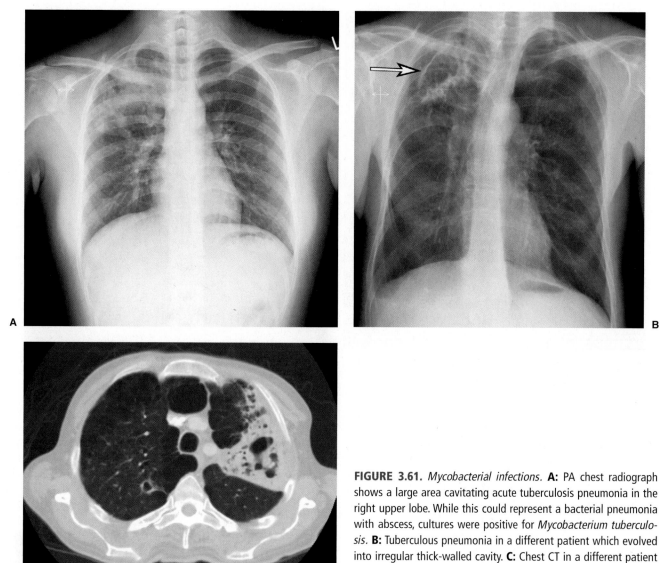

FIGURE 3.61. *Mycobacterial infections.* **A:** PA chest radiograph shows a large area cavitating acute tuberculosis pneumonia in the right upper lobe. While this could represent a bacterial pneumonia with abscess, cultures were positive for *Mycobacterium tuberculosis.* **B:** Tuberculous pneumonia in a different patient which evolved into irregular thick-walled cavity. **C:** Chest CT in a different patient shows a left upper lobe cavitary pneumonia due to *M. tuberculosis.*

extensive fibrosis in the upper lobes. *Miliary TB* is characterized by a multisystem dissemination any time after primary infection and occurs in immunosuppressed patients. The lesions are small (1 to 3 mm) discrete granulomata detectable on CT before a chest film. It is very unlikely that a calcified tuberculous granuloma will progress to active TB.

Pneumocystis pneumonia (PCP) or *pneumocystosis* is caused by a yeast-like fungus *Pneumocystis jirovecii,* a pathogen which is specific to humans. Pathologically the alveolar septa become thickened in combination with the development of an eosinophilic alveolar exudate. Both the thickened septa and the exudate contribute to the reduced oxygen diffusion which is characteristic of this pneumonia. Initially, chest imaging shows bilateral, diffuse, often perihilar, fine, reticular or reticulonodular *interstitial* pattern. This interstitial pattern progresses to *airspace* pattern disease over several days, which may then be followed by coarse reticulation as the infection resolves. Chest films

are normal in up to 20% of PCP patients, with HRCT and Gallium-67 imaging being more sensitive in making the diagnosis. On HRCT, PCP is seen as ground-glass attenuation, which refers to parenchymal opacification which does not obscure the underlying pulmonary architecture and represents an exudative alveolitis. Pneumothorax is a well-known complication of PCP.

PULMONARY NODULES, MASSES, AND CARCINOMA

A *solitary pulmonary nodule* (SPN) is defined as a discrete, rounded lung opacity less than or equal to 3 cm in diameter, and is not associated with adenopathy, collapse, or pleural effusion. The most common causes are listed in Table 3.7. Lesions larger than 3 cm are considered *masses* and are treated as malignancies until proven otherwise. The workup of an SPN depends on a variety of factors

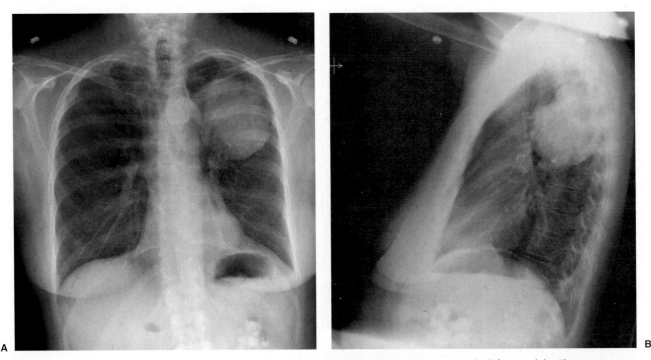

A   **B**

FIGURE 3.62. *Squamous cell lung carcinoma.* PA **(A)** and lateral **(B)** radiographs show a large mass in the left upper lobe. The risk of malignancy increases with lesion size.

including the pretest probability of malignancy, size, and morphology of the nodule, and the age of the patient, as it is known that 50% of smokers over the age of 50 have lung nodules on screening CTs.

Clearly, there is considerable difference in the likelihood of malignancy when dealing with a smooth 1-cm nodule in a 30-year-old nonsmoker compared to a 2-cm spiculated nodule in a 60-year-old lifetime smoker. First, the larger the nodule, the greater the chance that it will be malignant (Fig. 3.62). Second, any growth of a pre-existing nodule suggests a malignancy, so review of previous imaging is essential. Other features which increase the likelihood of malignancy include pleural effusions, hilar or mediastinal adenopathy, or presence of bone, adrenal gland, or liver lesions indicating potential sites of metastatic disease (Fig. 3.63). Primary lung carcinomas, especially squamous cell, may present as a cavity which may be mistaken as nonmalignant lung lesions such as a lung abscess (Fig. 3.64).

Imaging has not proven reliable in distinguishing benign from malignant lesions. While spiculation suggests malignancy, many malignant lung nodules, particularly metastases are smoothly marginated (Fig. 3.65). Dystrophic

calcification of a lung nodule suggests a benign process, specifically granulomatous disease (Fig. 3.66). Calcifications within granulomas are variable including solid, centrally located nidus, or laminar patterns. If there is doubt as to whether or not a nodule contains calcification, CT can be used to measure the density of the nodule. When the CT density of a pulmonary nodule measures greater than 200

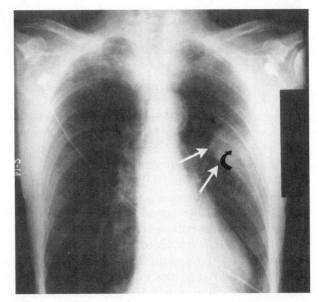

FIGURE 3.63. *Carcinoma of the lung with rib destruction.* AP chest radiograph shows a carcinoma in the left upper lobe (*white arrows*) with destruction of an adjacent rib due to local erosion (*black arrow*). Note that the lungs are overexpanded, secondary to COPD. A monitoring electrode runs across the thorax from left to right.

Table 3.7	
Causes of Pulmonary Nodules	
Single	**Multiple**
Granuloma	Metastases
Carcinoma	Histoplasmosis
Hamartoma	Sarcoidosis

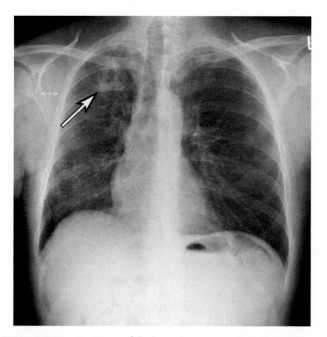

FIGURE 3.64. *Carcinoma of the lung.* There is a small cavitary right upper lobe pulmonary nodule (*arrow*). While the differential includes other nonmalignant diseases such as infection especially TB, or abscess, and subsequent biopsy revealed that this lesion was a squamous cell carcinoma.

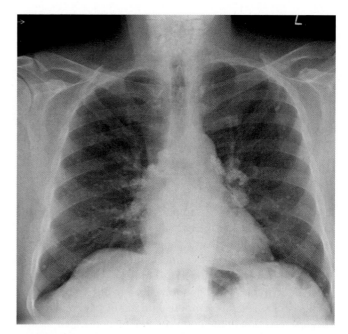

FIGURE 3.66. *Histoplasmosis.* PA chest radiograph shows numerous small calcified pulmonary nodules in both lungs due to *Histoplasma capsulatum.* Also note the calcified bilateral hilar lymph nodes.

Hounsfield units, and the calcification composes most of the nodule, a benign entity is confirmed and no further evaluation or surveillance is required. A 9-mm SPN with a (volume) doubling time of 100 days will measure 1.1 cm at 3 months and 1.4 cm at 6 months. Therefore, radiographic

surveillance necessitates accurate measurement. It has also been noted that as a nodule grows, it may become less well defined, and ironically appear smaller on subsequent chest films. CT which has better contrast resolution, provides better delineation if the margins of the nodule are unclear

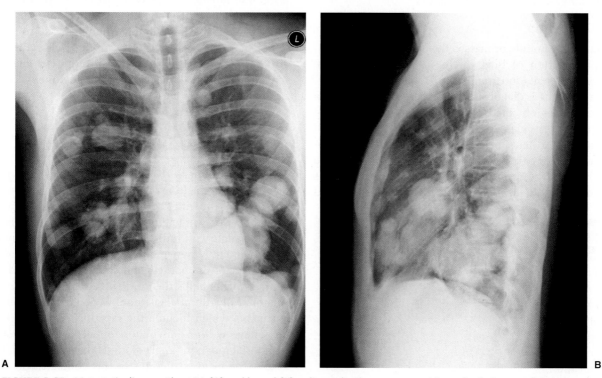

FIGURE 3.65. *Metastatic disease.* Chest PA **(A)** and lateral **(B)** radiographs show numerous bilateral soft tissue nodules consistent with metastases in a patient with testicular cancer.

on conventional chest films. A solitary noncalcified nodule which does not change in size or appearance over a 2-year period is considered benign. This rule should be applied however with caution, as there are exceptions, especially when the pretest probability for malignancy is high.

A panel of chest radiology experts (The Fleischner Society) have published guidelines for the management of SPNs and more recently "semisolid" pulmonary nodules (2,3). As a general rule, *biopsy* of an SPN is not indicated in the initial course of management because the results will be either positive (requiring surgical resection), or "nondiagnostic," that is, no evidence of tumor cells (which could be a false negative due to sampling error). A nondiagnostic biopsy would then leave two alternatives, namely surgical resection of the nodule or radiographic surveillance. When the pretest probabilities for cancer and the nodule are small, the best initial course of action should be surveillance with serial radiographs every 6 months for 2 years. Conversely, if the level of suspicion or pre-test probability is so high that surgical resection of the nodule would be performed regardless of the outcome of the biopsy, then, surgical resection rather than biopsy is the best course of action. Biopsy of any solitary nodule in this scenario only adds an intermediate step that has no real value. There are two exceptions to this rule when biopsy of a solitary nodule can be considered: (1) Patients who are either non-surgical candidates (due to coexisting morbidities) and a tissue diagnosis is needed prior to instituting therapy, or (2) a new pulmonary nodule is discovered in the setting of a known primary cancer. In the latter case, biopsy determines whether the nodule is a primary lung carcinoma or a metastasis.

Lung Carcinoma

A solitary lung nodule or mass is the most common radiologic presentation of lung carcinoma. Other radiologic findings at presentation are listed in Table 3.8.

The definitive diagnosis of lung cancer is based on a tissue diagnosis obtained by biopsy. Histologically lung carcinoma may be classified into small cell and nonsmall cell which is further subclassified into squamous, adenocarcinoma, and large cell carcinoma. *Small-cell lung carcinoma* (SCLC) should be regarded as a systemic disease and is rarely operable at diagnosis. It is classified as "limited

---

Table 3.8
Radiological Presentation of Lung Carcinoma
Solitary pulmonary nodule
Central/mediastinal/hilar mass
Persistent infiltrate
Cavity
Atelectasis
Pleural effusion
Calcification
Bone erosion (Rib/vertebral body)

---

stage" (confined to one-half of the chest) or "extensive stage" (more widespread disease). *Nonsmall-cell lung cancer (NSCLC)* is staged based on the size of the Tumor, Node involvement, and presence of Metastasis (TNM) with stages up to 3A being operable. A malignant pleural effusion indicates a stage T4 lung carcinoma, which precludes curative surgery. Genetic mutations (EGFR, KRAS, and ALK), which are found in up to 50% of adenocarcinomas of the lung, are predictive of successful treatment with newer chemotherapeutic agents such as thyrosine kinase inhibitors. Testing for these mutations requires a large sample of tissue which can be obtained with a core biopsy.

One-half of all patients are asymptomatic when diagnosed with lung carcinoma, and the aim of screening patients for lung carcinoma is to diagnose and treat them at an earlier stage, improving survival. Regular chest radiography examination programs have not been effective in reducing mortality from lung cancer. The International Early Lung Cancer Action Project (I-ELCAP) published the results of CT screening on over 31,000 high-risk patients in late 2006 (4). The vast majority of lung carcinomas detected were stage 1 and treatable. In 2007, another study in which 3,200 current or former smokers were screened for 4 years and offered three or four CT scans, found no mortality benefit from CT-based lung cancer screening (5). Although lung cancer diagnoses were three times as high, and surgeries were ten times as high, as predicted by a model, there were no significant differences between observed and expected numbers of advanced cancers or deaths. A third study which is ongoing, the *National Cancer Institute's National Lung Screening Trial* involves over 53,000 heavy smokers who either received three CT scans or three x-rays annually (6). Preliminary findings of the study have found that deaths in the CT scan group of patients were 20.3% lower than in the x-ray group. The benefits of screening still have to be balanced against the risks associated with false positives.

MEDIASTINAL COMPARTMENTS AND PATHOLOGY

The mediastinum is the space in the chest between the pleural sacs of the lungs that contains all the viscera of the chest except the lungs and pleurae. On a chest film, mediastinal masses characteristically form an *obtuse* rather than an acute angle with lung tissue and they do not show an air bronchogram. When presented with a mediastinal mass, knowledge of the borders and contents of the mediastinal compartments helps the differential diagnosis (Table 3.9). Anatomically, the mediastinum is divided into four compartments which include the *superior mediastinum* which lies above a line drawn horizontally from the sternal–manubrial junction (angle of Louis) back to the T4/T5 disc space. The major structures in this compartment include the thyroid gland, esophagus, trachea, and great vessels of the head and neck as well as the aortic arch. Radiologically,

Table 3.9

Mediastinal Mass by Location

Anterior
1. Thyroid and parathyroid masses
2. Thymic gland tumors (thymomas, cysts, thymic carcinoma/sarcoma)
3. Teratoma
4. Lymphadenopathy/lymphoma and leukemia
5. Aneurysms, especially of ascending thoracic aorta
6. Chest wall/bone tumor (i.e., sarcomas, metastatic disease)

Middle Mediastinum (90% of masses are malignant)
1. Bronchogenic carcinomas and bronchogenic cyst
2. Lymphadenopathy/lymphoma/leukemia
3. Pericardial fat pad and pericardial cyst
4. Diaphragm (Morgagni) hernia
5. Aneurysms
6. Esophageal neoplasms and masses

Posterior Mediastinum
1. Neurogenic tumors (30% are malignant)
2. Duplication cysts
3. Lymph node enlargement
4. Esophageal lesions
5. Diaphragmatic (Bochdalek) hernias
6. Extramedullary hematopoiesis

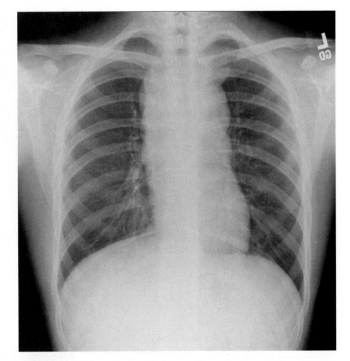

FIGURE 3.67. *Lymphoma.* PA chest radiograph shows bulky adenopathy producing a generalized widening of the mediastinum in a 24-year-old man with chest discomfort.

the contents of the superior mediastinum are incorporated in the respective anterior, middle, and posterior compartments as follows: The *anterior mediastinum* extends from the posterior margin of the sternum back to the anterior surface of the pericardium and includes mediastinal fat, thymic gland, anterior chest wall muscle and bone, lymphoid tissue, and the ascending thoracic aorta. Retrosternal extension of the thyroid gland must also be occasionally considered in this compartment as well. A useful mnemonic for anterior mediastinal masses is the "terrible T's" which include thymoma, thyroid tumors, terrible lymphoma, and occasionally germ cell tumors such as teratomas (Figs. 3.67–3.69).

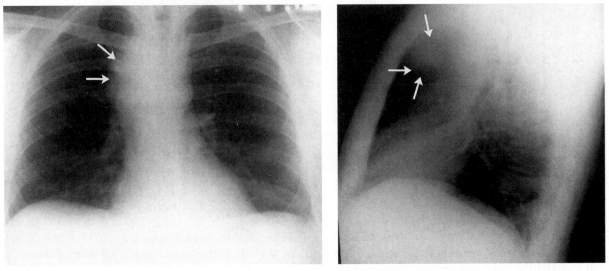

A   B

FIGURE 3.68. *Anterior mediastinal mass*: *Thymoma.* PA **(A)** and lateral **(B)** chest radiographs. There is an anterior mediastinal mass (*arrows*) in a patient with myasthenia gravis. This mass was surgically removed and revealed a benign thymoma. Malignant thymic lesions and lymphoma however would have a similar radiographic appearance.

FIGURE 3.69. *Vascular calcification.* PA **(A)** and lateral **(B)** chest radiographs show a calcified ascending thoracic aortic aneurysm (*straight arrows*) which is visible on both views. On the PA radiograph, the heart appears enlarged but on the lateral view it is within normal limits. Note the old healed right rib fracture deformities (*curved arrows*). The lungs are hyperinflated. Note the surgical clips (*arrowheads*) and the artifact (*) appearing on the right shoulder.

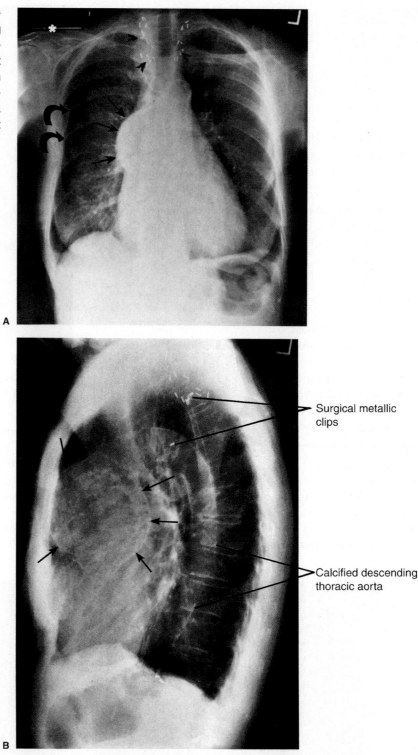

Surgical metallic clips

Calcified descending thoracic aorta

The *middle mediastinum* extends from the ventral pericardial surface posteriorly to the ventral surface of the thoracic spine and includes the heart pericardium, aortic arch, hila, esophagus, lymph nodes, and nerves (Fig. 3.70). The *posterior mediastinum* extends from the ventral border of the thoracic spine posteriorly to the chest wall and includes the spine and the descending thoracic aorta (Fig. 3.71). While CT is useful for workup of anterior and middle mediastinal masses, MRI is more helpful for posterior masses because the majority of these turn out to be neurogenic in nature.

When the hilar vessels are visible through a mediastinal mass, it is unlikely that the mass arises from the hilum.

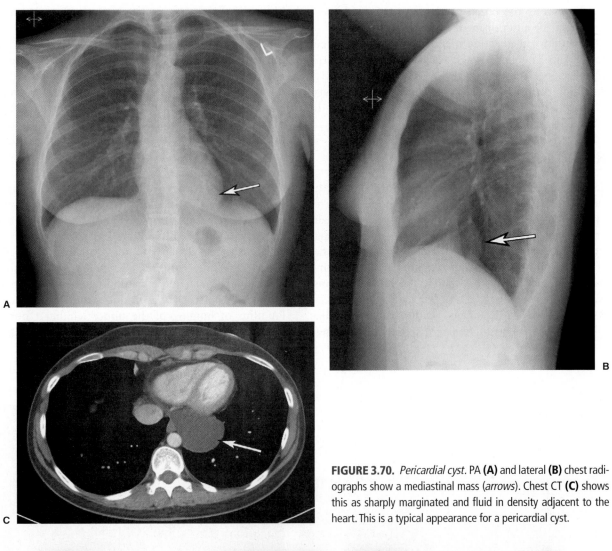

FIGURE 3.70. *Pericardial cyst.* PA **(A)** and lateral **(B)** chest radiographs show a mediastinal mass (*arrows*). Chest CT **(C)** shows this as sharply marginated and fluid in density adjacent to the heart. This is a typical appearance for a pericardial cyst.

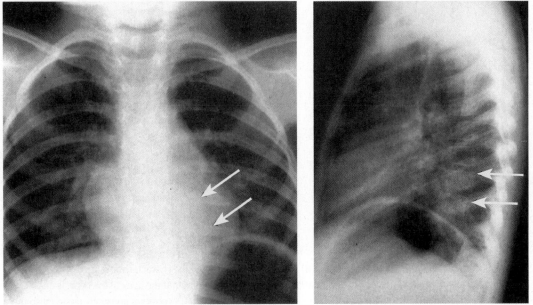

FIGURE 3.71. *Posterior mediastinal mass*: *Neuroblastoma.* **A:** On the PA view, a paraspinal mass can be seen projecting through the cardiac shadow (*arrows*). **B:** On the lateral film, the mass is posterior in location along the spine, producing a small "spine sign."

This is known as the *hilum overlay sign*. Most of these masses are in the anterior mediastinum.

The anterior mediastinum ends at the upper margin of the clavicle. Therefore, when a mass extends above the clavicle, it is located either in the neck or in the posterior mediastinum. When lung tissue is seen between the mass and the neck, the mass is probably in the posterior mediastinum. This is known as the *cervicothoracic sign*.

CARDIAC CHAMBER ENLARGEMENT

While cardiac enlargement may be global or of a specific chamber, the radiographic appearance of the heart correlates poorly with cardiac function. More advanced modalities such as echocardiography, MR imaging, nuclear imaging, and CT provide much better anatomical and functional information from which accurate quantitative data relating to myocardial perfusion and viability, ejection fractions, and valvular morphology and function can be obtained.

As discussed earlier, identification of the cardiac chambers on the PA and lateral projections of the chest films is useful in diagnosing certain cardiopulmonary and/or valvular heart diseases. The most commonly enlarged cardiac chamber in routine practice is the *left ventricle*. On the frontal (PA) projection, not only will the heart size appear enlarged but the cardiac apex is typically displaced down and out (Fig. 3.72A). On the lateral projection, expect to see posterior displacement of the left ventricular border toward the spine (Fig. 3.72B). Left ventricular dilatation can be seen with systemic hypertension, aortic valvular disease, and ischemic cardiomyopathies. When the *right ventricle* dilates, the cardiac apex is displaced upward and the heart appears somewhat boot-like in configuration (Fig. 3.73A). On the lateral film, expect to see some increased retrosternal opacity reflecting the dilated right ventricle (Fig. 3.73B). Right ventricular dilatation in adults can be seen in patients with pulmonary valvular disease or long standing pulmonary hypertension. *Left atrial* dilatation is most commonly seen in patients with mitral valve disease and produces the classic findings on PA films of bulging of the upper left heart border, the double density sign (Figs. 3.74 and 3.8), and occasionally

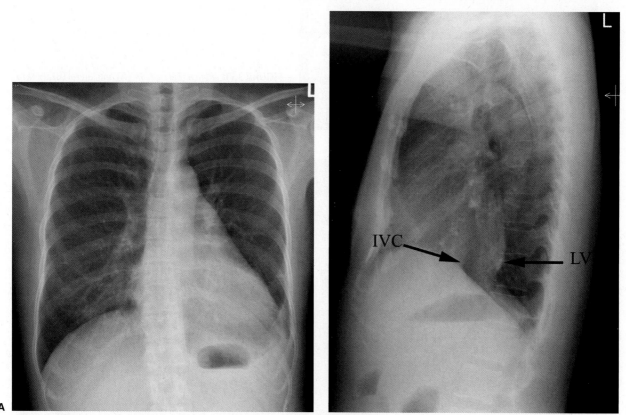

FIGURE 3.72. *Left ventricular dilatation.* PA **(A)** and lateral **(B)** views of the chest show the characteristic morphologic changes in the cardiac silhouette in a patient with left ventricular dilatation. **A:** Note on the PA film that the apex of the heart is displaced down and out. **B:** On the lateral film, note how the posterior margin of the left ventricle (LV) projects unusually posterior to the IVC. Normally, the posterior border of the left ventricle should be within 2 cm of the posterior border of the IVC.

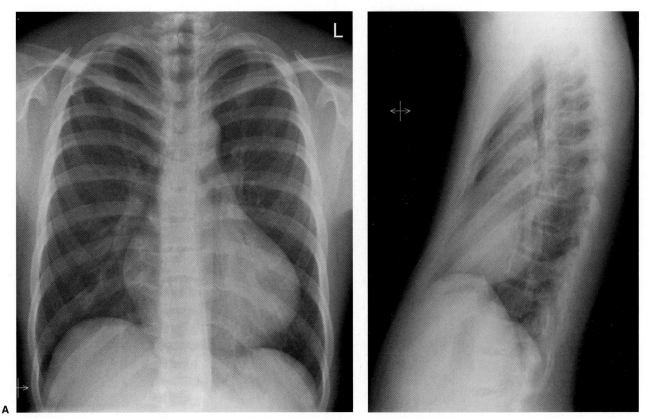

FIGURE 3.73. *Right ventricular enlargement.* **A:** PA film of the chest shows the characteristic upward pointing of the cardiac apex characteristic of right ventricular dilatation. **B:** On the lateral film, note how the retrosternal region is more opacified than usual reflecting the corresponding dilatation of the right ventricle.

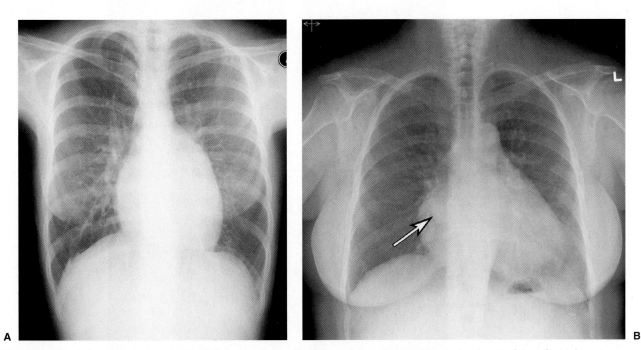

FIGURE 3.74. *Left atrial enlargement.* **A:** PA film shows convexity of the left heart border due to enlargement of the left atrial appendage. **B:** The double density sign of left atrial enlargement can be seen, which corresponds to the overlap of the right atrial shadow and the right lateral wall of the left atrium (*arrow*). Also see Figure 3.8.

FIGURE 3.75. *Multichamber enlargement: Mitral stenosis.* PA **(A)** and lateral **(B)** chest films show severe cardiomegaly and a prosthetic mitral valve (*straight arrows*). On the PA view, the enlarged left atrium creates the double density indicated by the *curved arrows,* and the left atrial appendage is prominent along the left cardiac border. Also, on the PA view, there is right atrial and left ventricular enlargement. On the lateral view, right ventricular enlargement results in fullness of the retrosternal space. Also, on the lateral view, there is enlargement of the left atrium and ventricle.

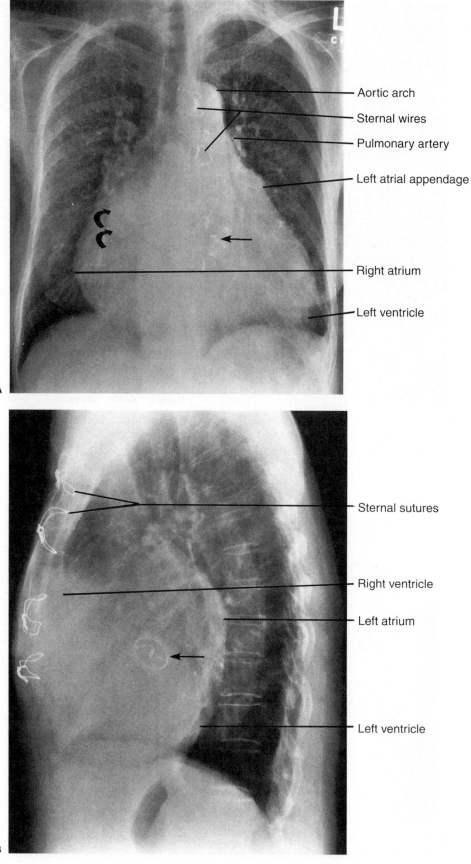

Aortic arch

Sternal wires

Pulmonary artery

Left atrial appendage

Right atrium

Left ventricle

Sternal sutures

Right ventricle

Left atrium

Left ventricle

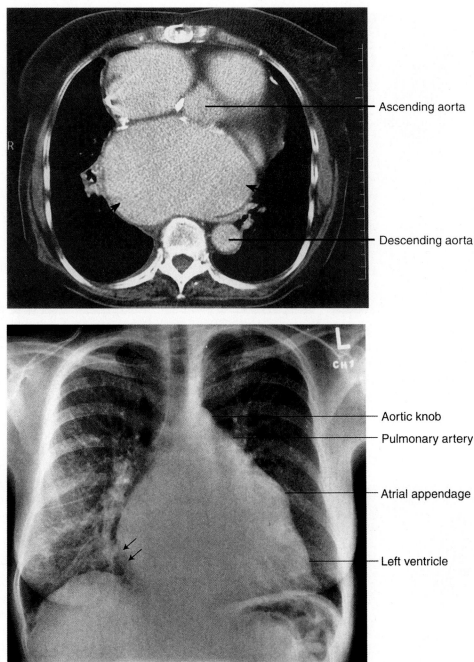

FIGURE 3.75. (*Continued*) **C:** Chest axial CT image through the atrial level. Left atrial enlargement (*straight arrows*). **D:** Shows typical changes in the morphology of the heart of left atrial enlargement in a patient with mitral stenosis. Again note the bulging left heart border and the double density sign (*arrows*).

displacement of the left mainstem bronchus. Examples of mitral and aortic valvular disease are illustrated on Figures 3.75 and 3.76, respectively. *Right atrial* enlargement will produce a conspicuous protuberant right heart shadow (Fig. 3.9) and can be most commonly seen in patients with tricuspid valve disease or right heart failure.

ANEURYSMS AND VASCULAR CALCIFICATIONS

Pulmonary arterial aneurysms may present as hilar enlargement which is a common finding in patients with pulmonary hypertension (Fig. 3.77). Atherosclerotic calcification of thoracic vessels occurs commonly with advancing age,

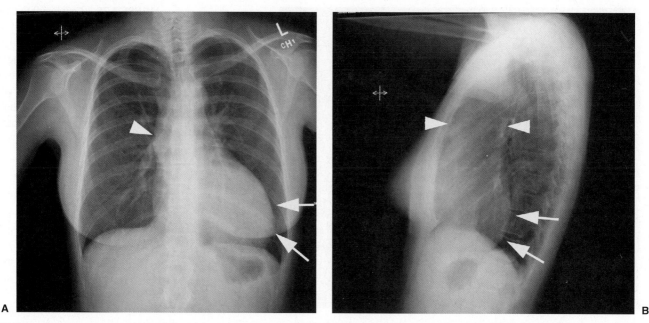

A   B

FIGURE 3.76. *Aortic stenosis.* PA **(A)** and lateral **(B)** radiographs show left ventricular enlargement (*straight arrows*) manifested by rounding of the cardiac apex on the PA view, and on the lateral view the enlarged left ventricle projects more than 2 cm posterior to the inferior vena cava). The ascending aorta is dilated (*arrowheads*), and this is often encountered in patients with severe aortic stenosis reflecting poststenotic dilatation.

usually without associated vascular aneurysm. Premature vascular calcifications, especially when discovered in younger patients can be indicators of hyperlipidemia or diabetes mellitus.

PULMONARY EDEMA

While there are many causes of pulmonary edema (Table 3.10), the most common cause, is left ventricular failure (*cardiogenic pulmonary edema*). Normally on upright films, most blood flow is seen in the lower one-third of each lung while the upper lobe vessels are normally usually collapsed

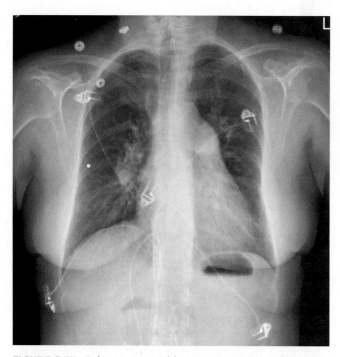

FIGURE 3.77. *Pulmonary arterial hypertension.* PA chest film showing enlargement of both pulmonary arteries. Since this finding however is present in only approximately 30% of patients with pulmonary hypertension, lack of pulmonary arterial enlargement on chest films does not exclude a diagnosis of pulmonary hypertension.

Table 3.10
Causes of Pulmonary Edema

1. Cardiogenic (heart failure)
2. Neurogenic (head injury)
3. Noncardiogenic (increased permeability > injury > edema)
   a. Toxic gas or smoke inhalation
   b. High-altitude sickness
   c. Aspiration
   d. Contusion
   e. Fat embolism
   f. Sepsis

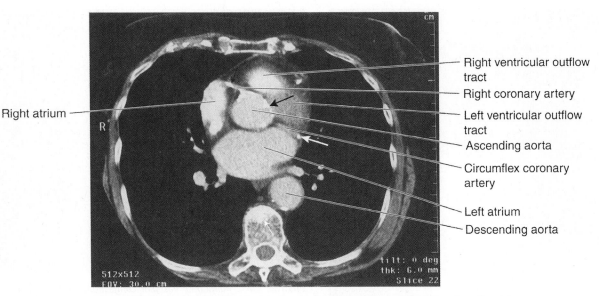

Right atrium

Right ventricular outflow tract
Right coronary artery
Left ventricular outflow tract
Ascending aorta
Circumflex coronary artery
Left atrium
Descending aorta

FIGURE 3.78. *Vascular calcification.* Axial CT with contrast image through the level of the left atrium. The right coronary artery, the circumflex coronary artery, and ascending and descending aorta all contain atherosclerotic calcifications (*white arrow*). Also note the aortic valve calcifications (*black arrow*).

and fairly inconspicuous. The radiographic appearances depend on the hydrostatic effects of left ventricular failure and pulmonary venous hypertension (Table 3.11). The first radiographic sign of congestive heart failure is *cephalad redistribution* of pulmonary blood flow to the upper lobes which is in response to impaired oxygen diffusion across the capillary–alveolar interface. In an attempt to improve oxygenation, pulmonary blood flow is diverted to the upper lobes. The pulmonary vessels at this stage should still remain sharp in outline (Fig. 3.78).

With further deterioration in left ventricular function, there is transudation of intravascular fluid into the adjacent perivascular connective tissues (interstitium). This phenomenon produces *interstitial edema* or *Kerley lines*, which are identified on chest films as small parallel linear shadows in the periphery of lungs, usually best seen in lower lobes (Fig. 3.79). In addition, since interstitial fluid also surrounds the pulmonary vessels and smaller bronchi, the borders of these structures appear less sharp

causing *vascular congestion and peribronchial cuffing*, respectively (Fig. 3.80). In cases of severe left ventricular failure, extravascular fluid eventually flows into the alveoli (*pulmonary edema*) and pleural spaces. Cardiogenic pulmonary edema is represented as bilateral symmetric airspace pattern disease which may be initially in a perihilar

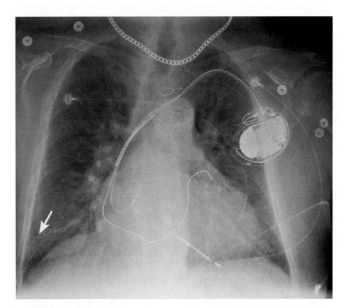

FIGURE 3.79. *Pulmonary venous hypertension.* Vascular redistribution in a patient with mild congestive heart failure. Portable chest film showing generalized dilatation of the pulmonary arteries in both lungs, especially in the upper lobes. Note that the pulmonary vessels in both lungs remain sharply defined, so there is no associated pulmonary vascular congestion. There is early interstitial edema (Kerley lines) bilaterally best appreciated in the right lung (*arrow*). Also, note the automatic defibrillator generator in the upper left chest wall with three leads extending into the heart.

Table 3.11

Radiographic Findings in Congestive Heart Failure

1. Vascular redistribution (increase size of vessels in the upper lobes)
2. Kerley B lines (interstitial edema)
3. Vascular congestion
4. Central peribronchial cuffing
5. Airspace disease/edema (batwing or diffuse and gravitational)
6. Pleural effusions (usually bilateral and symmetric in size)

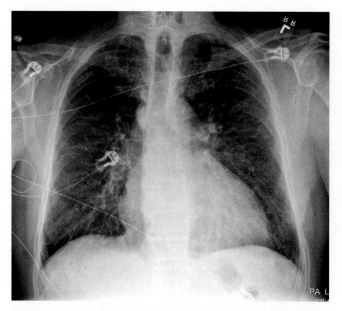

FIGURE 3.80. *Interstitial edema.* PA chest film showing diffuse linear markings throughout both lungs representing fluid in the interstitial spaces of the lungs. These markings are known as Kerley lines.

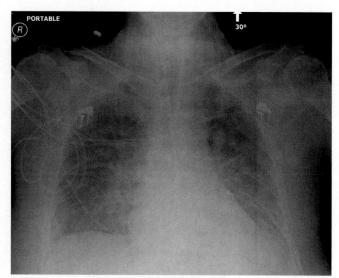

FIGURE 3.81. *Pulmonary vascular congestion.* AP chest radiograph in a patient in mild to moderate congestive heart failure demonstrates loss of sharpness of the borders of the pulmonary vasculature in both lungs reflecting the accumulation of fluid around these vessels. This is known as pulmonary vascular congestion.

or batwing distribution, and eventually becoming more diffuse in cases of severe heart failure (Fig. 3.81). Pleural effusions are common in congestive heart failure and are usually bilateral and symmetric in size. Additional helpful radiographic findings in congestive heart failure (or fluid overload) include widening of the vascular pedicle, which anatomically reflects excessive intravascular volume within the SVC and azygos vein. The vascular pedicle width is measured from the lateral aspect of the SVC at the insertion of the azygos vein horizontally to a line drawn vertically from the origin of the left subclavian artery (Fig. 3.9). On upright films, the azygos vein is usually collapsed measuring no wider than 1 cm. Distension or changes of the azygos vein diameter correlates well with changes in intravascular volume.

In contrast, *noncardiogenic pulmonary edema,* such as *Adult Respiratory Distress Syndrome (ARDS)* lacks most of the features characteristic of hydrostatic edema. In ARDS, pulmonary edema results directly from lung injury where the gap junctions of capillaries and the tight junctions of alveolar epithelium become diastatic, allowing vascular fluid and cellular constituents to accumulate within the alveoli. There is neither vascular redistribution nor interstitial edema. Furthermore, the development of pulmonary edema with lung injury is often patchy and asymmetric at onset, eventually becoming more uniform in distribution. This syndrome (ARDS) is also associated with considerable respiratory dysfunction, stiff lung compliance, and higher levels of morbidity. Because of the highly cellular composition of alveolar fluid, the overall course of the disease is protracted taking weeks to months to resolve in contrast to cardiogenic pulmonary edema which typically responds promptly to appropriate treatment.

TRAUMA

Chest radiographs allow a rapid evaluation for the presence of pneumothorax, pleural effusion, mediastinal hematoma, and lung contusion (Fig. 3.82). In patients who sustain significant chest trauma, especially those with rib fractures or rapid deceleration injury, lacerations or tears of lung tissue may occur. *Pulmonary lacerations* may be difficult to detect on routine chest radiographs but are readily apparent on CT (Fig. 3.83). These patients may

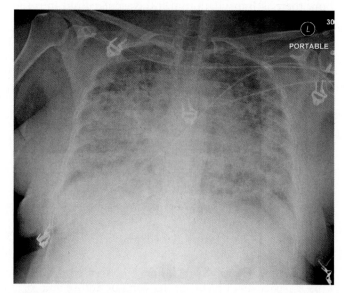

FIGURE 3.82. *Pulmonary edema.* AP chest film on a patient with severe congestive heart failure following acute myocardial infarction demonstrates widespread symmetric areas of airspace disease (edema) in both lungs.

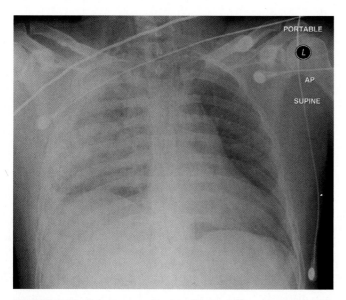

FIGURE 3.83. *Pulmonary contusion.* AP chest film on a patient following blunt trauma shows extensive unilateral airspace disease in the right lung reflecting pulmonary contusion or hematoma. Also, note the associated pleural effusion on the right reflecting a right hemothorax.

also have pulmonary contusions and pneumothoraces. Mediastinal widening in a trauma patient may be due to a hematoma and it suggests an aortic injury such as potentially fatal *transection* (traumatic aortic dissection) which most commonly occurs adjacent to the origin of the left subclavian artery (Fig. 3.84).

Rib fracture is the most common blunt thoracic injury and it is an indicator of trauma severity (Fig. 3.85). Studies have correlated the number of ribs fractured with a higher morbidity and mortality. A *first rib fracture* is significant

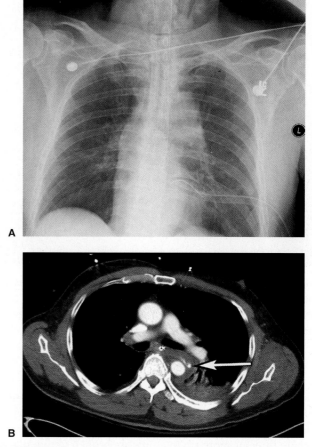

FIGURE 3.85. *Aortic transection (traumatic dissection).* Patient involved in a motor vehicle collision. **A:** AP chest radiograph obtained in the emergency room shows widening of the mediastinum suspicious for mediastinal hematoma. **B:** Contrast CT image at the level of the aortic arch showed a transection or traumatic dissection of the level of the ligamentum arteriosum with extravasation of contrast (*arrow*) from the aorta.

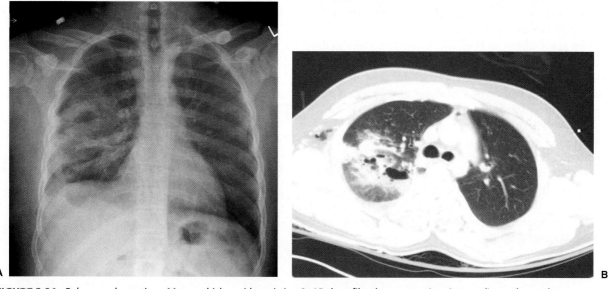

FIGURE 3.84. *Pulmonary lacerations.* Motor vehicle accident victim. **A:** AP chest film shows extensive airspace disease/hemorrhage in the right lung consistent with pulmonary contusion. Careful examination of the right lung also shows multiple lucencies. **B:** CT shows both the contusion (airspace opacities) with associated lacerations, which appear as lucencies or tears within the lung tissues.

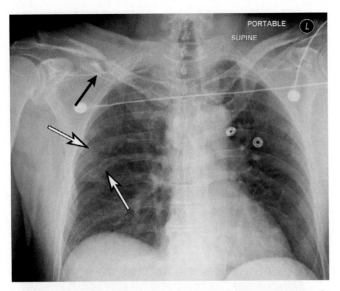

FIGURE 3.86. *Blunt chest trauma.* Patient involved in a motorcycle accident. AP chest film obtained in the emergency room shows a comminuted fracture of the right clavicle (*black arrow*) as well as several acute right rib fractures (*white arrows*).

because of the force necessary for it to occur which may also have caused thoracic visceral and vascular injury. A *flail chest* is described as a free floating segment of ribs where three or more rib fractures are broken in two places and results in paradoxical chest wall motion.

Key Points

- PA and lateral views are the routine standard chest radiographs and every attempt should be made to acquire these projections in preference to portable AP chest films which are less desirable.
- If rib or spine abnormalities are suspected, then dedicated views are necessary.
- Develop a simple systematic approach for viewing chest radiographs to avoid errors of omission. Practice and experience are paramount in developing a "good eye." Also remember that you only see what you know so knowledge of normal anatomy is a key to successful film interpretation.
- The cardiac transverse diameter should not exceed 50% of thoracic cage transverse diameter on the PA view. This is called the *cardiothoracic ratio.*
- Cardiac size appears larger on the AP than the PA view because of magnification.

- The right atrium forms the convex right cardiac border and the left ventricle forms the cardiac apex on AP or PA radiographs.
- Excessive translucency on a chest radiograph generally indicates too much air.
- Border definition is lost whenever two similar densities abut each other. This is known as the *silhouette sign* and represents a key observation for identifying pathologic processes within the chest.
  - It is useful to distinguish airspace from interstitial lung opacification.
  - Collapse/pneumonia of the various lobes has a unique appearance.
  - Atypical pneumonias result in inflammation of the interstitium rather than the alveoli.
  - Twenty percent of lung nodules are malignant.
  - CT is the best technique for diagnosis of PE in most patients.
  - The appearances of noncardiogenic edema generally take longer to resolve than cardiogenic edema.

REFERENCES

1. Appropriateness Criteria. The American College of Radiology. http://acsearch.acr.org
2. MacMahon H, Austin JH, Gamsu G, et al. Solitary pulmonary nodules. Guidelines for management of small pulmonary nodules detected on CT scans: A statement from the Fleischner Society. *Radiology.* 2005;237:395–400.
3. Naidich DP, Bankier AA, MacMahon H, et al. Recommendations for the management of subsolid pulmonary nodules detected at CT: A statement from the Fleischner Society. *Radiology.* 2013;266(1):304–317.
4. Henschke CI, Yankelevitz DF, Libby DM, et al. Survival of patients with stage I lung cancer detected on CT screening. *N Engl J Med.* 2006;355(17):1763–1771.
5. Bach PB, Jett JR, Pastorino U, et al. Computed tomography screening and lung cancer outcomes. *JAMA.* 2007;297(9): 953–961.
6. National Lung Screening Trial Research Team. The National Lung Screening Trial: Overview and study design. *Radiology.* 2011;258(1):243–253.

FURTHER READINGS

El-Khoury GY, Bergman RA, Montgomery WJ. *Sectional Anatomy by MRI,* 2nd ed. New York, NY: Churchill Livingstone, 1995.
Collins J, Stern EJ. *Chest Radiology: The Essentials.* Philadelphia, PA: Lippincott, Williams and Wilkins, 2007
Mergo PJ. *Imaging of the Chest: A Teaching File.* Philadelphia, PA: Lippincott Williams & Wilkins, 2002.
Kazerooni EA, Gross BH. *Cardiopulmonary Imaging.* Philadelphia, PA: Lippincott Williams & Wilkins, 2004.

QUESTIONS

1. A pulmonary nodule is considered benign if it remains unchanged in size over a surveillance period of how many months?
   a. 6 months
   b. 12 months
   c. 16 months
   d. 24 months

2. The silhouette sign refers to
   a. the presence of air within the mediastinum
   b. loss of normal radiographic borders due to adjacent areas of abnormal lung or pleural opacity
   c. enlargement of the cardiac silhouette
   d. tension pneumothorax

3. A 47-year-old male presents with a 1.3-cm diameter smoothly marginated pulmonary nodule. Which of the following would be the best next course of action?
   a. Surgical resection
   b. Biopsy
   c. Radiographic surveillance with serial chest films
   d. Comparison with old films

4. A 55-year-old male presents with an anterior mediastinal mass on chest film. Which of the following would not be included in the differential diagnoses?
   a. Thymoma
   b. Lymphoma
   c. Aortic aneurysm
   d. Pericardial cyst

5. A 65-year-old male presents with an acute myocardial infarction. His first chest radiographs are normal. As this patient goes into congestive heart failure (CHF), the first radiographic evidence of CHF would be
   a. Kerley lines
   b. pleural effusions
   c. cephalad redistribution of blood flow
   d. vascular congestion

6. Which of the following radiographic findings would not be associated with a tension pneumothorax?
   a. Displacement of the heart and mediastinum toward the side of the pneumothorax
   b. Depression of the ipsilateral diaphragm
   c. Tracheal deviation away from the side of the pneumothorax
   d. Pulmonary laceration

7. The double density sign indicates which of the following?
   a. Right atrial enlargement
   b. Left atrial enlargement
   c. Left ventricular enlargement
   d. Pulmonary hypertension

8. A 35-year-old female presents to the emergency room with acute shortness of breath. The attending physician suspects acute pulmonary thromboembolic disease. Which of the chest films finding might be expected?
   a. A normal chest film
   b. Pleural effusion
   c. Hampton hump
   d. Pulmonary hemorrhage
   e. All of the above

9. Which of the following would be the best radiographic sign of postobstructive left lung collapse?
   a. Total opacification of the left lung
   b. Bronchial cut-off sign
   c. Hyperinflation of the contralateral right lung
   d. Volume loss

10. A 37-year-old female presents with a solitary pulmonary nodule on her chest film. CT confirms that the nodule is densely calcified. Which of the following would be the best next step in management?
    a. Follow-up chest film in 6 months
    b. PET scan to establish the metabolic activity of the lung nodule
    c. Biopsy
    d. No additional tests

Abdomen

David M. Kuehn

Careful history and physical examination allow diagnosis of most abdominal complaints. When diagnosis remains uncertain following these procedures, an abdominal radiograph is often the first diagnostic imaging procedure requested. Recall that in women of childbearing age, consideration of possible pregnancy should precede a radiograph.

The anteroposterior (AP) radiograph (often referred from "KUB," i.e., kidney, ureter, bladder), the most frequently performed abdominal imaging study, is performed with the patient supine (Fig. 4.1A). An upright radiograph (Fig. 4.1B) is useful in searching for free intraperitoneal air and/or intestinal air–fluid levels. If the patient cannot stand, a decubitus radiograph obtained with the patient lying on either the right or, preferably, the left side (Fig. 4.1C) can be substituted.

VIEWING ABDOMINAL RADIOGRAPHS

Step 1 is to position the radiograph correctly on the imaging reader device, with the film R (right side) marker opposite the viewer's left side and the patient's head toward the top of the film. On the AP upright radiograph, there should be a sign indicating an upright view, usually an arrow near the R or L marker, pointing toward the patient's head. Similarly, decubitus radiographs should be clearly labeled as such and should note which side is up or down.

Step 2 is to glance at the entire radiograph in a relaxed manner to allow an obvious abnormality to jump out at you. When you do discover an abnormality, do not terminate your subsequent search.

Step 3 is to evaluate the radiograph systematically. Any system or checklist will suffice. Table 4.1 will work, until you develop your own. First, locate the water density liver and spleen silhouettes. One clue to locating liver and spleen edges is the presence of bowel gas in the right and left upper abdominal quadrants. Such bowel gas permits an indirect estimate of the location of the hepatic and splenic borders, because the gas is located at the lower edges of the liver and spleen. With a little experience, you will recognize a normal-sized liver. When the liver shadow

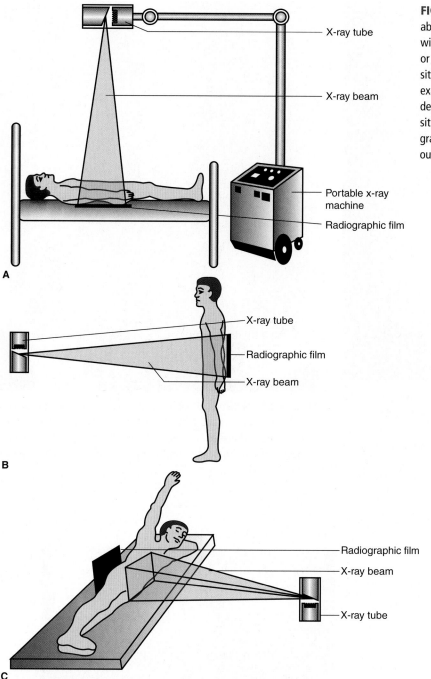

FIGURE 4.1. A: Patient positioning for an AP supine abdomen radiograph. This examination is performed with the patient supine, either on a radiographic table or in bed (using a portable x-ray unit). **B:** Patient positioning for an AP upright abdomen radiograph. This examination is usually accomplished in the radiology department, with the patient standing. **C:** Patient positioning for a left lateral decubitus abdomen radiograph. The patient's arms are positioned comfortably out of the way.

Table 4.1

Routine for Evaluating Abdominal Radiographs

1. Once-over glance
2. Liver and spleen
3. Psoas shadows
4. Renal contours and position
5. Abdominal calcifications
6. Intestinal gas pattern
7. Bones

extends to the iliac crest, it is usually enlarged. Also with more experience, you will readily detect an enlarged spleen (splenomegaly; Fig. 4.2).

In the normal radiograph, psoas muscle margins are usually visible. A nonvisible psoas margin should alert you to a possible abnormality adjacent to that structure. As your eyes drift toward the renal shadows, evaluate their size, shape, and position. The renal silhouettes are visible because they are water density structures (gray) surrounded by variable amounts of retroperitoneal fat (black). You should attempt to locate the upper and lower renal

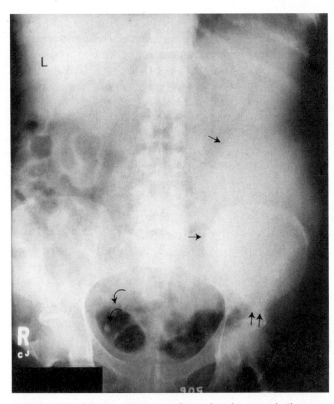

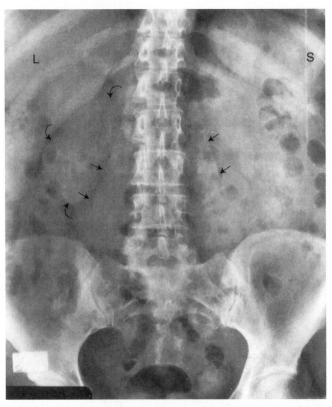

FIGURE 4.2. Abdomen AP supine radiograph. Splenomegaly. The water density spleen is enlarged (*single straight arrows*), and the inferior margin projects just above the left hip (*double straight arrows*). The large spleen has displaced the intestinal gas into the right abdomen. The liver size is normal (L, liver). Incidentally noted are phleboliths (*curved arrows*), small intravenous stones secondary to calcified thrombi.

FIGURE 4.3. Abdomen AP supine radiograph. Normal. The psoas muscles (*straight arrows*) and the right kidney (*curved arrows*) are visible. The left renal silhouette is obliterated by intestinal gas. It is common to have intestinal gas and contents obliterating the renal shadows (L, liver; S, spleen).

FIGURE 4.4. Abdomen AP supine radiograph. Classic appearance of tablets or pills (*arrows*) in the GI tract. All the tablets are the same size and shape with homogeneous density. (Not all tablets or pills can be visualized on a radiograph.)

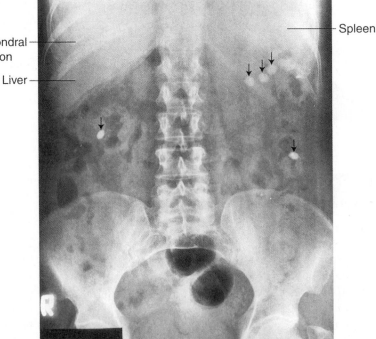

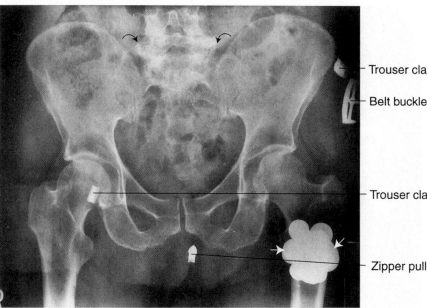

- Trouser clasp
- Belt buckle
- Trouser clasp
- Zipper pull

FIGURE 4.5. Abdomen AP supine radiograph. Metal coins (*white arrows*) in the left trouser pocket. The patient was not completely disrobed prior to obtaining the radiographs. Note the degenerative or osteoarthritic changes in the lower lumbar spine (*black arrows*).

poles as well as their medial and lateral borders. If the renal long axis is not parallel with the psoas muscle margin, you should consider a mass or other water density abnormality in the kidney or the retroperitoneum. Always look for calcifications (white) in the abdomen, especially in the region of the kidneys, ureters, urinary bladder, and the gallbladder (discussed later).

The term *Aunt Minnie,* coined by the late Dr. Ben Felson, refers to the unmistakable and unforgettable appearance of your Aunt Minnie, or Uncle Al, or any other family character. A radiologic Aunt Minnie describes an image appearance so classic that, once you see it, you never forget it. The following abdominal radiographic

Aunt Minnies (Figs. 4.3–4.9) are commonly encountered. File them away in your visual-cerebral computer, and your ability to recognize them will make you a star in the eyes of your colleagues, teachers, and patients.

Now, evaluate the bowel gas pattern (see the next section). Last but not least, look at the bones systematically, beginning with the visible ribs and spine (Fig. 4.10). Study the pedicles of the lower dorsal and lumbar spine, proceeding from head to foot. They resemble automobile headlights on an AP radiograph. A missing pedicle indicates a destructive process, such as metastatic disease. Evaluate all visible bones, including the pelves, hips, and femurs, for their overall density and any abnormalities.

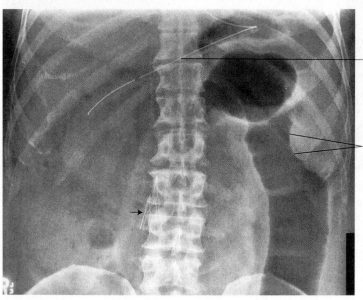

- Nasogastric tube
- Splenic impression on descending colon

FIGURE 4.6. Abdomen AP supine radiograph. An umbrella-shaped inferior vena cava filter (*arrow*), placed in the inferior vena cava by angiographic technique, entraps venous thromboemboli originating in the lower extremities and pelvis.

FIGURE 4.7. Abdomen AP upright radiograph. Surgical laparotomy pad in a postoperative abdomen. The radiograph was obtained when the patient experienced severe postoperative abdominal pain and distention. The *straight arrow* indicates the opaque strip in the laparotomy pad, and the *curved arrow* indicates the metallic ring attached to the laparotomy pad. Note the mottled black appearance of the air trapped in the laparotomy pad. The air–fluid level in the gastric fundus gives a clue to the upright position of the patient.

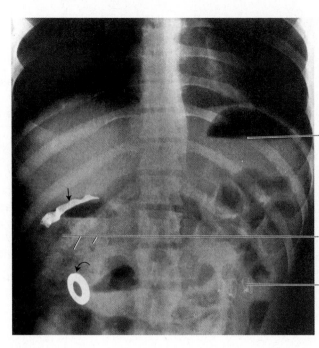

Gastric air–fluid level

Air trapped in laparotomy pad

Opaque sutures

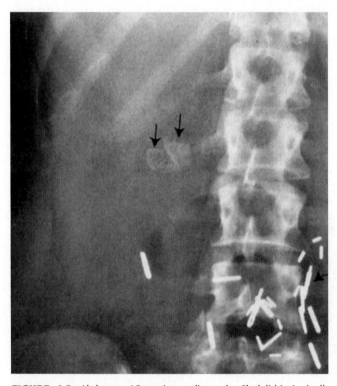

FIGURE 4.8. Abdomen AP supine radiograph. Cholelithiasis (gallstones). The calcified calculi (*arrows at center*) are faceted. Surgical metallic clips (*arrow at right*) are secondary to previous abdominal surgery.

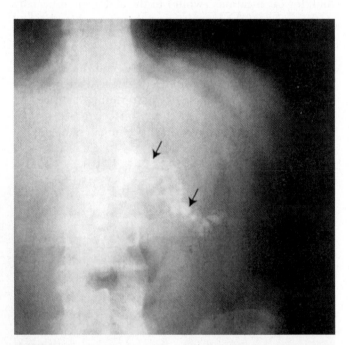

FIGURE 4.9. Abdomen AP supine radiograph. Calcifications (*arrows*) in the body and tail of the pancreas owing to chronic pancreatitis.

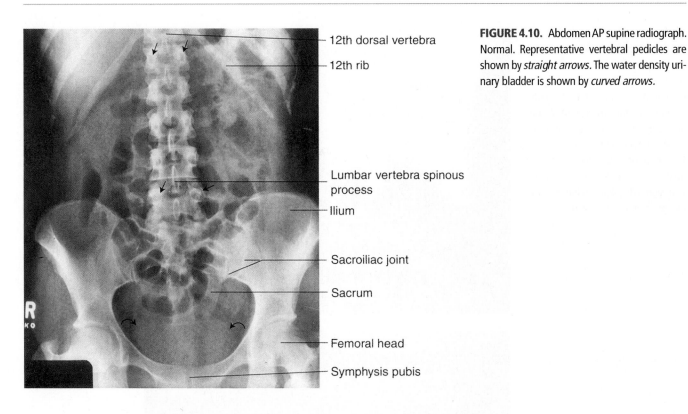

FIGURE 4.10. Abdomen AP supine radiograph. Normal. Representative vertebral pedicles are shown by *straight arrows*. The water density urinary bladder is shown by *curved arrows*.

12th dorsal vertebra

12th rib

Lumbar vertebra spinous process

Ilium

Sacroiliac joint

Sacrum

Femoral head

Symphysis pubis

Use a similar search system for the AP upright abdominal radiograph while being especially alert for free air beneath the diaphragms. Free intraperitoneal air is usually visualized only on an upright radiograph, because only this position allows free air to rise to the subdiaphragmatic regions.

EVALUATING THE INTESTINAL AIR OR GAS PATTERN

Intestinal gas (black) provides a natural contrast medium that can be useful for detecting abdominal disease. When evaluating the intestinal gas pattern, ask yourself several important questions. Is the bowel gas pattern normal? Remember that there is normally some air or gas in the stomach, small intestine, colon, and rectum. With experience, you will begin to recognize abnormal amounts of air in the gastrointestinal (GI) tract. This is similar to recognizing a normal heart on a chest radiograph. If the gas pattern is not normal, ask more questions. Is there too much or too little air? Is the air in the wrong place?

Too Much Bowel Gas

Here, where differential diagnosis includes adynamic ileus and bowel obstruction, we need a systematic approach to arrive at the correct diagnosis. In adynamic ileus (also referred to as *paralytic ileus* or just *ileus*), there is too much bowel gas in the entire GI tract, including the small and large intestines (Fig. 4.11). Adynamic ileus may arise from

intra-abdominal cases or as a reflex phenomenon from disease elsewhere. The multiple causes are listed in Table 4.2. If you identify comparable amounts of gas in the small and large intestines and in the rectum, this generally indicates adynamic ileus. Air in the rectum may be a key differential point.

In intestinal obstruction, another reason for too much bowel gas, there is usually air-filled, dilated intestine proximal to the point of obstruction and little or no air distal to the obstruction (Fig. 4.12). In both ileus and obstruction, often the dilated small and large bowels containing too much air will have air–fluid levels noted on upright and decubitus radiographs.

If a diagnosis of obstruction versus adynamic ileus is not readily apparent, it is necessary to obtain additional studies to arrive at the correct diagnosis. These include barium studies, computed tomography (CT) (Fig. 4.13), and ultrasound (US). Note the relative ease of identifying small versus large bowel using CT.

If you diagnose intestinal obstruction, you next need to determine the location of the obstruction. Is the obstruction in the small or large bowel? In small bowel obstruction, there are loops of dilated small bowel proximal to the obstruction site and little or no gas in the colon or the rectum. In large bowel obstruction, there is dilated colon proximal to the obstruction site but little or no air distally and minimal air in the rectum.

Sometimes it is difficult to differentiate dilated small bowel from large bowel. One way is to identify the valvulae conniventes and colon haustra. *Valvulae conniventes* are

FIGURE 4.11. A: Abdomen AP supine radiograph. Postoperative adynamic ileus. Air is present throughout the entire GI tract, including the rectum (not shown). Note the haustrations in the transverse colon. **B:** Lower abdomen AP supine radiograph 24 hours later in the same patient. A considerable amount of intestinal air has moved into the rectum and sigmoid colon, confirming the diagnosis of adynamic ileus.

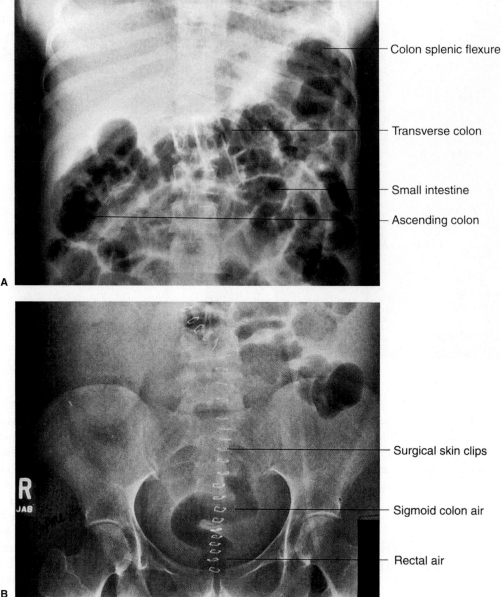

Colon splenic flexure

Transverse colon

Small intestine

Ascending colon

A

Surgical skin clips

Sigmoid colon air

Rectal air

B

Table 4.2
Adynamic Ileus: Major Causes

Intra-abdominal
- Postoperative or posttraumatic
- Postinflammatory: Pancreatitis, enteritis, colitis
- Pain-related: Renal colic, epidural disease

Extra-abdominal
- Septicemia
- Metabolic disease: Hyperkalemia, uremia
- Medications (especially narcotics)
- Prolonged bed rest

regularly spaced, thin mucosal folds that extend across the entire small bowel lumen (see Fig. 4.12). On the other hand, the colon can usually be identified by the somewhat irregularly spaced transverse bands, called *colon septa* or *haustral folds,* that do not extend completely across the colon lumen (see Fig. 4.11).

Sigmoid volvulus is a dramatic clinical event that occurs predominantly in elderly patients with a long history of constipation. The chronic constipation results in a redundant sigmoid mesentery that has the potential to twist on itself like a garden hose. If twisting occurs, there is complete or partial obstruction, and an abdominal radiograph shows a dramatically dilated sigmoid colon. Barium enema is

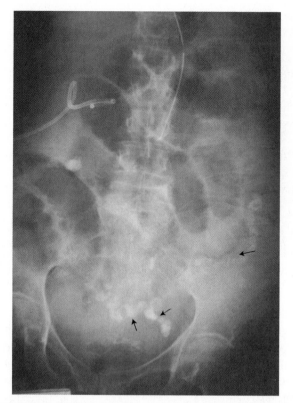

FIGURE 4.12. Abdominal radiograph. Small bowel obstruction. There are many dilated loops of small bowel in the midabdomen. They are identified as small bowel by their position, semihorizontal orientation, and valvulae conniventes traversing the entire transverse diameter. There is a small amount of residual barium in a collapsed descending colon (*arrows*). Incidentally noted are the nasogastric and abdominal drainage tubes. (Courtesy of Bruce Brown, M.D.)

confirmatory with complete obstruction to the retrograde flow of barium at the site of the twist (Fig. 4.14). The obstruction can often be relieved by gently passing a sigmoidoscope past the point of the obstruction or twist.

Too Little Bowel Gas

When the abdominal radiographs show a paucity or absence of bowel gas, the differential diagnosis listed in Table 4.3 should be entertained.

Gas in the Wrong Places

There are several situations in which air is found outside of the intestinal lumen (Table 4.4). Free air in the perito-

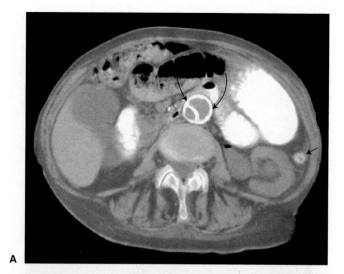

A

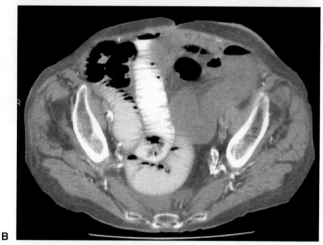

B

FIGURE 4.13. Abdominal axial CT. Small bowel obstruction. **A:** Here are many dilated loops of small bowel, some of which contain barium. The only colon visualized (*straight arrow*) in the left lower abdomen is tiny. (The aortic image (*curved arrows*) shows a segment of calcified intima, indicating previous aortic dissection.) **B:** CT at the level of the pelvis confirms the dilated small bowel extending into the pelvis (the rectum is surgically absent). (Courtesy of Gerald Decker, M.D.)

neal cavity results from any process that perforates the intestinal tract. AP supine and upright abdominal radiographs should be performed if there is clinical suspicion of gut perforation. The upright position allows free intraperitoneal air to rise to the subdiaphragmatic regions of the

Table 4.3

Too Little Bowel Gas

- Enlarged abdominal organs
- Intra-abdominal tumor
- Fluid-filled intestines
- Gastroenteritis
- Neurologic deficit (with reduced swallowing)

Table 4.4

Abdominal Air or Gas in the Wrong Place

- Pneumoperitoneum from ruptured intestines: Ulcer, trauma, cancer, enteritis
- Abscess
- Pneumatosis intestinalis

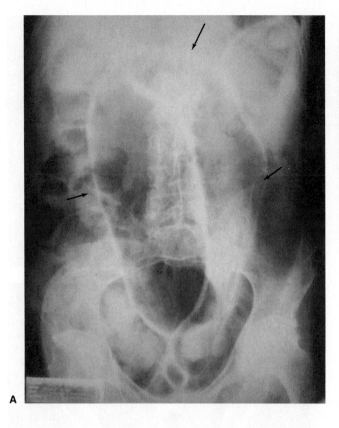

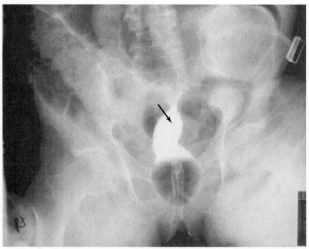

FIGURE 4.14. Sigmoid volvulus. **A:** Abdominal radiograph. The air-filled, obstructed sigmoid colon (*arrows*) arises from the pelvis. **B:** Barium enema. Contrast introduced per rectum shows obstruction and a twist (*arrow*) at the sigmoid colon. (Courtesy of Bruce Brown, M.D.)

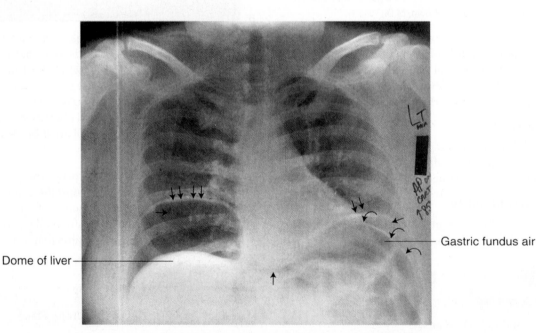

FIGURE 4.15. Chest AP upright radiograph. Free intraperitoneal air. The right and left hemidiaphragms (*double straight arrows*) are elevated owing to bilateral subdiaphragmatic air (*single straight arrows*). The black zone between the right hemidiaphragm and the dome of the liver represents free intraperitoneal air. On the left, there is air in the gastric fundus as well as free air surrounding the gastric fundus, allowing visualization of both sides of the stomach wall (*curved arrows*). When you see both sides of the gut wall, this represents free intraperitoneal air (Rigler's sign).

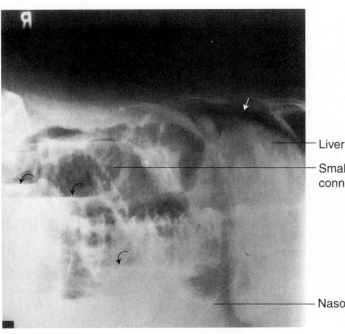

Liver

Small intestine (valvulae conniventes)

Nasogastric tube

FIGURE 4.16. Abdomen left lateral decubitus radiograph (left side down). Free intraperitoneal air in a patient with small bowel obstruction and perforation. The free intraperitoneal air (*white arrow*) is between the right rib cage and the liver. The dilated small bowel contains multiple air–fluid levels (*black arrows*).

abdomen (Fig. 4.15). If the upright view is not possible owing to the patient's condition, a decubitus radiograph will suffice. On a decubitus radiograph, the air rises to the nondependent portion of the peritoneal cavity (Fig. 4.16). Either technique has the potential to identify as little as 2 cc of free intraperitoneal air, as long as the patient is in the upright or decubitus position approximately 5 minutes prior to the radiograph.

Another example of air in the wrong place is pneumatosis intestinalis (Fig. 4.17). Causes of this are listed in Table 4.5. Gas-filled abscesses can be found in any location, including the abdomen (Fig. 4.18).

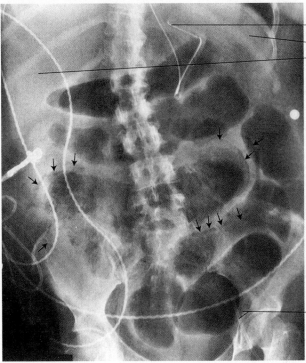

Nasogastric tube

Spleen

Liver

Femoral line

FIGURE 4.17. Abdomen AP supine radiograph. Pneumatosis intestinalis (air in the bowel wall). There is widespread bubbly air within the small intestine walls (*arrows*).

FIGURE 4.18. Abdomen AP supine radiograph. Right subdiaphragmatic abscess. The black areas along the right lateral aspect of the liver represent air in the abscess cavity (*straight arrows*). Incidentally noted is contrast material in the common bile duct, gallbladder, and small bowel, injected during an endoscopic retrograde cholangiopancreatography (ERCP). Some of the contrast spilled into the small intestine. The filling defect (*curved arrow*) in the gallbladder is probably a calculus.

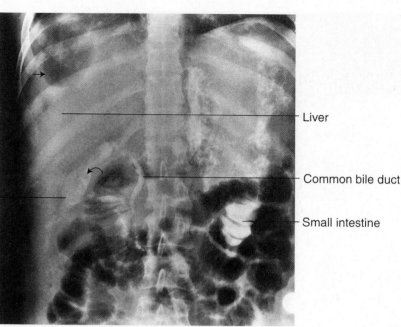

Liver

Common bile duct

Small intestine

Gallbladder

GASTROINTESTINAL CONTRAST STUDIES

For inspection of the mucosal surface of the esophagus, stomach, and duodenum, endoscopy is often preferred. To evaluate the gut lumen and wall, traditional radiologic GI contrast studies are accurate, safe, and less expensive than the endoscopic studies and enjoy excellent patient acceptance. These studies consist of fluoroscopy and radiographs obtained following introduction of barium sulfate (metallic density or white) and/or air (black) into the GI tract.

Upper Gastrointestinal Series

For an upper GI series, the patient swallows liquid barium, often combined with gas-producing crystals, under fluoroscopy to visualize the esophagus, stomach, and small intestine (Fig. 4.19). When both barium and air are used, the process is referred to as a double-contrast study. When barium is used alone, it is a single-contrast study. Preparation for an upper GI series consists simply of nothing by mouth (non per os [NPO]) for 8 to 12 hours prior to the study. When perforation of the upper GI tract is suspected, water-soluble contrast media is used.

Table 4.5
Pneumatosis Intestinalis

- Bowel ischemia
- Steroid and immunosuppressive therapy
- Proximal to intestinal obstruction
- Collagen diseases
- Neonatal necrotizing enterocolitis
- Benign idiopathic pneumatosis

Antegrade Small Bowel Examination

The usual small bowel examination is performed after an upper GI series by having the patient drink additional barium. Serial radiographs of the abdomen are performed at 15- to 30-minute intervals thereafter to evaluate the small bowel as barium passes through (Fig. 4.20). Fluoroscopy is commonly used as a supplement to study

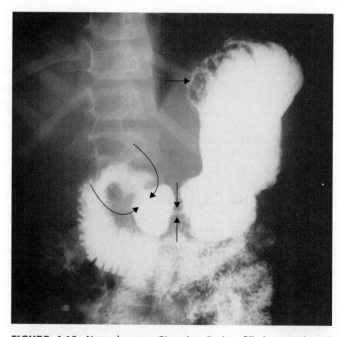

FIGURE 4.19. Normal upper GI series. Barium-filled stomach and duodenum. The patient is in the prone position. Gas (*horizontal arrow*) is seen in the gastric fundus, a peristaltic wave (*vertical arrows*) crosses the gastric antrum, the pylorus (*curved arrows*) separates the duodenal bulb and stomach.

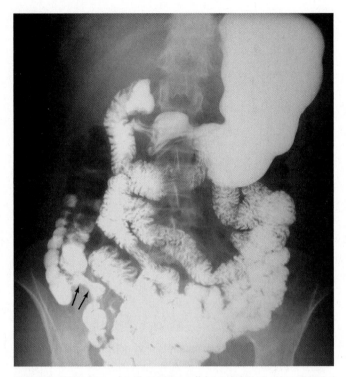

FIGURE 4.20. Normal antegrade small bowel examination. Barium was administered by mouth, and this radiograph was done about 30 minutes later. Note the barium-filled stomach, duodenal C-loop, feathered jejunum in the upper abdomen, and relatively formless mucosa of the ileum in the lower and right abdomen. The terminal ileum (*arrows*) entering the cecum can be identified. (Courtesy of Bruce Brown, M.D.)

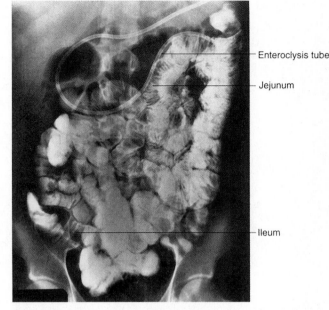

FIGURE 4.21. Small bowel enteroclysis. Normal. The nasointestinal tube has been positioned just beyond the duodenal–jejunal junction. Barium fills the entire small bowel.

the terminal ileum when barium begins to enter the colon or to further investigate abnormalities seen on the serial radiographs.

Enteroclysis

Enteroclysis is a focused examination of the small intestine, wherein air and barium sulfate are introduced directly into the small intestine via a nasointestinal tube. Under fluoroscopy, the tip of the tube is placed just beyond the duodenal–jejunal junction and contrast is injected (Fig. 4.21). Advantages of this procedure are that the small bowel can be distended and the stomach and duodenum do not obstruct visualization. The main disadvantages are the discomfort associated with a nasal tube and the radiation exposure.

Retrograde Small Bowel Examination

On occasion, especially when disease of the terminal ileum is suspected and previous examinations are nondiagnostic, barium can be refluxed from a filled colon into the ileum. Although the procedure is useful, there is considerable patient discomfort alleviated slightly by antispasmodic agents.

Barium Enema

Introduction of barium sulfate and/or air into the colon via a rectal tube is called a lower GI series or barium enema. For this study, it is important to have a clean colon; this is best

accomplished with laxatives and large amounts of orally ingested fluids. Barium and often air are administered via a rectal tube under fluoroscopic observation. When both air and barium are used, it is called a double-contrast study (Fig. 4.22), whereas barium alone is a single-contrast study. A properly performed barium enema has minimal associated discomfort. The double-contrast study is preferred to evaluate intraluminal and mucosal diseases, such as small ulcers and polyps. Again, if colon perforation is suspected, a water-soluble contrast medium is used.

Colonoscopy, an expensive alternative to colon barium studies, can directly visualize the mucosa. However, it requires conscious sedation because of patient discomfort. Virtual colonoscopy is an examination of the entire colon using multidetector CT and a dedicated software program so that the colon is displayed throughout its length with stacked images created to form a three-dimensional (3D) picture of the colon at each level. The examination is usually performed after administration of an agent that tags fecal material, which can then be subtracted from the viewed images. Before the examination begins, the colon is insufflated with air so that the images resemble the interior view of the colon as would be seen by endoscopy. Virtual colonoscopy has the ability to discover almost all colon cancers (Fig. 4.23) as well as larger polyps (Fig. 4.24) (which are premalignant). The examination takes but a few minutes and does not require the sedation and analgesics required for optical colon endoscopy. As experience with the technique has increased, it seems more accurate than barium enema techniques and perhaps as good as optical colonoscopy. Its disadvantages are the use of radiation and probably reduced detectability of flat mucosal lesions. It is

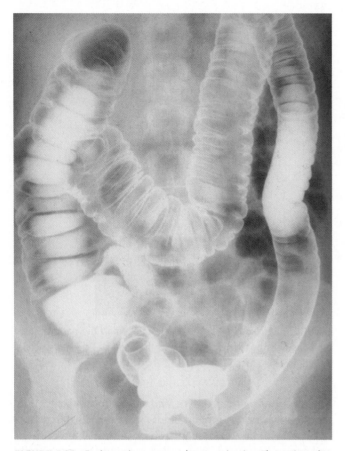

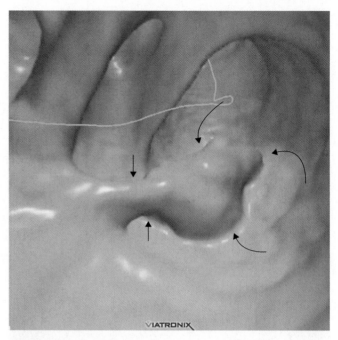

FIGURE 4.24. Virtual colonoscopy. Colon polyp detected in virtual colonoscopy. The stalk (*short arrows*) and the polyp (*curved arrows*) are readily apparent. (Courtesy of Wei Chang, M.D.)

FIGURE 4.22. Barium–air contrast colon examination. The entire colon is filled with barium and air. Films are made in prone, supine, and both decubitus positions so that different parts of the colon can be visualized with the air-contrast techniques. (Courtesy of Bruce Brown, M.D.)

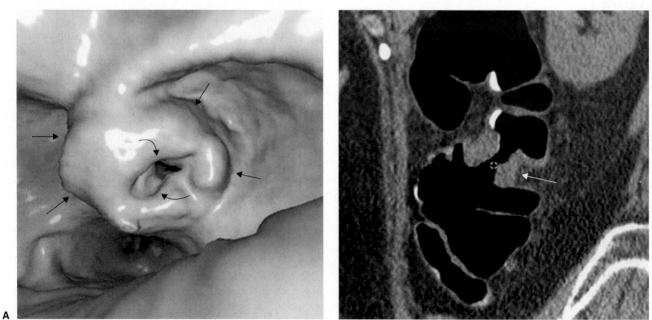

FIGURE 4.23. "Apple core" invasive cancer discovered on virtual colonoscopy. **A:** The virtual colonoscopy image shows a large endoluminal mass (*straight arrows*), associated with narrowing of the colon lumen (*curved arrows*). **B:** Coronal CT reconstruction of the colonoscopic image. The tumor (*arrow*) is noted on both sides of the colon lumen and extrudes into the pericolic space. (Courtesy of J.G. Fletcher, M.D.)

much less expensive than optical colonoscopy. At the time of this writing, indication for its use as a substitute for screening optical colonoscopy is imprecise, but considerable improvement of the technique is anticipated.

STUDY OF GALLBLADDER AND BILIARY TRACT

In years past, the oral cholecystogram was performed to visualize the gallbladder following the oral ingestion of special iodinated compounds that are excreted into the biliary system and subsequently concentrated in the gallbladder. The study is seldom performed now because of the greater accuracy of US. With US, one can examine the liver and biliary tract as well as the gallbladder. CT and magnetic resonance imaging (MRI) are needed in certain situations to complement US.

In endoscopic retrograde cholangiopancreatography (ERCP), the endoscopist passes a fiberoptic scope under fluoroscopic control antegrade through the esophagus, stomach, and duodenum and retrogrades into the common bile duct. The pancreatic ducts can also be cannulated. Contrast media can be injected into any of these structures and appropriate radiographs obtained (Fig. 4.25). ERCP is usually performed when less-invasive studies (CT, US, MRI, or contrast studies) are indeterminate or nondiagnostic or as part of a therapeutic endoscopic procedure.

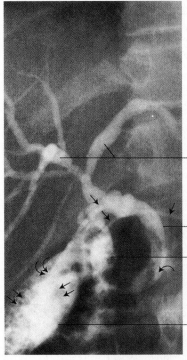

Right and left hepatic ducts

Common bile duct

Duodenum

Gallbladder

FIGURE 4.25. Endoscopic retrograde cholangiopancreatography (ERCP). Cholelithiasis and choledocholithiasis. The gallbladder is filled with calculi (*double straight arrows*), and there is a large calculus in the distal common bile duct (*single curved arrow*). A nasobiliary drain (*single straight arrows*) is in place with the tip (*double curved arrows*) in the gallbladder.

URINARY TRACT EXAMINATIONS

The first methodology to examine the urinary tract directly (about 1,900 present) was to inject radiopaque material directly into the bladder or other urinary structures (retrograde cystography or pyelography) at the time of cystoscopy. It was later discovered that intravenous contrast material that is excreted by the kidneys could be given with relative safety; excretory urography (EU) was developed shortly thereafter. Other names given for EU are intravenous urogram and intravenous pyelogram. Multislice CT has now evolved as the new standard, CT urography (CTU). A multifaceted radiologic approach to genitourinary (GU) problems is now possible, with supplemental US and MRI examination.

EU with traditional radiographs, although still a useful technique, is performed much less frequently in the investigation of GU disease than is CTU, principally because the renal parenchyma, pelvicalyceal system, ureter, and bladder can be more accurately visualized with multislice techniques. US remains a valuable technique to complement radiographic investigation.

Excretory Urography and Computed Tomography Urography

Both EU and CTU involve the administration of an intravenous contrast medium that is excreted by the kidneys. In CTU the contrast medium is delivered in bolus fashion to maximize renal parenchymal visualization. In EU one recognizes the urinary structures as seen through overlying bowel gas, soft tissue, and so on. In CTU, multidetector CT is utilized, permitting visualization of urinary structures without overlying structures. A further advantage is the ability to reconstruct images in any plane—axial, coronal, or sagittal. A final advantage of CTU is a reconstruction technique so that the urinary tract is viewed in 3D with all other structures subtracted.

Disadvantages of CTU include a higher patient radiation dose (about double) and additional cost. Three-dimensional reconstruction requires image manipulation by a specially trained technologist. Thus, EU remains an accepted technique for most children, for many follow-up studies, and at sites without multidetector CT. Both types of examinations are featured in this chapter.

EU and CTU do not require special patient preparation, merely abstaining from food and liquids for several hours before contrast administration.

The timing of EU and CTU radiographs can be varied, depending upon the patient's clinical problems. Nevertheless, both techniques usually require examination during the nephrographic phase (for visualization of the renal cortex), followed by image(s) of the pelvicalyceal system and bladder, which are opacified later. Delayed films can be obtained for hours, or even days, in situations such as ureteral obstruction or renal failure.

Viewing an Excretory Urogram or Computed Tomography Urogram

An EU study begins with a preliminary or scout radiograph that includes the entire abdomen. You can evaluate this preliminary radiograph using the same system as described previously. The radiographs obtained immediately following intravenous contrast media demonstrate the nephrogram phase wherein the contrast media is located in the renal capillaries, glomeruli, and proximal convoluted tubules (Fig. 4.26A). Compare the nephrograms for symmetry, as size discrepancy is suspicious for unilateral renal disease.

Next, evaluate the later postcontrast injection radiographs, at which times the contrast media is normally present in the calyces, renal pelves, portions of the ureters, and urinary bladder (Fig. 4.26B). Normal calyces are sharp in outline with various numbers and geometry. Oblique, prone, and abdominal compression radiographs are often obtained to better display portions of the urinary tract.

The CTU is evaluated for the same factors as the EU, albeit in different fashion. A computed abdominal radiograph is performed, followed by axial scans of the abdomen before, immediately after, and at a later time following the bolus of contrast material (Fig. 4.27). In

FIGURE 4.26. Abdomen AP EU. Normal. **A:** There are symmetric nephrograms 1 minute postinjection of contrast media. The renal outlines (*arrows*) are clearly defined owing to the presence of the contrast media within the kidneys. **B:** Note that it is possible to see the calyces, infundibula, renal pelves, portions of ureters, and urinary bladder on this 15-minute radiograph.

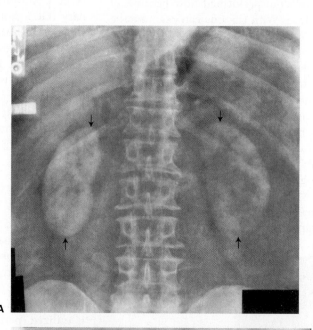

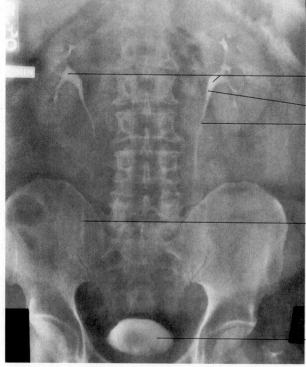

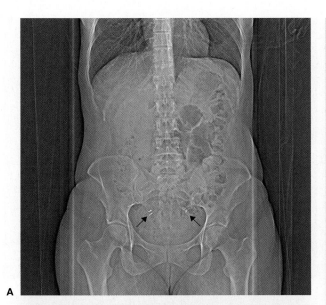

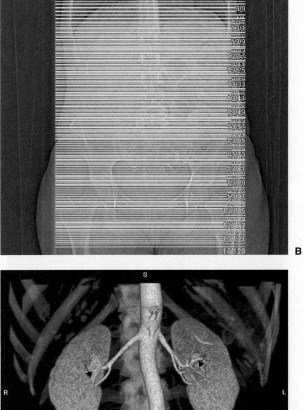

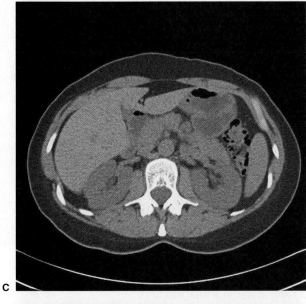

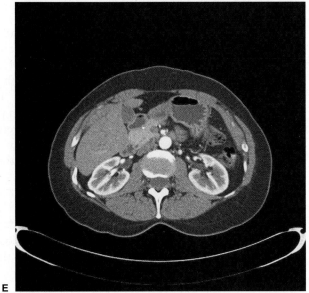

FIGURE 4.27. Normal CT urogram in a potential renal donor. **A:** Preliminary scout image of the abdomen is normal except for benign small calcifications (*arrows*) in the pelvis. **B:** Scout image with superimposed lines indicating the many axial slices performed to create the image data. **C:** One slice of the nonenhanced scan of the abdomen before administration of contrast. No abnormalities of the kidneys or other areas are noted. **D:** Coronal CT images after contrast administration shows aorta, single bilateral renal arteries (*arrows*), and normal size kidneys. **E:** Axial scan early after contrast demonstrates well demarcation of renal cortex and medulla. (*continued*)

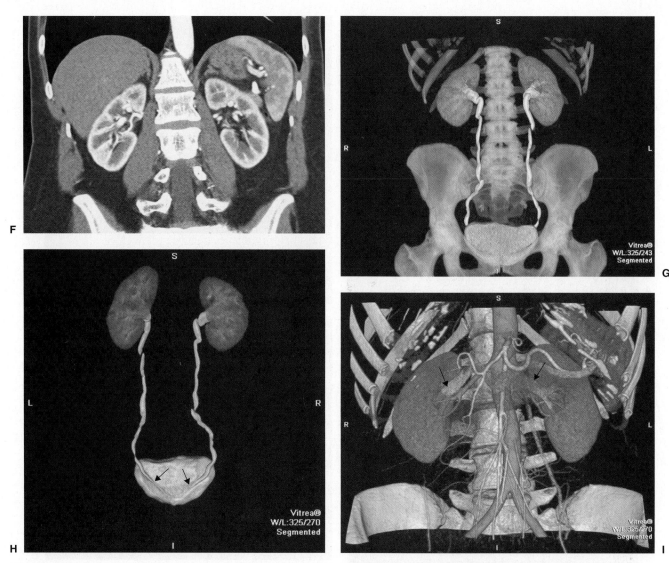

FIGURE 4.27. (*Continued*) **F:** Coronal reconstruction at the same time as **(E)**. **G:** Later reconstructed coronal image showing normal kidneys, ureters, and bladder. **H:** Coronal image of the urinary tract viewed from posterior showing entry of the ureters into the bladder (*arrows*). **I:** Later coronal image showing both renal veins (*arrows*) as well as arterial structures.

special situations (e.g., study of renal donor), immediate postcontrast scans can be obtained to visualize renal arteries and later the veins. As in EU, pay attention to size and symmetry of the kidneys, pelvicalyceal systems, and bladder.

Other Urinary Tract Examinations

Direct injection of contrast material into the bladder or ureter (retrograde pyelogram) is of value when a detailed view of a portion of the ureter or pelvicalyceal system is necessary. It is often an adjunct to endoscopy.

Vesicoureteral reflux, a condition in which bladder urine refluxes in retrograde fashion into the ureters, is a common phenomenon in children but infrequent in adults. It can be associated with urinary tract infection. With the voiding cystourethrogram, contrast medium is introduced via a urethral catheter into the bladder. Subsequent fluoroscopy and filming allow one to identify and quantitate vesicoureteral reflux if present (Fig. 4.28). At the completion of the study, the patient voids, with the voiding sequence recorded in some imaging form. This allows detection of urethral abnormalities, which can produce bladder obstruction and secondary vesicoureteral reflux. Cystography and retrograde urethrography are examinations usually performed to detect urinary extravasation in trauma cases.

ABDOMINAL ULTRASOUND

US, being a different modality from x-rays, shows abdominal organs in a different fashion. There are roughly three patterns of reflected US.

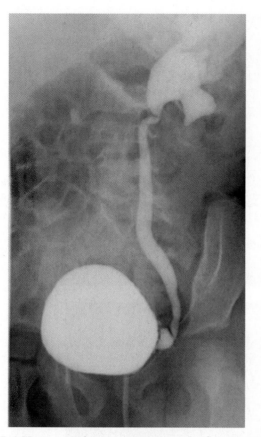

FIGURE 4.28. Cystourethrogram. Vesicoureteral reflux. Contrast introduced via urethral catheter into the bladder fills the bladder and refluxes into the left ureter.

1. No reflection of the sound wave. Almost all of the sound passes through the area. This is termed sonolucent and is traditionally viewed as black on images. Fluid, such as in ascites or abdominal cysts, is sonolucent.
2. Reflection and transmission of some sound. Solid organs, such as the kidney or liver, are examples. US waves are reflected, particularly at boundaries of organs of differing echogenicity, such as the boundary between the liver and the kidney.
3. Reflection of all sound. Bone, other calcifications, and air in the gut are examples. One can make use of this by noting such shadowing and the absence of echoes distal to a lesion to help diagnose gallstones and like abnormalities.

There are two major problems in learning to read US images.

1. It requires one to think differently. You are looking at differences in transmission and reflection of US rather than transmitted x-rays.
2. Orientation of the image. This is the chief stumbling block. One may consider the US image as representing a roughly pie-shaped wedge of tissues, less than 1 cm thick, below the US transducer.

Even experienced radiologists and clinicians have considerable difficulty figuring out the nature of the US image if they did not perform the study. Orientation must be provided by the person who performed the scan. In most situations, there is a relatively fixed method of performing abdominal US. In general, one evaluates each area of interest in at least two dimensions, typically axial (transverse) and longitudinal (sagittal). For technical reasons, the direction of the scan beam shows the anatomy best if it is perpendicular to the organ of interest. As few abdominal organs are 100% oriented anterior–posterior or medial–lateral, the scanned images are, to varying degrees, oblique.

Probably the best method to be introduced to US is to attend an imaging session with a knowledgeable mentor who discusses the anatomy as it is being scanned. Combined with this, learn the usual routines for US scanning in your institution and try to figure out how each image was performed. Conventionally, images are labeled as to the method by which they are done, for example, kidney—transverse.

There are many abdominal applications of US related to its widespread availability and cost (it is about half the cost of CT and about one-third that of MRI). Ultrasonography is valuable in the workup of diseases involving the liver, biliary tract, kidneys, abdominal aorta, and abdominal masses. It is particularly useful in defining fluid versus solid (e.g., cyst vs. solid mass) as well as in imaging fluid-filled structures, such as the gallbladder, urinary bladder, and renal pelvis. The various abdominal organs and pathologic processes have their own characteristic echo patterns, as shown in Figure 4.29.

Obstetric and gynecologic US is particularly important because of the absence of significant biologic risk to the fetus or maternal genital structures. In obstetric US, the fetus is surrounded by amniotic fluid, making visualization easier (Fig. 4.30). In addition, one can use real-time US images to evaluate the beating heart. For gynecologic examinations, both transabdominal (Fig. 4.31) and transvaginal techniques are used. Transvaginal imaging has the technical advantage of eliminating echoes from the abdominal wall from the area of interest, allowing better definition of genital organs (Fig. 4.32).

Diagnostic US of the prostate has been disappointing, as it is relatively insensitive to identifying abnormalities of this organ. In the scrotum, US is superb. It localizes the site of disease (e.g., testis vs. epididymis) and often allows specific diagnosis of the abnormality present (Fig. 4.33). Correct diagnosis of epididymitis versus testicular torsion versus orchitis is possible, separating those who need surgery from those who require only medical treatment. Hydrocele and varicocele are easily identified with US. Identification of testicular tumors is good, although identifying tumor type is less reliable.

FIGURE 4.29. A: Longitudinal (sagittal) abdominal sonogram. Normal liver and right kidney echo patterns. The *cross marks* indicate the longitudinal (sagittal) liver dimension. The right kidney borders are demarcated by the *straight arrows* and the right hemidiaphragm by the *curved arrows*. **B:** Transverse (axial) abdominal sonogram. Normal spleen echo pattern. The side-to-side spleen dimension lies between the *X marks,* and the cephalocaudal dimension lies between the *crosses*. The left hemidiaphragm is indicated by the *arrow* (S, spleen). Note the labels on the images (**A,** Rt long; **B,** Lt trans spl). Such labels are helpful in orienting the images for the observer.

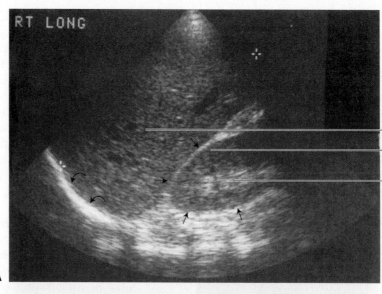

Liver

Right kidney cortex

Right kidney upper collecting system

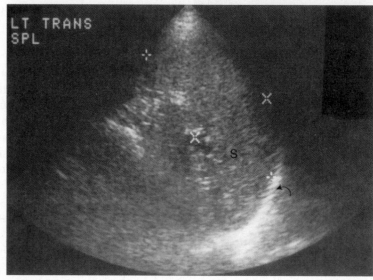

COMPUTED TOMOGRAPHY AND MAGNETIC RESONANCE IMAGING OF THE ABDOMEN

Both CT and MRI are useful in the diagnosis and management of abdominal disease. CT is usually the favored procedure because of its wide availability and lower cost. Patient motion is seldom a problem in CT but is a frequent occurrence in MRI. Both techniques have the ability to produce images in any dimension (axial, sagittal, coronal, or oblique).

Except in emergencies, the patient for CT has usually fasted for several hours. In most cases (suspected renal disease is the usual exception), a dilute contrast material (such as barium or iodine containing) is given orally before the study begins to demarcate the GI tract. This allows one to identify bowel loops, distinguishing them from masses and solid organs.

Immediately before (or sometimes during) abdominal CT, contrast material is injected intravenously to allow identification of arteries and veins (the enhanced CT). The intravenous contrast is excreted by the kidneys so that the kidneys (and later the urinary collecting systems and bladder) will be opacified (see CTU).

A relatively new examination is the positron emission tomography (PET)-CT (see nuclear medicine). A special machine combines CT and PET scanning so that the patient is not moved between examinations. Software programs fuse the CT and PET images into a single image. The advantage is to combine the PET-increased sensitivity of small tumors with the improved anatomical localization of CT.

The abdominal MRI examination is tailored to the suspected abnormality, the technical details being beyond the scope of this discussion. Intravenous contrast agents, such as gadolinium, which can change the MR signal in

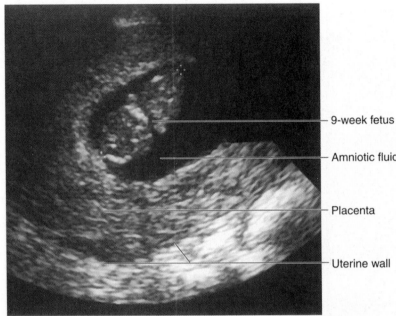

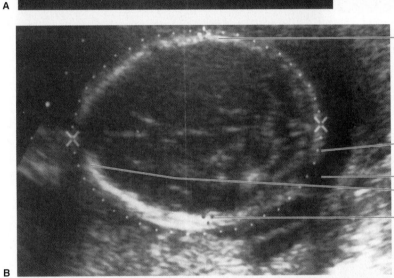

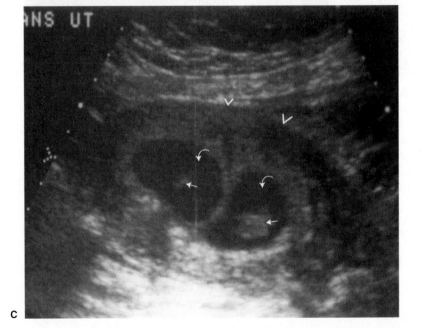

FIGURE 4.30. Obstetric sonograms. **A:** Study in a 9-week fetus. The *caliper markers* indicating crown to rump distance confirm the 9-week gestation. **B:** Skull of a fetus near term. The *white dotted lines* outline the skull, and the biparietal diameter confirms the fetal age. The cerebral ventricles are vaguely seen within the skull. **C:** Twin pregnancy. The uterine wall is marked by the *arrowheads.* Each fetus (*straight arrows*) is surrounded by amniotic fluid (*curved arrows*). There are separate sacs.

A (labels): 9-week fetus · Amniotic fluid · Placenta · Uterine wall

B (labels): Parietal bone · Posterior skull · Amniotic fluid · Anterior skull · Parietal bone

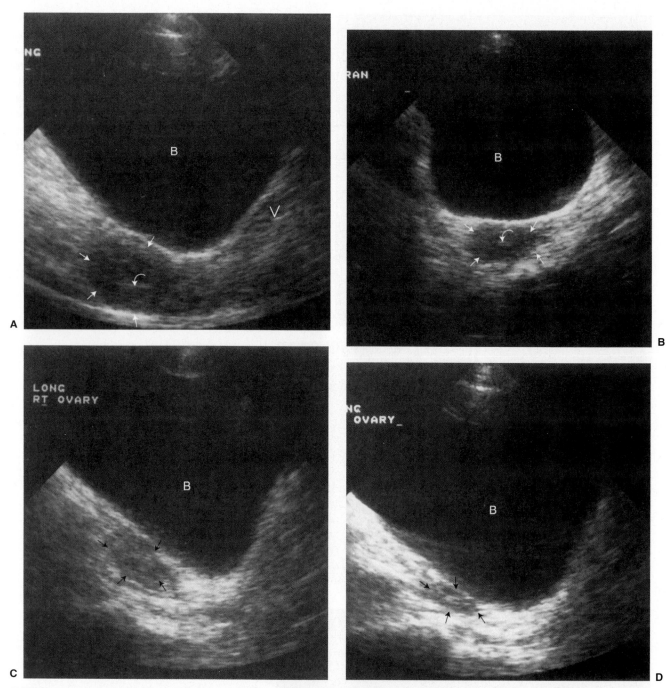

FIGURE 4.31. A: Transabdominal midline longitudinal (sagittal) sonogram. Normal uterus (*straight arrows*). The urine-filled bladder is essentially echo free and thus serves as an acoustic window to the pelvis. Notice the characteristic homogeneous echo pattern of the normal uterus. The endometrial stripe (*curved arrow*) represents the layers that line the endometrial cavity. The presence of the endometrial stripe indicates the absence of an intrauterine pregnancy or other intrauterine mass (B, urinary bladder; V, vagina). **B:** Transabdominal transverse (axial) sonogram. Normal uterus. The uterine fundus is outlined by the *straight arrows;* the endometrial stripe (*curved arrow*) appears smaller on the transverse image. **C:** Transabdominal right longitudinal (sagittal) sonogram. Normal right ovary (*arrows*). **D:** Transabdominal left longitudinal (sagittal) sonogram. Normal left ovary (*arrows*).

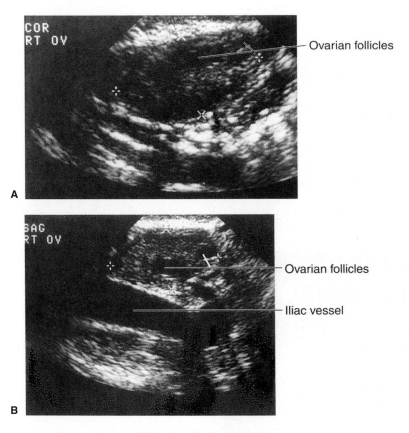

A

B

FIGURE 4.32. Transvaginal sonograms of the right **(A)** and left **(B)** ovaries. The dimensions of the ovaries are indicated by the *X marks* and *crosses*. Note the better definition of the ovaries, so that follicles are visible, when compared with the transabdominal images in Figure 4.31.

many organs and diseases, are frequently given as part of the MR study.

How to Read Abdominal Computed Tomography and Magnetic Resonance Imaging

Reading cross-sectional images of the abdomen is not particularly difficult for the neophyte radiologist *if* one's anatomical knowledge is adequate. You will find the system for

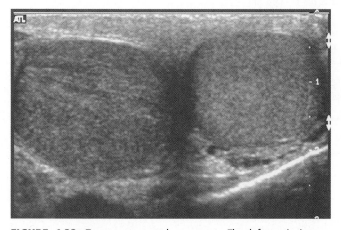

FIGURE 4.33. Transverse scrotal sonogram. The left testis is normal. The right testis is enlarged, has reduced echogenicity, and shows streaky, black linear echodensities. These findings indicate orchitis. (Courtesy of Monzer Abu-Yousef, M.D.)

axial images described herein to be time consuming but rewarding. First, arrange the images in order, from top (toward the head) to bottom. In many circumstances, this is already done for you electronically. Next, look at all the images (using the cine mode if available) in gestalt fashion to discover any obvious abnormalities. Then, look at each organ individually, from top to bottom (i.e., all CT slices containing the organ of interest). In each organ, evaluate the size and shape of each area of reduced or increased density. Do this for visible lung, liver, gallbladder, spleen, pancreas, adrenals, both kidneys and ureters, the bladder, and genitals. Evaluate the stomach, duodenum, small bowel, colon/appendix, and mesentery. Study the retroperitoneum from top to bottom—aorta, vena cava, and mesenteric vessels, also looking for adenopathy or other masses. Check the peritoneal cavity for fluid or masses. Look at the vertebrae (and spinal cord within) and bony pelvis. Finally, concentrate on the abdominal wall, hips, and adjacent soft tissues. Thoroughness leads to success in reading abdominal CT scans. The same methodology applies to evaluation of coronal and sagittal images.

The same system can also be applied to abdominal MRI but—unfortunately for the nonradiologist—there are usually many more images, often with oblique planes and several pulse sequences, often later supplemented with intravenous magnetic contrast material. Normal abdominal CT and MRI anatomy is illustrated in Figures 4.34 to 4.45.

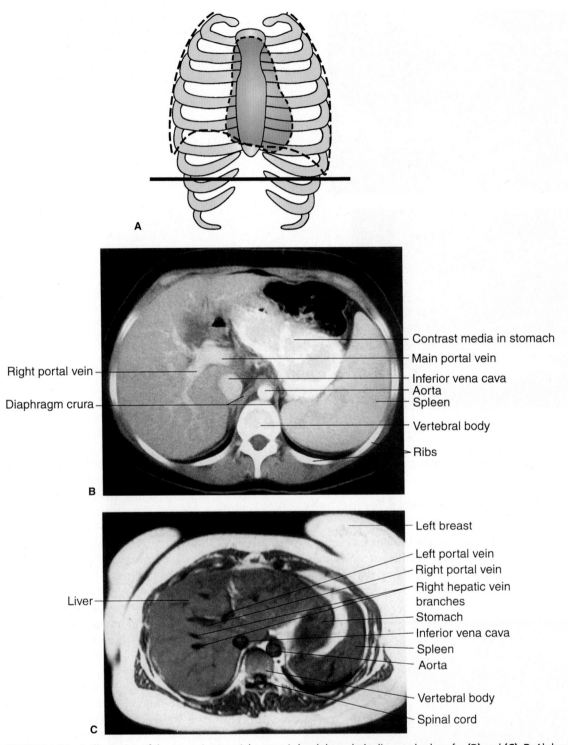

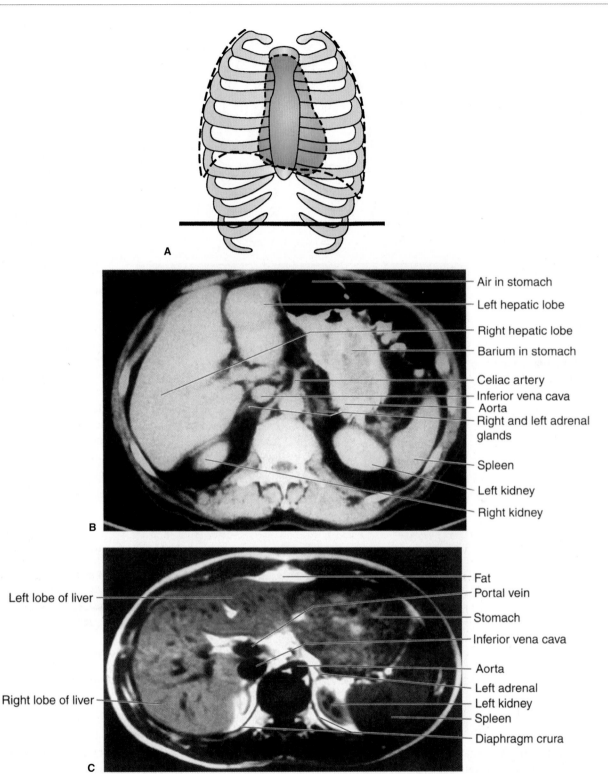

FIGURE 4.35. **A:** Illustration of the approximate axial anatomic level through the liver and spleen for **(B)** and **(C)**. This level is just caudad to the level in Figure 4.34. **B:** Abdomen axial CT image through the liver and spleen. Normal. **C:** Abdomen axial MR image through the liver and spleen. Normal.

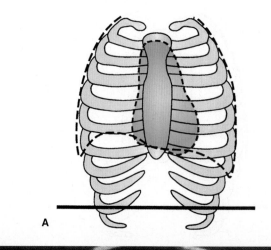

A

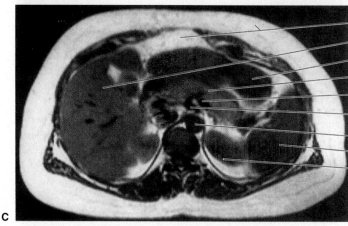

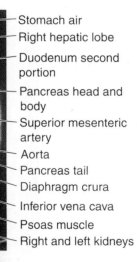

Stomach air

Right hepatic lobe

Duodenum second portion

Pancreas head and body

Superior mesenteric artery

Aorta

Pancreas tail

Diaphragm crura

Inferior vena cava

Psoas muscle

Right and left kidneys

Superior mesenteric vein-portal vein confluence

B

Fat

Liver

Gastric body

Pancreas body

Splenic vein

Celiac artery

Aorta

Spleen

Left kidney

C

FIGURE 4.36. A: Illustration of the approximate axial anatomic level through the pancreas for **(B)** and **(C)**. **B:** Abdomen axial CT image through the pancreas level. Normal. **C:** Abdomen axial MR image through the pancreas level. Normal.

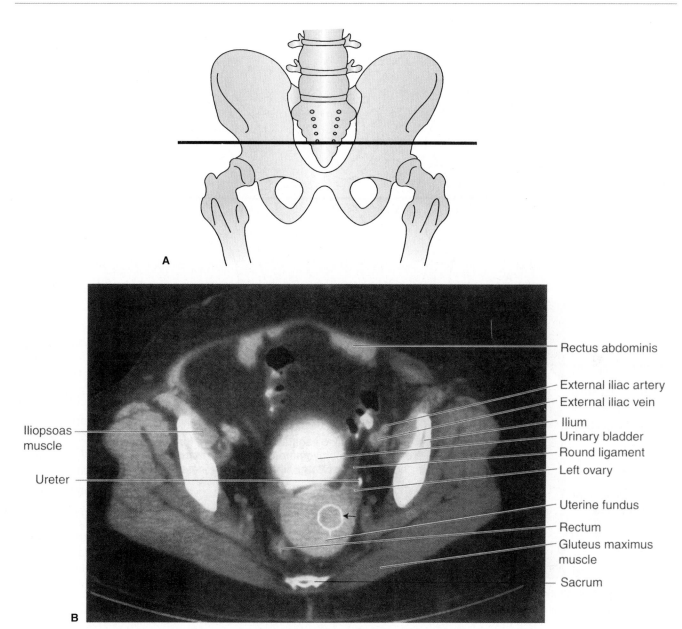

A

B

Iliopsoas muscle

Ureter

Rectus abdominis

External iliac artery

External iliac vein

Ilium

Urinary bladder

Round ligament

Left ovary

Uterine fundus

Rectum

Gluteus maximus muscle

Sacrum

FIGURE 4.37. A: Illustration of the approximate axial anatomic level for **(B)**. **B:** Female pelvis axial CT image through the uterus after intravenous contrast media. Normal. The white metallic density ring (*straight arrow*) that projects over the uterus is merely a region of interest cursor for measuring tissue density.

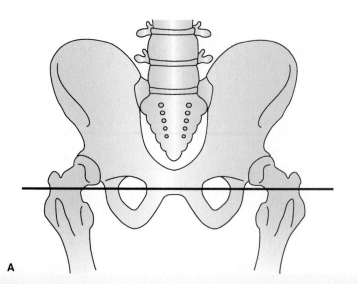

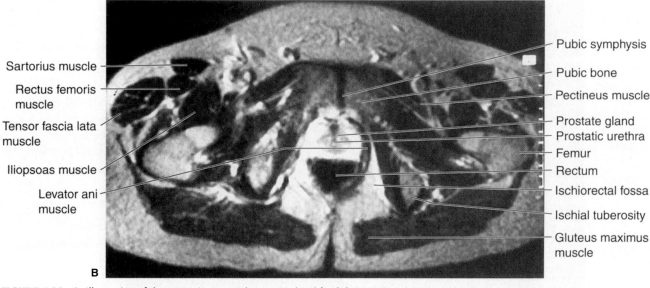

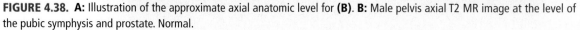

A

Sartorius muscle

Rectus femoris muscle

Tensor fascia lata muscle

Iliopsoas muscle

Levator ani muscle

B

Pubic symphysis

Pubic bone

Pectineus muscle

Prostate gland
Prostatic urethra

Femur

Rectum

Ischiorectal fossa

Ischial tuberosity

Gluteus maximus muscle

FIGURE 4.38. A: Illustration of the approximate axial anatomic level for **(B)**. **B:** Male pelvis axial T2 MR image at the level of the pubic symphysis and prostate. Normal.

ANGIOGRAPHY

Aortography (catheter injection into the abdominal aorta) and selective arteriography of individual vessels in the abdomen are sometimes performed for diagnostic reasons, particularly in trauma or with GI hemorrhage. With rapid CT imaging, visualization of the arteries and/or veins can be obtained using this modality after intravenous contrast material, thus avoiding the necessity for placing an intra-aortic catheter.

Recall that moving tissue, such as intravascular blood, has less MRI signal than surrounding tissue. Various tech-

nical manipulations are possible using this phenomenon, with or without the addition of magnetic contrast material, to allow excellent visualization of almost all of the major abdominal vessels without direct aortic catheterization (Figs. 4.46 and 4.47). The choice of CT angiography versus MR angiography is largely dependent on the expertise of the radiologist and the type of equipment available at individual institutions.

Conventional angiography was used in the past to delineate tumors of the solid organs. CT and MRI are now more effective and less invasive methods for characterizing masses.

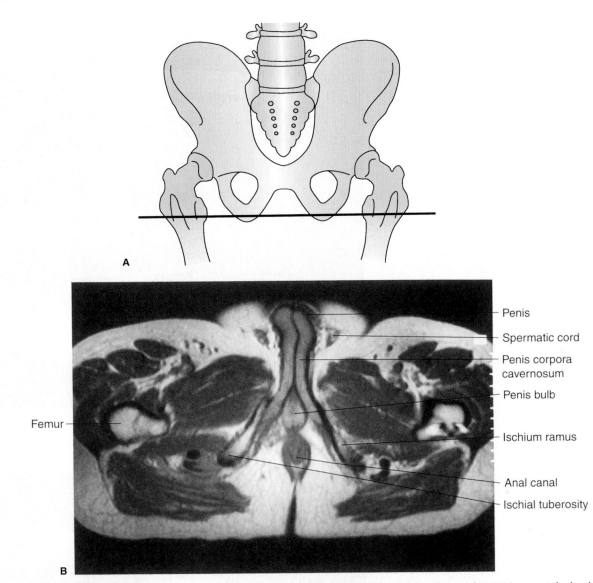

FIGURE 4.39. A: Illustration of the approximate axial anatomic level for **(B)**. **B:** Male pelvis axial T2 MR image at the level of the penile structures. Normal.

IMAGING FEATURES OF GASTROINTESTINAL ABNORMALITIES USING TRADITIONAL CONTRAST RADIOGRAPHS

The gut, being a hollow organ extending from the mouth to the anus, has a basic structure and radiographic appearance throughout. If contrast material (barium) fills the gut, one obtains information about the lumen and gut wall. Visualization of the mucosal surface is improved by double-contrast techniques, as barium coating the mucosal surface contrasts with the intraluminal air. Thus, there are only a few basic patterns that are much alike within the esophagus, stomach, and small or large bowel (Fig. 4.48). They are the following.

1. Intraluminal lesion. Examples include a polyp, foreign body, or exophytic tumor.
2. Mucosal diseases. Examples include inflammation of the mucosa and adjacent musculature, indicative of enteritis.
3. Mural lesion. The abnormality is in the bowel wall (with or without concomitant mucosal involvement). Examples include tumor, transmucosal inflammation, and edema. If the abnormality encircles the bowel wall (as is often seen in colon cancer), a napkin-ring appearance results.
4. Extrinsic lesions. Here, both the bowel wall and lumen are displaced by an extrinsic force. Examples include enlarged mesenteric nodes adjacent to the gut.
5. Extraluminal projections beyond the bowel lumen. Typical abnormalities are ulcerations and diverticula.

FIGURE 4.40. Female pelvis axial T2 MR image. Same anatomic level as Figure 4.38 (R, rectum; U, uterine wall; E, endometrial cavity; C, cervix; O, ovary). (Courtesy of Alan Stolpen, M.D.)

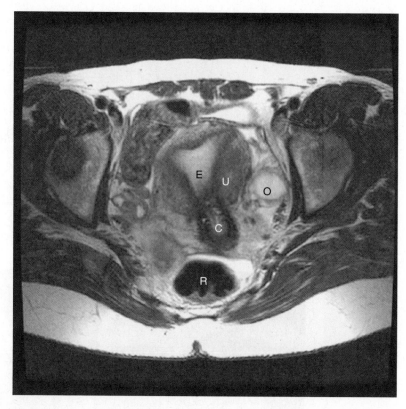

FIGURE 4.41. Female pelvis axial T2 MR image. Same anatomic level as Figure 4.39. (Courtesy of Alan Stolpen, M.D.)

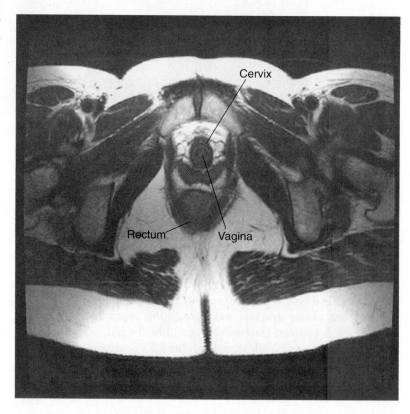

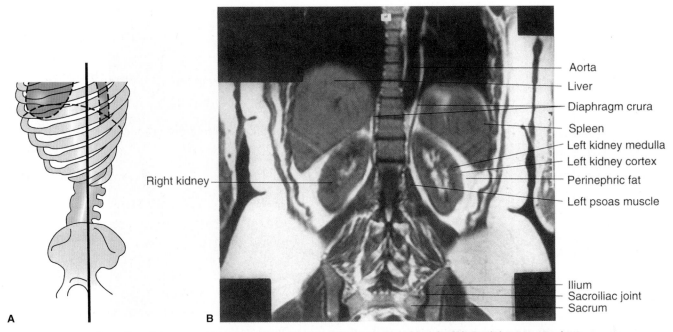

FIGURE 4.42. A: Illustration of the approximate coronal anatomic level through the kidneys for **(B)**. **B:** Abdomen coronal MR image through the kidneys. Normal.

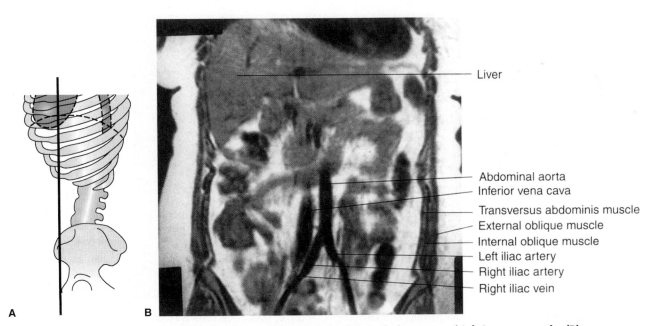

FIGURE 4.43. A: Illustration of the approximate coronal anatomic level through the aorta and inferior vena cava for **(B)**. **B:** Abdomen coronal MR image through the abdominal aorta and inferior vena cava. Normal.

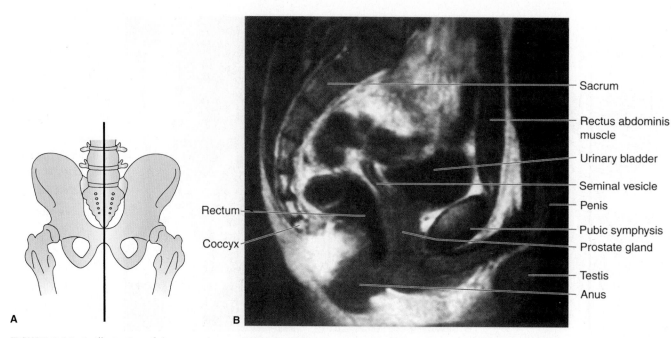

FIGURE 4.44. A: Illustration of the approximate midline sagittal anatomic level for **(B)**. **B:** Male pelvis midline sagittal T2 MR image at the level of the urinary bladder and pubic symphysis. Normal.

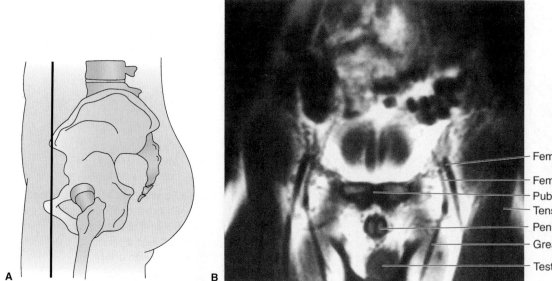

FIGURE 4.45. A: Illustration of the approximate coronal anatomic level for **(B)**. **B:** Male pelvis coronal T1 MR image through the pubic symphysis. Normal.

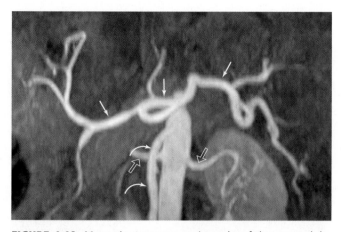

FIGURE 4.46. Magnetic resonance angiography of the upper abdomen. This MR image clearly defines the celiac (*straight arrows*) and superior mesenteric (*curved arrows*) arteries and their branches. The origins of the renal arteries (*open arrows*) from the aorta are noted. (Courtesy of Alan Stolpen, M.D.)

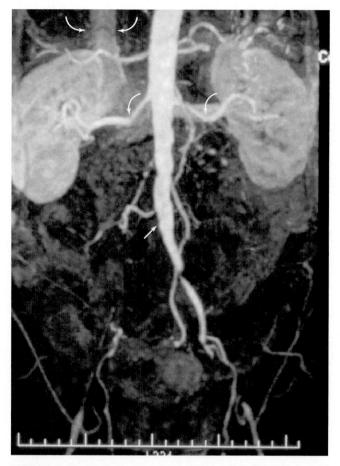

Symptoms arising from esophageal disease include heartburn and dysphagia (difficulty swallowing). In gastroesophageal reflux disease, common in elderly patients, heartburn and later dysphagia occur, owing to reflux of gastric contents into the esophagus, with resultant esophagitis and eventual stricture. Hiatal hernias often accompany gastroesophageal reflux. The barium esophagram easily detects hiatal hernia and stricture (Fig. 4.49). The esophagram is less sensitive in the diagnosis of esophagitis when compared with endoscopy. Esophageal cancer typically has an intraluminal and an intramural component with abnormal mucosa and narrowing of the esophageal lumen (Fig. 4.50). Esophagography is useful in studying motility disorders of the esophagus.

FIGURE 4.47. Magnetic resonance angiography of the aorta and its branches in a patient with arteriosclerosis. The right iliac artery is occluded at its origin (*straight arrow*). Both renal arteries (*curved arrows*) are intact. The inferior vena cava (*curved arrows at top*) can be seen. (Courtesy of Alan Stolpen, M.D.)

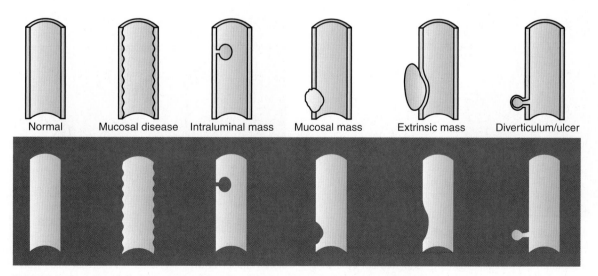

FIGURE 4.48. Types of GI abnormalities (*above*) and their radiographic appearance (*below*).

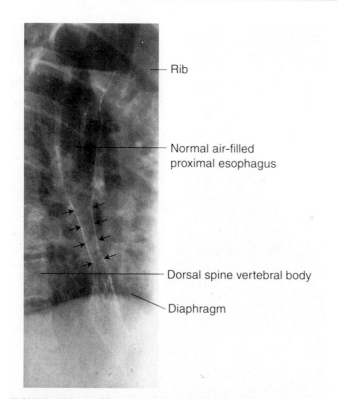

FIGURE 4.49. Double-contrast esophagram. Distal esophageal stricture. The smooth, long, tapered appearance of the narrowed distal esophagus (*arrows*) is typical of a benign stricture owing to reflux of gastric contents into the esophagus.

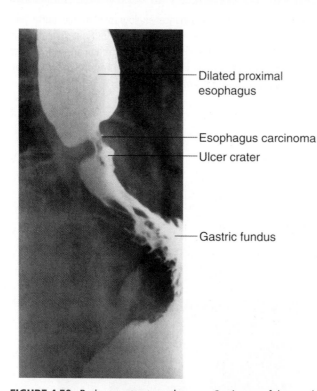

FIGURE 4.50. Barium-contrast esophagram. Carcinoma of the esophagus. The cancer produces a narrowed segment with irregular mucosa and ulceration. The proximal esophagus is dilated but otherwise normal.

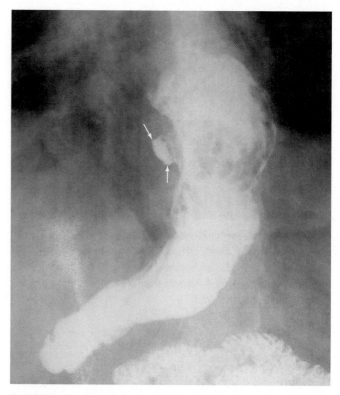

FIGURE 4.51. Gastric ulcer, upper GI series. The lesser curvature ulcer (*arrows*) protrudes from the stomach lumen.

The majority of upper GI series are performed to detect peptic ulcer disease in either the stomach or duodenum. Clearly protruding from the lumen, ulcers are most easily seen on double-contrast examinations (Fig. 4.51). If seen en face, the ulcer crater appears as a glob of increased density as barium fills the ulcer crater and the lumen is filled with air (Fig. 4.52). Often, mucosal folds radiate

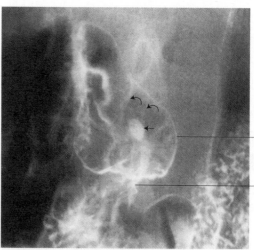

FIGURE 4.52. Double-contrast upper GI series. Central duodenal bulb ulcer (*straight arrow*). The duodenal mucosal folds (*curved arrows*) radiate toward the ulcer crater.

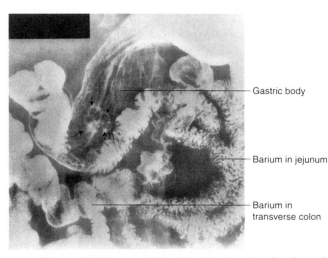

FIGURE 4.53. Double-contrast upper GI series. Gastric polyp. The stalk (*curved arrow*) of the benign polyp (*straight arrows*) is clearly visible.

Gastric body

Barium in jejunum

Barium in transverse colon

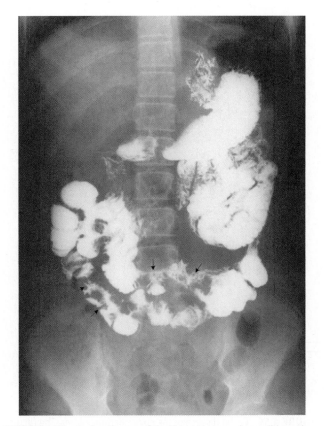

FIGURE 4.54. Crohn disease of the ileum. Antegrade small bowel examination. The affected small bowel (*arrows*) is narrowed; the adjacent space between small bowel loops indicates bowel wall thickening.

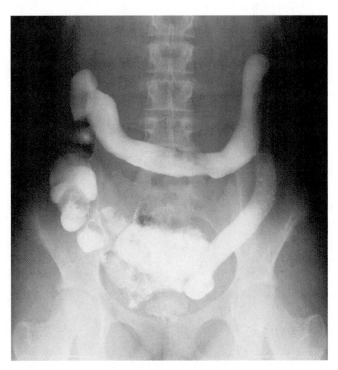

FIGURE 4.55. Ulcerative colitis. Barium enema. The entire colon, except the cecum, is uniformly narrowed, the mucosal surface is irregular, and the overall configuration suggests a lead pipe appearance.

toward the ulcer crater, aiding in its detection. With recurrent disease, deformity of the adjacent bowel, particularly in the duodenum, accompanies the ulcer.

Gastric tumors are uncommon in North America. Polyps (Fig. 4.53) are seen in the elderly. Stomach cancer usually appears as an ulcerated, irregular mucosal mass, often accompanied by concentric narrowing of the adjacent stomach.

Localized small bowel disease in North America is most often Crohn disease, which produces inflammation with mucosal ulcerations and thickening of the bowel wall (Fig. 4.54). Other localized lesions and primary small bowel tumors are rare.

A wide variety of metabolic, immune, and other disorders can involve the entire small bowel. The classic example is sprue (gluten hypersensitivity) with associated small bowel dilatation. Dilution of barium and prominence of the mucosal folds are also noted.

Barium enema studies are useful in the workup of inflammatory colon disease. Ulcerative colitis begins in the rectum and extends a variable distance proximally (Fig. 4.55). The mucosal surface shows tiny ulcerations in a uniform nature throughout the affected area, often accompanied by loss of haustrations (the lead pipe colon). Crohn disease affecting the colon (Fig. 4.56) often spares the rectum, skip lesions are common, and deeper ulcerations occur.

The barium enema, particularly with double-contrast technique, is valuable in detecting colon polyps as well as colon cancer. Intraluminal polyps (Fig. 4.57) are more easily detected than those that are sessile (along the colon wall). Evolution of polyps into colon cancer does occur; the larger the polyp, the greater the chance the histology will show a malignant change. There are approximately 150,000 new cases of carcinoma in the colon and rectum reported each year in the United States. Early detection of this

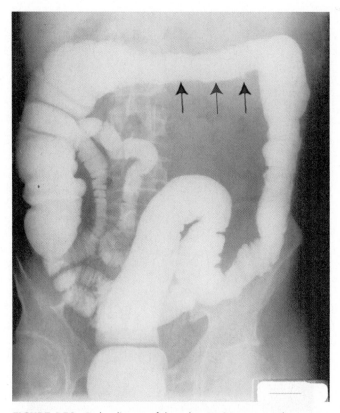

FIGURE 4.56. Crohn disease of the colon. Barium enema. The rectum, sigmoid, and ascending colon are normal. The descending and transverse colon are slightly narrowed, and the mucosa is nodular with small ulcerations (*arrows*) extending from the colon lumen.

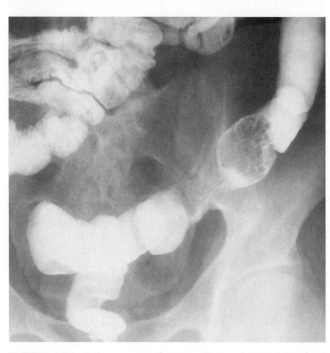

FIGURE 4.57. Barium enema showing villous adenoma with focal carcinoma in the polyp mucosa. A large, lobulated mass fills the lumen of the sigmoid colon.

disease improves survival dramatically. As colon cancer progresses in size, it often surrounds the bowel lumen in a fashion described as an apple core or napkin ring (Fig. 4.58). Large advanced cancers are evident on abdominal CT (Fig. 4.59).

There are a number of syndromes characterized by multiple colonic polyps, sometimes with additional polyps of the small bowel or stomach. Prominent among these is familial polyposis of the colon, which is characterized by multiple adenomas, all with malignant potential (Fig. 4.60).

As noted earlier, polyps and tumors of the colon may be identified with virtual colonoscopy (see Figs. 4.23 and 4.24).

Acute appendicitis is the most common surgical disease of the abdomen. If clinical history and physical examination are strongly suggestive of appendicitis, further imaging examinations are not needed, as the accuracy of clinical findings approaches 90%. Plain films of the abdomen are not particularly helpful in the diagnosis of appendicitis, unless a calcified appendicolith is noted. Imaging studies are most valuable in those individuals with low to moderate probability of a positive diagnosis (Fig. 4.61). In children, careful US examination performed by a skilled radiologist is frequently the study of choice; CT is sometimes difficult because of the small amount of periappendiceal fat in this age group. In adults, multislice CT of the right lower quadrant, with or without the use of contrast material, is recommended. The abnormal appendix can be identified in most cases as a small tubular structure with distended lumen, thickening of the periappendiceal wall, and inflammation of adjacent fat (Fig. 4.62). One can usually diagnose perforation of the appendix by changes adjacent to the organ.

IMAGING FEATURES OF GENITOURINARY ABNORMALITIES

Certain anomalies obstruct the flow of urine, producing proximal obstruction. Congenital ureteropelvic junction (UPJ) obstructions can sometimes be diagnosed in utero; less severe cases do not present until later in life. The UPJ obstruction can be unilateral or bilateral. US is an excellent technique for following UPJ obstruction, showing the amount of pelvicalyceal dilatation and its effect on the renal parenchyma (Fig. 4.63). Congenital vesicoureteral junction obstruction is less frequent but usually bilateral (Fig. 4.64).

Embryologically, the kidneys develop in the pelvis and migrate cephalad into the abdomen. The kidney that fails to migrate cephalad into the abdomen is called a pelvic kidney, sacral kidney, or simple ectopia (Fig. 4.65). In a horseshoe kidney, the lower poles of the right and left kidneys are connected by a bridge, or isthmus, of renal tissue (Fig. 4.66).

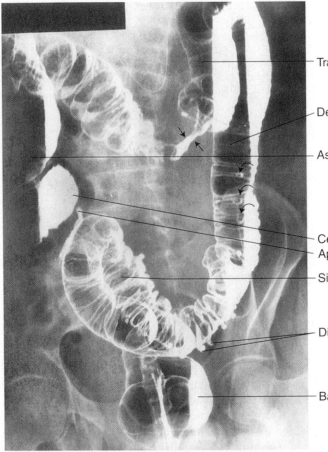

Transverse colon

Descending colon

Ascending colon

Cecum

Appendix

Sigmoid colon

Diverticula

Barium in rectum

A

FIGURE 4.58. A: Adenocarcinoma of the transverse colon. Double-contrast colon examination. Note the classic apple core appearance of the colon cancer. The core represents the patent portion of the bowel lumen (*straight arrows*). Diverticula of the descending colon are seen en face. **B:** Close-up view of the tumor mass in **(A)**. Note the irregular mucosa of the narrowed lumen of the apple core lesion (*white arrows*). The mass creates a shouldering (*black arrows*) deformity in the neighboring transverse colon both proximally and distally.

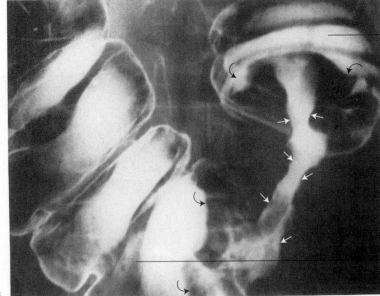

Normal transverse colon

Normal transverse colon

B

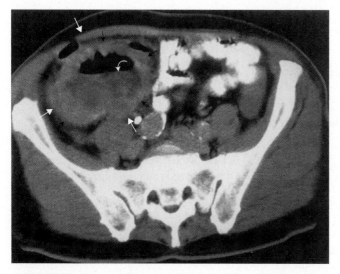

FIGURE 4.59. Lower abdomen axial CT image. The *white arrows* outline a large cecal neoplasm. The *curved arrow* shows an air–fluid level within the tumor mass secondary to necrosis.

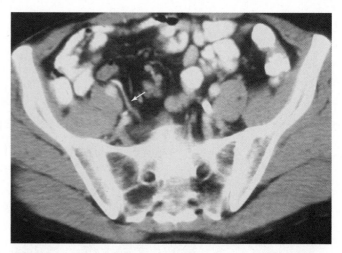

FIGURE 4.61. Normal appendix. Abdominal CT. The appendix is the wormlike, barium-filled density (*arrow*) in the right lower quadrant. (Courtesy of Bruce Brown, M.D.)

Ureterocele (Fig. 4.67) refers to a dilated intramural ureteral segment that protrudes into the bladder, simulating a cobra's head. Ureteroceles result from either congenital or acquired stenosis at the ureteral orifice and can cause partial ureteral obstruction.

Bladder diverticula are generally acquired but on occasion are congenital (Fig. 4.68).

Urolithiasis is one of the most common urologic problems encountered in the everyday practice of medicine. Most ureteral stones are less than 1 cm in diameter, and approximately 75% of acutely symptomatic stones are

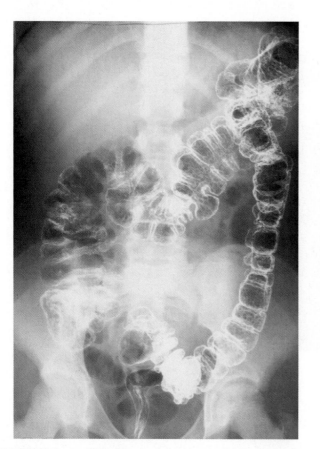

FIGURE 4.60. Familial polyposis of the colon. Double-contrast barium enema. There are innumerable tiny polyps throughout the colon.

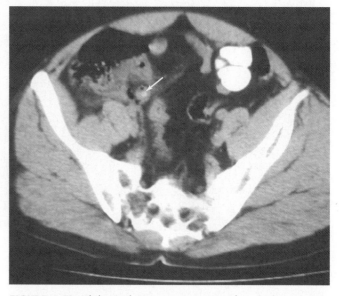

FIGURE 4.62. Abdominal CT transverse view of appendix. Appendicitis with perforation. A calcified appendicolith is in the lumen of the appendix (*arrow*). There is gas in the appendiceal wall and periappendiceal fluid. (Courtesy of Bruce Brown, M.D.)

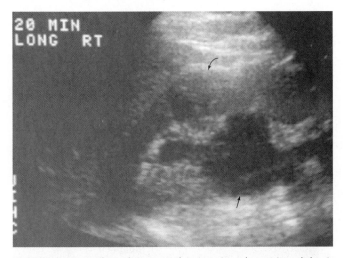

FIGURE 4.63. Unilateral ureteropelvic junction obstruction abdominal sonogram. The echo-free renal pelvis and associated calyces (*arrow*) are dilated. Renal–cortical borders are indicated by the *curved arrow*. (Courtesy of Monzer Abu-Yousef, M.D.)

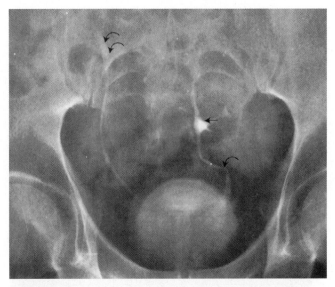

FIGURE 4.65. Abdomen AP EU. Pelvic kidney (simple ectopia). The left kidney is situated in the pelvis, just cephalad to the urinary bladder. The upper collecting system of the pelvic kidney is indicated by the *straight arrow*. Note the foreshortened left ureter (*single curved arrow*) and the normal right ureter (*double curved arrows*).

located in the distal third of the ureter. Approximately 90% of all GU calculi are radiopaque on plain film.

Some radiopaque renal calculi actually fill all or part of an upper collecting system and are called staghorn calculi (Fig. 4.69). When such calculi are bilateral, their appearance should not be mistaken for contrast media in the upper collecting systems. Although EU has been used to diagnose urolithiasis (it is valuable in quantitating the degree of ureteral obstruction), it is considerably less sensitive than

CT. Current protocol for patients with suspected ureteral stones calls for multislice CT through the regions of the kidneys and ureters without intravenous contrast material, usually followed by repeat examination with contrast material (Fig. 4.70). Obviously, calculi can occur at any location in the urinary tract. The differential diagnosis for a renal pelvis filling (nonradiopaque) defect is listed in Table 4.6.

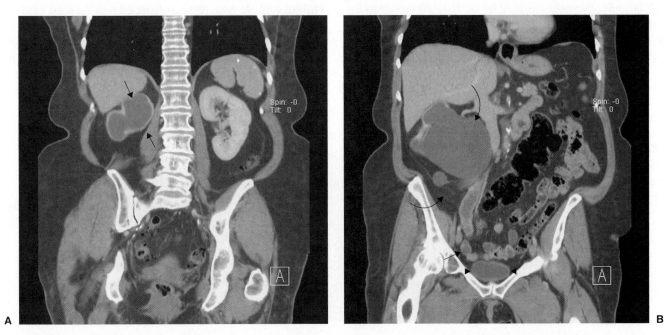

FIGURE 4.64. Unilateral vesicoureteral obstruction. **A:** Coronal CT. The left kidney is normal, but a urine-filled sac surrounded by renal cortex (*arrows*) is seen on the left. **B:** Later coronal CT shows the dilated right renal pelvis (*curved arrows*) and ureter (*straight arrows*) extending to the bladder (*arrowhead*). (Courtesy of Andrew Wu, M.D.)

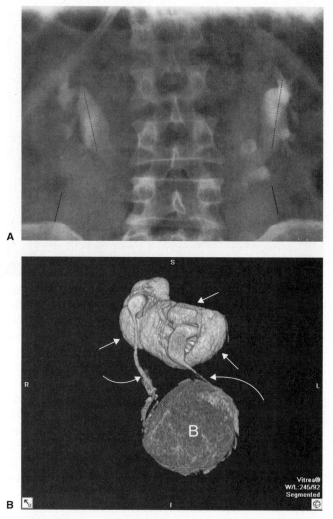

FIGURE 4.66. Horseshoe kidney. **A:** The excretory urogram shows the lower pole calyces closer to the midline than those of the upper poles. **B:** Three-dimensional reconstruction of **(A)** shows the fused kidneys (*straight arrows*), both ureters (*curved arrows*), and bladder **(B)**.

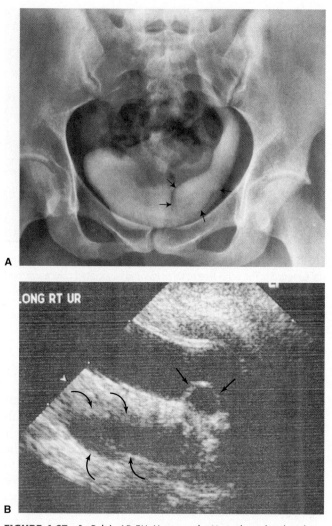

FIGURE 4.67. **A:** Pelvis AP EU. Ureterocele. Note the cobra head appearance (*arrows*) of the ureterocele. The left ureter is moderately dilated. **B:** Ureterocele, pelvic US. The wall of the ureterocele (*straight arrows*) is visualized by echo-free urine in the bladder and within the ureterocele. A dilated ureter (*curved arrows*) is noted posterior to the bladder.

FIGURE 4.68. Cystogram. Bladder diverticulum (*straight arrows*). There are unilateral pins traversing a left hip fracture (*curved arrow*).

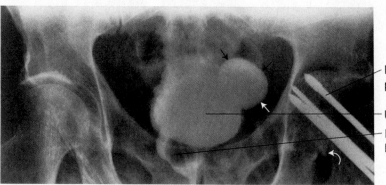

— Metallic orthopedic pins

— Urinary bladder

— Foley catheter balloon

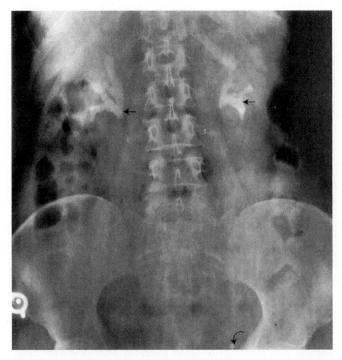

FIGURE 4.69. AP supine abdomen. Bilateral renal staghorn calculi. The calculi (*straight arrows*) closely resemble contrast media in upper collecting systems, demonstrating the importance of the preliminary radiograph. Incidentally noted is a left pelvic phlebolith (*curved arrow*).

Multiple unilateral or bilateral interstitial renal calcifications are referred to as nephrocalcinosis. Nephrolithiasis, or calcification in the renal tubules, occurs with metabolic abnormalities (hypercalcemia) or with congenitally dilated collecting tubules (medullary sponge kidney). The US and CT appearances (Fig. 4.71) are pathognomonic—another Aunt Minnie.

Therapeutic US has become a useful tool for breaking up calculi. This is called extracorporeal sound wave lithotripsy (Fig. 4.72). The fragmented calculi usually pass spontaneously without surgical intervention.

GU infections are a common occurrence in medicine and usually do not require diagnostic imaging procedures. In children, especially males, with documented urinary infection, study for vesicoureteral reflux is recommended (see Fig. 4.28) and US study of the kidneys is often of value. Severity of infection ranges from mild cystitis to

Table 4.6
Masses in the Renal Pelvis

- Stones
- Tumor
- Mycetoma (fungus ball)
- Blood clot
- Necrotic renal papillae

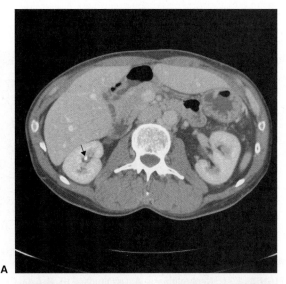

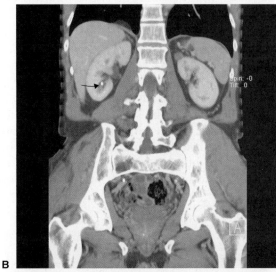

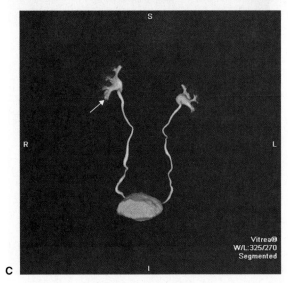

FIGURE 4.70. Renal calculus coronal. Axial **(A)** and coronal **(B)** CTs without contrast material. The stone (*arrows*) lies in a lower pole calyx of the right kidney. **C:** On reconstructed CT urogram, the stone (*arrow*) is more difficult to recognize. (Courtesy of Andrew Wu, M.D.)

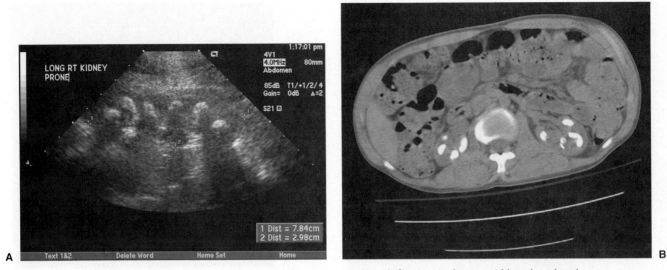

FIGURE 4.71. Nephrolithiasis. **A:** Longitudinal US. **B:** Axial CT. These are extensive calcifications in the pyramid (not the calyces) of the kidneys. (Courtesy of Simon Kao, M.D.)

perinephric abscess. Acute pyelonephritis usually causes renal enlargement, which may be focal (Fig. 4.73); with atrophic pyelonephritis, the kidney may shrink.

Renal cysts may be single, multiple, unilateral, or bilateral. These lesions are usually asymptomatic and often are an incidental finding on abdominal imaging performed for other reasons. Although cysts are of no clinical significance, they must be evaluated closely to

distinguish them from solid tumors. This is easily done with US (Fig. 4.74) or CT (Fig. 4.75) as the water density and sharp borders of cysts are apparent. Other benign renal tumors are uncommon.

Malignant renal tumors are solid masses. Approximately 90% are renal cell carcinomas. Patients with renal cell carcinomas may present with gross or microscopic hematuria, pain, or other symptoms. US (Fig. 4.76) determines the

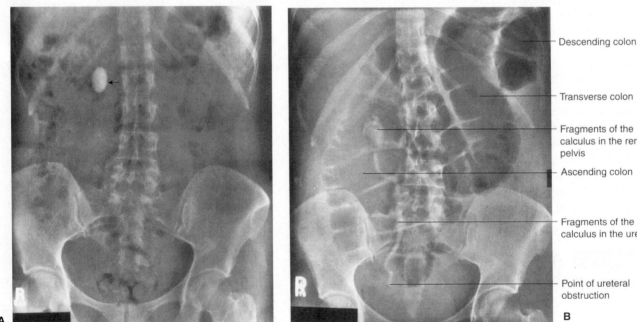

FIGURE 4.72. A: Abdomen AP radiograph. Solitary radiopaque calculus in the right renal pelvis (*arrow*). **B:** Abdomen AP radiograph 24 hours postextracorporeal sound wave lithotripsy. The obstructed ureter is filled with multiple small fragments of the calculus, referred to as "steinstrasse" (or "stone street"). The colon is air-filled and dilated (adynamic ileus) owing to pain of renal colic.

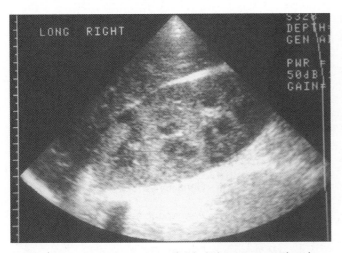

FIGURE 4.73. Sagittal sonogram of right kidney. Segmental pyelonephritis. Note the increased echogenicity of the upper pole. The foci of decreased lucency in both upper and lower poles are the renal pyramids. (Courtesy of Monzer Abu-Yousef, M.D.)

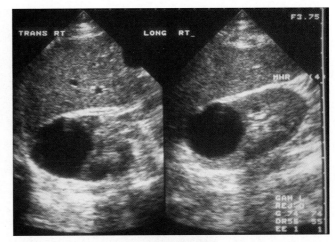

FIGURE 4.74. Transverse and longitudinal sonograms of the right kidney. Renal cyst of the upper pole. The cyst is echolucent, has sharp borders, and shows posterior enhancement. (Courtesy of Monzer Abu-Yousef, M.D.)

solid nature of the mass. CT or MRI is the proven method of diagnosis. EU is less sensitive and accurate. Some examples of renal malignancies are shown in Figures 4.76 to 4.79.

Malignant tumors of the urothelium occur in the renal pelvis, ureter, or bladder. As they often cause urinary obstruction, ureteral opacification displays them best (Figs. 4.80–4.82).

Extrinsic malignancies, such as retroperitoneal tumors, can displace or obstruct the ureter and kidneys

(Fig. 4.83). Primary and secondary neoplasms can also involve the ureter and the bladder (Fig. 4.84).

Prostatic cancer is the most common neoplasm of elderly males. Neither CT nor MRI is of particular value of screening for this malignancy, but both are beneficial in staging the disease. Specifically, MRI evaluates the possibility of spread of the tumor beyond the prostate capsule, and both CT and MRI allow demonstration of pelvic lymph node metastasis (Fig. 4.85).

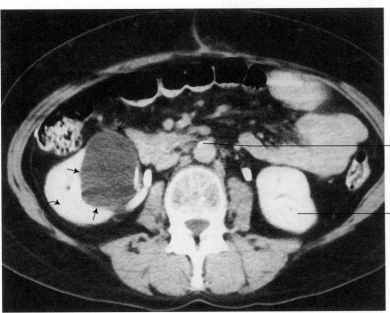

— Abdominal aorta calcification

— Normal left kidney

FIGURE 4.75. Abdomen axial CT image through the kidneys after intravenous contrast media. Right renal cyst. The cyst has sharp, smooth margins (*straight arrows*) and a low tissue density when compared with the remainder of the right kidney (*curved arrow*).

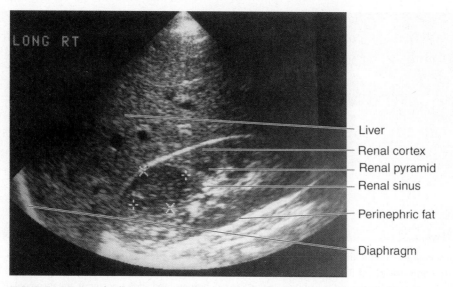

Liver
Renal cortex
Renal pyramid
Renal sinus
Perinephric fat
Diaphragm

FIGURE 4.76. Renal cell carcinoma. Right renal longitudinal sonogram. The electronic caliper *X marks* and *crosses* delineate an upper pole renal mass. The numerous internal echoes (hyperechoic) within the mass indicate that it is solid.

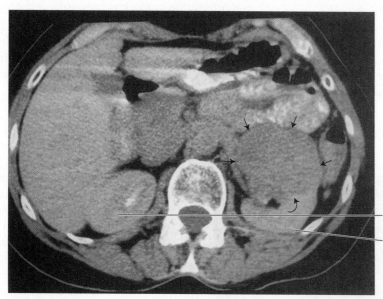

Normal right kidney
Normal portion left kidney

FIGURE 4.77. Abdomen axial CT. Left renal cell carcinoma (*straight arrows*). The mass lesion is solid, and its border with the normal kidney (*curved arrow*) is poorly defined.

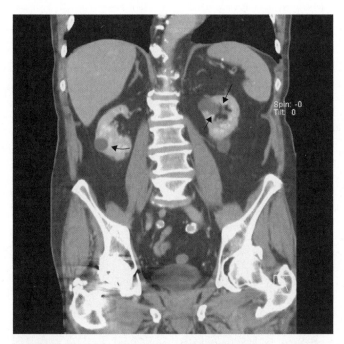

FIGURE 4.78. Renal cell carcinoma (*arrows*) left kidney and benign cyst (*arrow*) right kidney. CT. Note the smooth borders and spherical shape of the cyst versus the irregular border of the cancer.

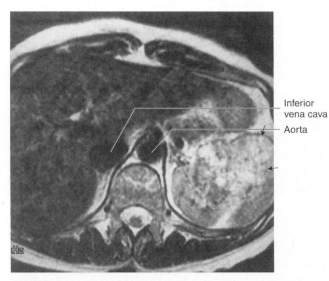

FIGURE 4.79. Abdomen axial T2 MR image. There is a large left renal cell carcinoma (*arrows*).

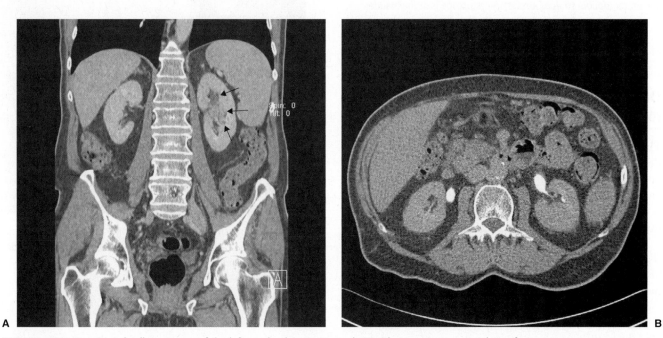

FIGURE 4.80. Transitional cell carcinoma of the left renal pelvis. **A:** Coronal CT without contrast material. A soft tissue mass (*arrows*) fills the central left renal pelvis (compare the right and left renal pelves). **B:** Axial CT with contrast. The upper pole tumor replaces contrast across the posterior kidney.

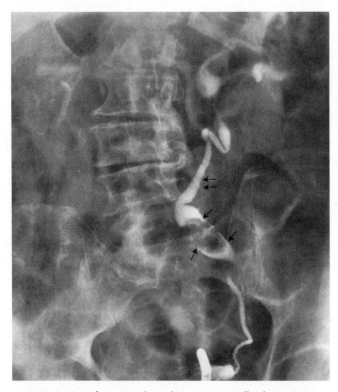

FIGURE 4.81. Left retrograde pyelogram. A partially obstructing ureteral carcinoma (*single straight arrows*) has resulted in a dilated proximal ureter (*double straight arrows*). A cystoscope is in the bladder.

OBSTETRIC AND GYNECOLOGIC IMAGING

There is seldom a need today for abdominal plain films in the diagnosis of pregnancy; however, when such a study is done (for necessity or by accident; Fig. 4.86), the risk of damage to the fetus from radiation is extremely low. Here is another Aunt Minnie—a radiograph showing an intrauterine contraceptive device (Fig. 4.87).

Routine US evaluation of the pregnant woman and her fetus, a standard practice in the developed world, is of considerable value in obstetrics. Fetal maturation, major anomalies, placental assessment, and many associated maternal conditions can be evaluated (Figs. 4.88 and 4.89). Ectopic (tubal) pregnancy is readily diagnosed with US (Fig. 4.90).

Uterine anomalies and tubal diseases affecting fertility are often studied with hysterosalpingography. In this examination, contrast material is injected into the cervix, outlining the uterine cavity and fallopian tubes (Fig. 4.91). In a normal woman, contrast spills into the peritoneal cavity. Uterine anomalies can be detected with US, CT, and MRI (Fig. 4.92). Infected fallopian tubes typically fill

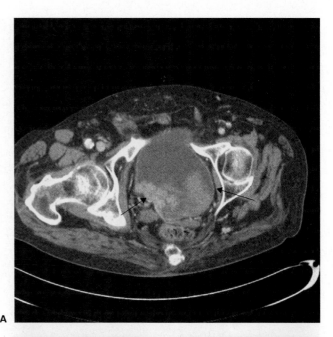

A

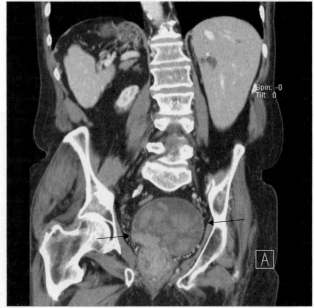

B

FIGURE 4.82. Transitional cell bladder cancer. Axial **(A)** and Coronal **(B)** CT. The bladder (*arrows*) is filled with polypoid masses surrounded by nonradiopaque urine.

with pus (pyosalpinx) and have characteristic US features (Fig. 4.93).

Benign uterine fibroids (leiomyomatosis), the most common gynecologic tumor, can (if calcified) be recognized by their classic appearance in the abdominal radiograph (Fig. 4.94). They are often seen on other imaging modalities (Figs. 4.95 and 4.96).

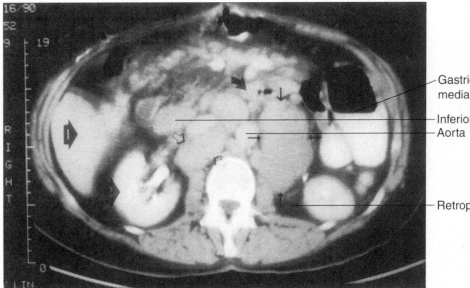

Gastric air–fluid (contrast media) level

Inferior vena cava

Aorta

Retroperitoneal fat

FIGURE 4.83. Abdomen axial CT image. Lymphoma. The tumor (*arrows*) involves lymph nodes in the retroperitoneum and surrounds the enhanced aorta and inferior vena cava. The arrow labeled *1* indicates the inferior aspect of the liver.

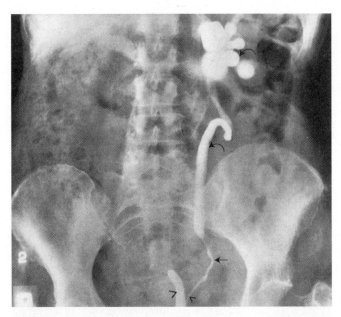

FIGURE 4.84. Left retrograde pyelogram. Encasement of the distal left ureter by cancer of the cervix has resulted in stricture and partial obstruction of the distal left ureter (*straight arrow*). The left ureter proximal to the stricture is dilated (*curved arrow*s). The cystoscope and retrograde catheter (*arrowheads*) can be seen.

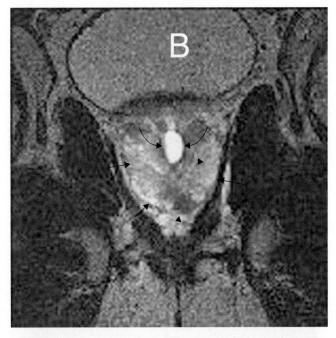

FIGURE 4.85. Coronal prostate MRI in an elderly man with prostate cancer extending into adjacent tissue. B, bladder, prostatic urethra (*curved arrows*), prostatic capsule (*straight arrows*), cancer spread beyond capsule (*arrowheads*). The spreading cancer is low signal as compared to the rest of the prostate and the capsule cannot be identified in the region of the cancer. (Courtesy of Eve Clark, M.D.)

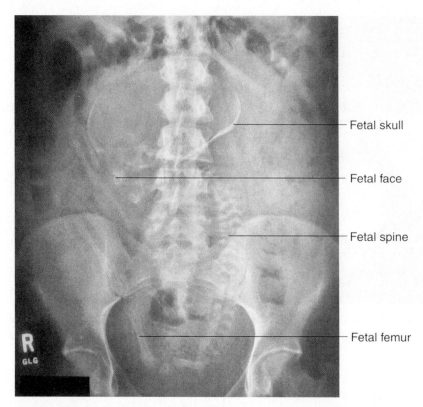

— Fetal skull

— Fetal face

— Fetal spine

— Fetal femur

FIGURE 4.86. Abdomen AP radiograph. Third-trimester intrauterine pregnancy in a breech presentation.

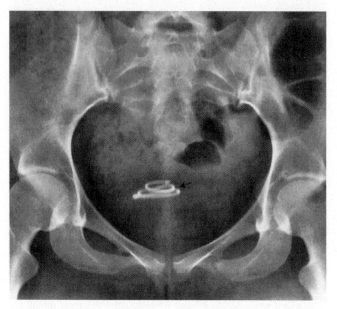

FIGURE 4.87. Pelvis AP radiograph. Normal position and appearance of an intrauterine contraceptive device (*arrow*).

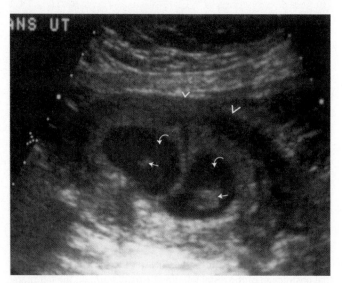

FIGURE 4.88. Transabdominal transverse obstetrical sonogram. Twin pregnancy. The twin fetuses (*straight arrows*) are located in separate sacs and are surrounded by amniotic fluid (*curved arrows*). The uterine wall is indicated by *arrowheads*.

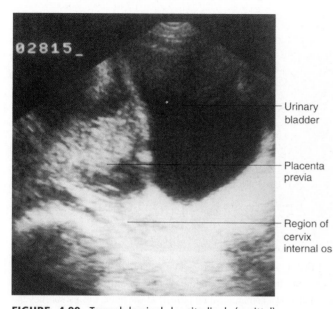

FIGURE 4.89. Transabdominal longitudinal (sagittal) sonogram. Placenta previa. The sonogram shows the placenta covering the internal cervical os, thus precluding vaginal delivery.

— Urinary bladder

— Placenta previa

— Region of cervix internal os

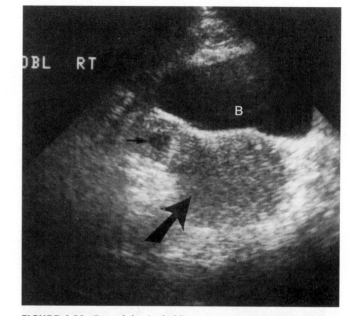

FIGURE 4.90. Transabdominal oblique sonogram. Ectopic pregnancy. The *large arrow* indicates the hyperechoic, blood-filled uterus. The *small arrow* indicates the gestational sac in the right fallopian tube (B, urinary bladder).

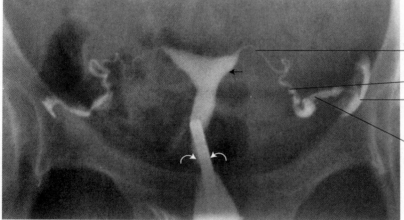

Isthmus of fallopian tube

Ampulla of fallopian tube

Peritoneal contrast media spill

Fimbriated portion of the fallopian tube

FIGURE 4.91. Hysterosalpingogram. Normal uterus (*straight arrow*) and fallopian tubes. Contrast media injected into the uterus via a cervical cannula (*curved arrows*) spills into the peritoneal space, indicating fallopian tube patency.

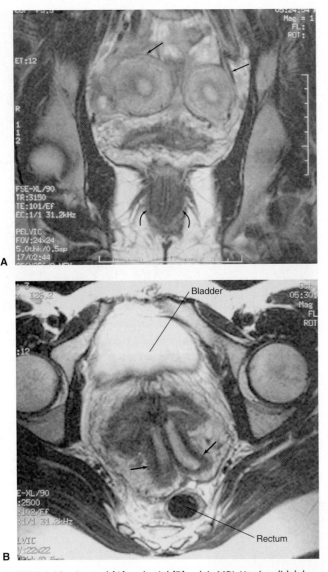

FIGURE 4.92. Coronal **(A)** and axial **(B)** pelvic MRI. Uterine didelphys, demonstrating two separate uteri (*straight arrows*) with their endometrial cavities, two uterine cervices, and two vaginas (*curved arrows*). (Courtesy of Alan Stolpen, M.D.)

Imaging has, to date, played a minor role in evaluating carcinoma of the endometrium. MRI may be useful in staging cervical cancer (Fig. 4.97).

Detectability of ovarian tumors is much better with imaging studies than with physical examination. Tumors are seldom diagnosed on plain film unless they are huge or have typical features (Fig. 4.98). Both benign and malignant neoplasms have characteristic features on US, CT, and MRI. As in the kidney, US separates solid and cystic (usually benign) masses (Fig. 4.99).

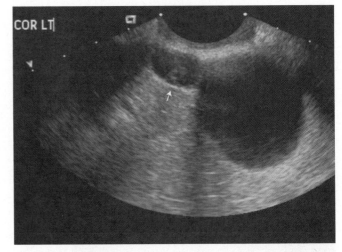

FIGURE 4.93. Coronal transvaginal sonogram. Hydro(pyo)salpinx. The fluid collection has some internal echoes; its configuration is oval with a smaller oval communication (*arrow*) at the apex; this establishes the fallopian tube as the locale of the abnormality. (Courtesy of Monzer Abu-Yousef, M.D.)

IMAGING ACCESSORY DIGESTIVE ORGANS

Almost all imaging modalities can be used for the evaluation of liver disease. In general, the plain film is relatively insensitive, although it will show calcifications or gas in the liver. Evaluation for hepatomegaly is probably best by CT or nuclear medicine scans, although US examinations are also useful. MRI of liver disease is usually reserved for circumstances in which a definitive diagnosis is not possible with another modality.

Cirrhosis in North America is most often related to chronic alcoholism or as a complication of hepatitis. The severity of cirrhosis is primarily evaluated by physical examination and laboratory tests, but imaging is often useful. Early changes include hepatomegaly with fatty infiltration of the liver, easily detected on CT (Fig. 4.100). As

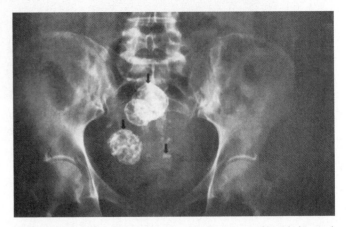

FIGURE 4.94. Pelvic radiograph. The calcified uterine fibroids (*arrows*) are an Aunt Minnie.

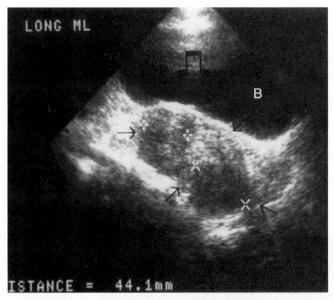

FIGURE 4.95. Transabdominal longitudinal (sagittal) sonogram. The uterus is outlined by the *arrows*. The electronic caliper *X marks* and *crosses* outline two large fibroids. The many internal echoes within the masses indicate that they are solid.

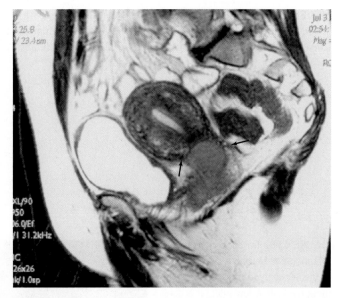

FIGURE 4.97. Sagittal pelvic MR image. Cervical carcinoma. There is abrupt transition of normal uterine mucosa at the tumor margin (*arrows*). Inferiorly, the tumor is more infiltrative. (Courtesy of Alan Stolpen, M.D.)

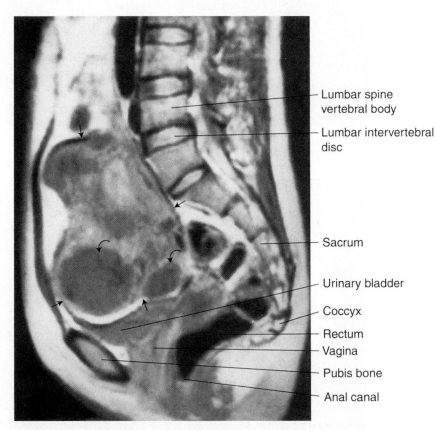

Lumbar spine vertebral body

Lumbar intervertebral disc

Sacrum

Urinary bladder

Coccyx

Rectum

Vagina

Pubis bone

Anal canal

FIGURE 4.96. Pelvis midline sagittal T1 MR image. The enlarged uterus is outlined by *straight arrows*. Two large fibroids are indicated by the *curved arrows*.

FIGURE 4.98. Pelvic radiograph. Bilateral ovarian teratoma. Each tumor contains teeth (*straight arrows*) and substantial intratumor fat (*curved arrows*) allowing the tumors to be better visualized. (Courtesy of Alan Stolpen, M.D.)

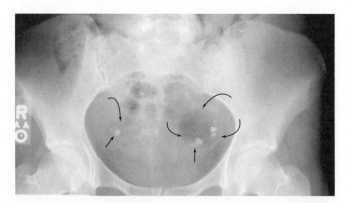

FIGURE 4.99. Transabdominal sagittal sonogram. Mucinous cystadenoma of the left ovary (*arrows*). The ovarian mass has only a few internal echoes and demonstrates posterior enhancement typical of a cyst.

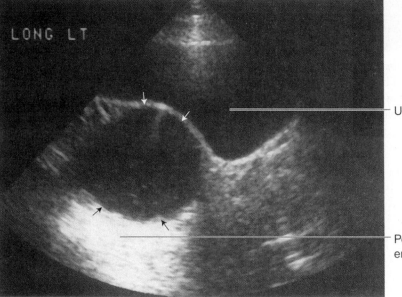

Urinary bladder

Posterior enhancement

FIGURE 4.100. Axial abdominal CT. Fatty liver (not in a cirrhotic patient). The *large arrow* indicates the fatty changes. The *small arrow* indicates vessels within the fat. The *open arrow* indicates a normal enhanced liver.

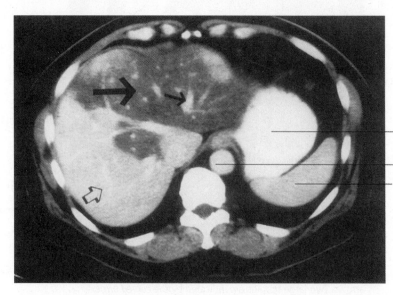

Stomach

Abdominal aorta

Spleen

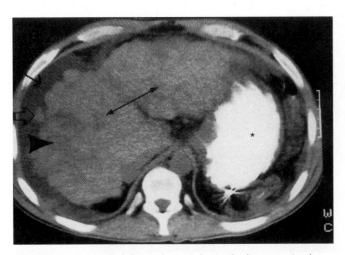

FIGURE 4.101. Axial abdominal CT. Cirrhosis. The liver margins (*open area*) are nodular. There are scattered fatty changes (*arrowhead*) and ascites (*short black arrow*). Both lobes (*two-headed arrow*) are involved.

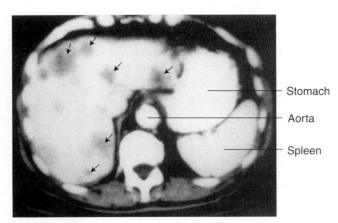

FIGURE 4.103. Abdomen axial CT. Right and left hepatic lobe metastases. The metastases (*arrows*) appear hypodense compared with the enhanced normal liver. Liver enhancement was accomplished by intravenous injection of contrast media.

cirrhosis progresses, there is diminution in the size of the liver and development of heterogeneous density of the liver parenchyma with a knobby surface related to coexisting scarring and regeneration of liver nodules (Fig. 4.101). Changes of portal hypertension (splenomegaly, ascites, and dilated portal veins and tributaries) can be found in severe disease. Portal venous flow may be reduced or even reversed in severe cirrhosis, and secondary hepatic venous occlusion can occur. These can be delineated with Doppler US examination (Fig. 4.102).

The liver is the most common site for metastases from intra-abdominal organs and often from tumors elsewhere in the body (lung and breast). Metastatic tumors in the liver are found 10 to 20 times more often than primary malignant tumors. Often, the hepatic metastatic disease is the first clinical indication of tumor. Imaging of metastatic liver disease is best done with CT using intravenous contrast material. Metastatic lesions are most often of reduced density when compared with the liver parenchyma (Fig. 4.103).

Benign primary tumors of the liver include hepatic cysts and cavernous hemangiomas; both are incidental findings and of no clinical significance. Larger hemangiomas or others with bizarre features may require MRI to be separated from malignant lesions (Fig. 4.104). Primary hepatoma occurs primarily in patients with pre-existing liver disease.

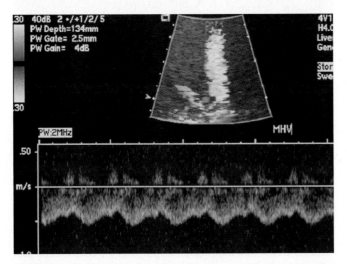

FIGURE 4.102. Hepatic venous Doppler US in a cirrhotic patient. The study shows patent hepatic veins converging. The up-and-down Doppler signal indicates normal venous flow. (Courtesy of Monzer Abu-Yousef, M.D.)

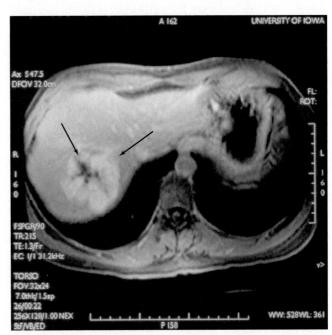

FIGURE 4.104. Axial MRI. Liver hemangioma. This study performed after intravenous administration of gadolinium shows a high signal mass (*arrows*) with bright walls characteristic of a hemangioma. (Courtesy of Alan Stolpen, M.D.)

FIGURE 4.105. Longitudinal decubitus sonogram. Cholelithiasis. Note how the dense gallstones (calculi, *curved arrows*) cast acoustic shadows (*straight arrows*) because the sound waves are unable to penetrate or traverse the dense calculi. This is similar to a shadow cast by a tree or building.

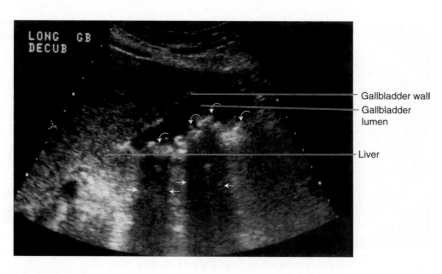

Gallbladder wall
Gallbladder lumen
Liver

Hepatoma is less dense than normal liver parenchyma and has ill-defined margins. CT and MRI are useful for defining hepatic anatomy to determine resectability of tumors.

There are many methods to image biliary tract abnormalities. US is the workhorse. Gallstones are the most common abnormalities of the gallbladder. About 10% of stones are calcified and visible on plain films (see Fig. 4.8). Ultrasonography is effective in detecting gallstones, as the highly echogenic stones are surrounded by echo-free bile. Failure to propagate the sound wave distally causes shadowing (Fig. 4.105). The common bile duct is also studied during gallbladder examinations.

Acute cholecystitis can be confirmed, if US shows gallstones, with thickening of the gallbladder wall and localized tenderness. In ambiguous cases, radionuclide cholescintigraphy is performed. In acute cholecystitis, there is obstruction of the cystic duct so that radioactive material secreted from the liver fills the biliary tract, including the common duct but not the gallbladder (see Chapter 9).

In distal obstruction, such as with common duct stones or pancreatic tumors, the proximal biliary tract dilates. Recent technical developments in MRI allow the evaluation of the biliary tract and pancreatic duct noninvasively. MRI offers spectacular imaging of biliary obstruction (Fig. 4.106).

Splenomegaly is sometimes evident on the abdominal radiograph (see Fig. 4.3) but is more reliably evaluated by US or CT. There are measurements available to separate the normal-sized from the enlarged spleen, although considerable overlap exists. Perhaps this is an appropriate time to again quote Ben Felson, "A radiologist with a ruler in his hand is a dangerous person."

Pancreatitis occurs as a complication of alcoholism, biliary tract disease, and sometimes trauma. Although the inflamed pancreas sometimes appears normal on US or CT examination (Fig. 4.107), more often there is diffuse or localized swelling of the gland and inhomogeneity of US signal and CT as well as adjacent fluid (Fig. 4.108). An important complication of acute pancreatitis is pseudocyst formation. The large, frequently multiloculated cysts are visible on either US or CT.

In pancreatic carcinoma, clinical manifestations are infrequent before metastases have occurred. Both US and CT are useful for detecting pancreatic neoplasms as well as for staging the extent of metastatic disease. Tumor involvement of the celiac or superior mesenteric vessels makes resection impossible (Fig. 4.109).

Abscess can occur anywhere in the abdomen—in a solid organ such as the liver or loculated anywhere in the peritoneal cavity (Fig. 4.110). CT is probably the best

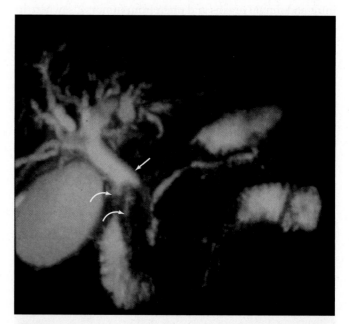

FIGURE 4.106. MRI cholangiopancreatogram. The common bile duct (*straight arrow*) and its proximal branches are dilated owing to obstruction (*curved arrows*) from pancreatic carcinoma. The pancreatic duct, gallbladder, and duodenal lumen are also visualized. (Courtesy of E. Scott Pretorius, M.D.)

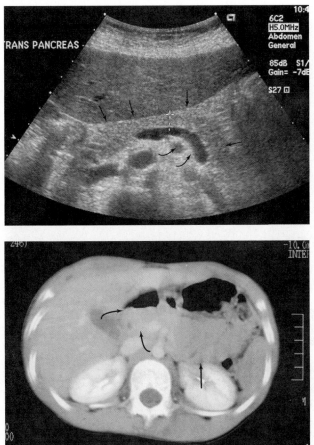

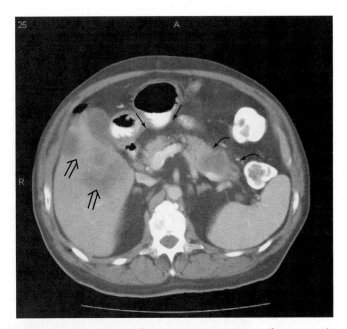

FIGURE 4.109. Abdominal CT. Pancreatic carcinoma. The pancreatic head and body (*straight arrows*) are normal. There is a poorly marginated hypodense mass (*curved arrows*) in the pancreatic tail. Several hypodense metastases (*open arrows*) are noted in the liver.

FIGURE 4.107. A: Transverse abdominal sonogram. Normal pancreas. The pancreas (*straight arrows*) is posterior to the liver (*L*) and anterior to the splenic vein (*curved arrows*). *Crosses* are in place to measure transverse pancreatic diameter. (Courtesy of Monzer Abu-Yousef, M.D.) **B:** Abdominal CT. Traumatic pancreatitis. The pancreatic body and tail (*straight arrow*) are enlarged and of uneven density. The mass (*curved arrows*) in the region of the pancreatic head is a hematoma.

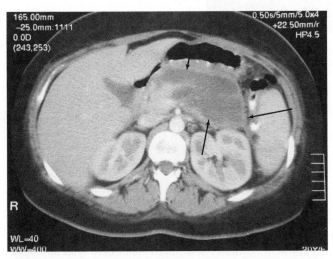

FIGURE 4.108. Pancreatic pseudocyst. Abdominal CT. The hypodense pseudocyst (*arrows*) replaces the body and tail of the pancreas. (Courtesy of Bruce Brown, M.D.)

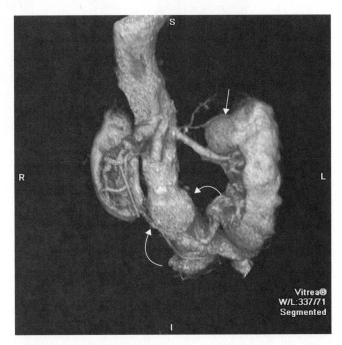

FIGURE 4.110. Abdominal aneurysm and renal cell carcinoma. CT angiogram. The cancer (*straight arrow*) extends from the superior pole of the left kidney. The abdominal aneurysm (*curved arrows*) is evident by the convexity of the aorta distal to the renal arteries.

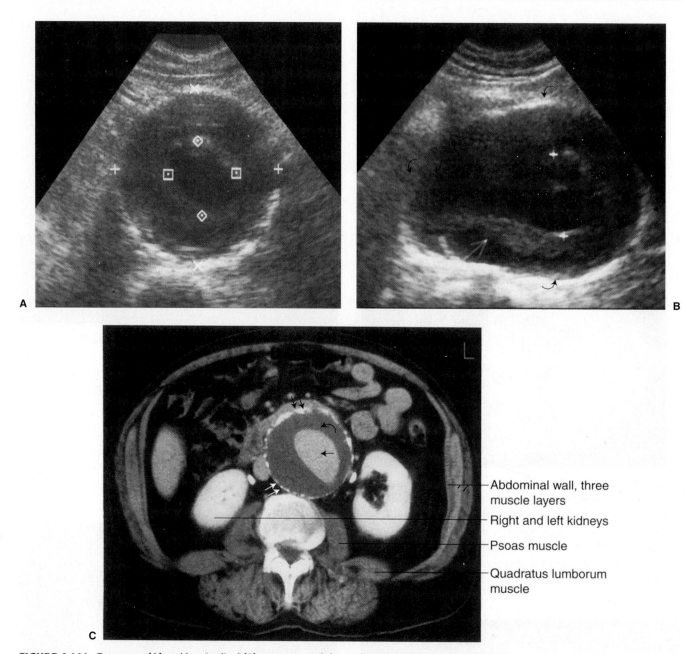

FIGURE 4.111. Transverse **(A)** and longitudinal **(B)** sonograms. Abdominal aortic aneurysm. Thrombus extends from the aortic wall, restricting blood flow to the midportion (outlined by *markers*) of the aorta. **C:** Axial abdominal CT. The *single straight arrow* indicates the patent central lumen with thrombus (*curved arrow*) peripherally. The aortic wall (*double straight arrows*) is partially calcified.

modality to detect and locate an intra-abdominal abscess. Percutaneous drainage with CT guidance is often possible.

Abdominal aortic aneurysm is a common malady, particularly of the elderly. Calcification of the wall of the aneurysm is occasionally seen on plain films or the aneurysm detected incidentally on CT (Fig. 4.110). Abdominal US detects abdominal aneurysms, often when they are relatively small. In such circumstances, serial US examinations to evaluate the progression of disease may ultimately

determine the need for repair. In larger aneurysms, extensive thrombosis occurs (Fig. 4.111). Dissection of an aneurysm occurs as a complication of atherosclerosis or other disease of the aortic wall. Here, blood dissects into the vessel media, producing a false channel and compromising the true lumen. As dissection progresses, there is hemorrhage into the retroperitoneum with shock and substantial mortality. CT (Fig. 4.111C) is a valuable method of diagnosing and staging this disease.

SPECIAL PROBLEMS IN ABDOMINAL IMAGING

Trauma

In all age groups, trauma is the most common cause of preventable disease. Major types of abdominal trauma include motor vehicle accidents, falls, and assault. Imaging studies are important in the evaluation of abdominal trauma as clinical evaluation is unreliable.

The first decision in dealing with a trauma victim is, "Is there any clinical evidence of abdominal abnormality?" Unless there is at least some clinical suspicion (e.g., abdominal pain, contusion, or guarding), the likelihood of finding significant disease with special studies is very low.

If there is concern about abdominal injury, minimal imaging examination includes plain film with supplemental horizontal beam film (upright, decubitus, lateral). Although not a particularly sensitive examination, it is useful for orientation in subsequent studies and allows diagnosis of pneumoperitoneum, massive intraperitoneal fluid, or large soft tissue masses. Contrast studies of the gut, particularly with barium, are less sensitive than other imaging modalities, can cause significant imaging artifacts, and play no major role in acute trauma. US, although useful in diagnosing large amounts of intraperitoneal fluid, is less sensitive than CT. Angiography plays a minor role, unless there is strong suspicion for vascular injury (e.g., a cold leg after pelvic trauma); it may have a therapeutic role in trauma patients, such as those with embolization of a bleeding spleen.

Focused assessment with sonography for trauma (FAST) has been suggested as a screening tool in abdominal trauma. The FAST scan is a US examination, usually performed in the trauma suite by an operator with basic US training. Although highly touted at the time of its introduction, current reports of its accuracy are very variable. Although specificity for diagnosis of hemoperitoneum is good, false-negative events (missing significant trauma) are quite common.

CT, particularly with multislice equipment, is the study of choice for evaluating abdominal trauma. With current equipment, the examination can be completed in less than 1 minute. Previously, most radiologists regarded patient hemodynamic stability necessary before CT could be performed. With the rapid procedure time available today, some compromise in the degree of stability is possible. Most examinations are done with administration of intravenous material. Oral contrast is customarily not given, because of the time involved for it to pass through the gut and its lesser value in diagnosis, unless bowel or pancreatic injury is suspected.

Hemoperitoneum from any source can be identified on CT, and the amount of blood can be quantified (Fig. 4.112). Multiple organ injuries are common; the liver, spleen, and kidney are affected more than other structures. Injuries to these organs are diagnosed with an accuracy of well over 95%. CT detects both the type and the

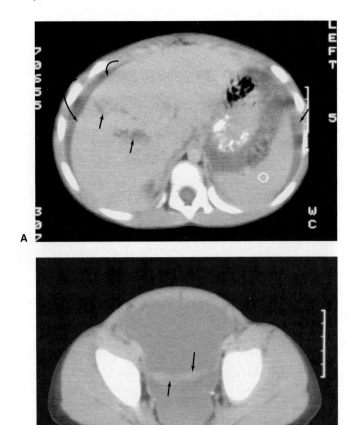

FIGURE 4.112. Abdominal CT. Hemoperitoneum, owing to liver laceration in a child. **A:** An irregular laceration (*straight arrows*) is seen in the hepatic parenchyma. Blood (*curved arrows*) surrounds the borders of the liver and spleen. **B:** In the pelvis, blood fills the peritoneal cavity, outlining the infantile uterus (*arrows*).

severity of injury, an aid in determining which patients need immediate surgery versus nonoperative treatment (Figs. 4.112–4.114).

Gastrointestinal Bleeding

In acute GI bleeding, a major concern is to decide whether the source of blood loss is from the upper or lower GI tract. Statistically, about two-thirds of patients have upper GI bleeding. Some common causes are listed in Table 4.7. Clinical clues are hematemesis, seen in bleeding from the upper GI tract, and hematochezia, from the colon. Melena can occur in either group but is more often associated with upper GI bleed.

Endoscopy is the procedure of choice for evaluating upper GI bleeding. It allows better localization than imaging examinations, and endoscopic treatment of the bleeding site is often possible. Imaging studies are used when bleeding is so massive that endoscopy is not practical. In these circumstances, angiography is often diagnostic and

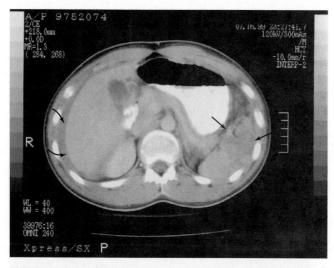

FIGURE 4.113. Abdominal CT after intravenous contrast material. Splenic laceration. The anterior portion of the spleen (*straight arrows*) has irregular density and does not opacify. Hemoperitoneum is evident by the hypodense fluid at the margins of the liver (*curved arrows*).

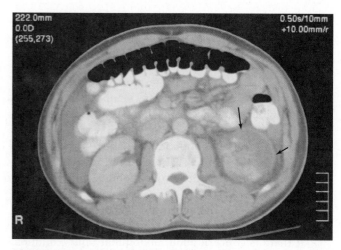

FIGURE 4.114. Abdominal CT after intravenous contrast material. Left kidney, traumatic laceration. Renal density is irregular anteriorly (*arrows*), indicating renal parenchyma admixed with blood.

can be used therapeutically to occlude sites of bleeding (Fig. 4.115). Multislice CT can be valuable for acute bleeding, but barium is seldom indicated. For acute lower GI bleeding, proctosigmoidoscopy is the first procedure, followed by angiography, if needed.

In chronic GI bleeding, nuclear medicine studies are more sensitive than other imaging studies. Either technetium-labeled sulfur colloid or red cells can be used. These examinations allow detection of active bleeding as low as 0.05 to 0.1 cc/min, and the examination can be done in less than an hour. Technical reasons favor one over the other in specific situations.

Acute Abdomen

A rough definition of *acute abdomen* is a situation involving a patient with acute abdominal pain and related signs wherein emergency surgery is being considered. Some common

causes are listed in Table 4.8. In years past, exploratory surgery in the acute abdomen was often necessary, causing considerable morbidity and often unnecessary surgery. Imaging allows discrimination of nonsurgical disease (e.g., acute regional enteritis) versus diseases requiring surgery. It is of considerable value in delineation of the type of surgical disease—for instance, appendicitis versus ectopic pregnancy.

Traditionally, abdominal plain film and horizontal beam film are performed in all but those with the most urgent abdominal disease. Evaluation of the gas pattern and detection of pneumoperitoneum are its strong points. US is of value in certain situations, especially for gynecologic diagnosis; CT is generally more accurate in other areas.

Table 4.7

Etiology of Gastrointestinal Bleeding

Esophagus, Stomach, Duodenum
- Varices with portal hypertension
- Peptic ulcer

Small Bowel
- Duplication
- Mesenteric vascular disease
- Meckel diverticulum

Colon
- Angiodysplasia
- Polyp or tumor
- Colitis

Table 4.8

Common Causes of Acute Abdomen

Medical
Chest disease—pneumonia, infarct, pleurisy
Cardiac disease—myocardial infarct, pericarditis
Mesenteric adenitis
Ileitis, colitis
Renal colic
Drugs
Metabolic disease

Surgical
Appendicitis
Cholecystitis
Bowel perforation
Intestinal obstruction
Pancreatitis
Mesenteric vascular ischemia
Salpingitis
Ectopic pregnancy
Leaking abdominal aneurysm

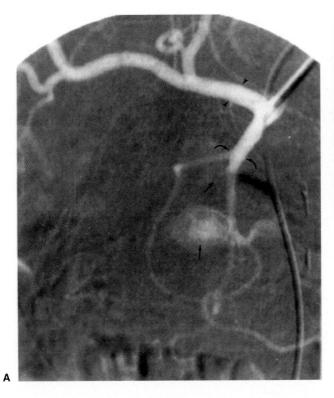

A

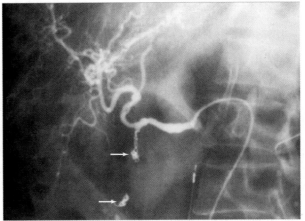

B

FIGURE 4.115. A: Selective angiogram opacities of hepatic (*arrowheads*) and gastroduodenal (*curved arrows*) arteries. Bleeding duodenal ulcer. Contrast material (*straight arrows*) extravasates into the duodenal lumen, indicating an actively bleeding ulcer. **B:** Coils were introduced into the gastroduodenal artery. The follow-up angiogram shows the coils (*arrows*) in place with occlusion of the gastroduodenal artery. There was immediate cessation of the gastrointestinal bleeding. (Courtesy of Shiliang Sun, M.D.)

Multislice CT is performed in most patients with acute abdomen, except those in whom clinical diagnosis is certain without imaging. These cases are done with the use of intravenous contrast (exception: Suspected urolithiasis). Oral contrast and rectal contrast use have their proponents in the patient with acute abdomen, but others point out their disadvantages, particularly the increased time involved in the study.

The technique of CT examination is somewhat modified by the likely diagnosis suspected. Some common surgical causes of acute abdomen diagnosable on CT include appendicitis, bowel obstruction, urolithiasis, bowel perforation (most often peptic ulcer), gynecologic disease, pancreatitis, and aortic aneurysm. Less frequent causes include small bowel and colon disease, ischemic gut disease, and infections of solid organs.

Key Points

- Imaging evaluation of the abdomen usually begins with an AP supine abdominal radiograph. This is particularly helpful in evaluating the gas pattern.
- Small bowel obstruction is characterized by dilated small bowel proximally with collapsed colon and minimal rectal gas.
- In adynamic ileus, there is proportional dilatation of both small and large bowels with gas throughout the gut.
- If bowel perforation is suspected, it is critical to perform horizontal beam films (upright, decubitus, or cross-table lateral) in as much as little as 2 cc of free intraperitoneal air can be identified.

- Contrast studies of the gut remain a valuable method to detect intraluminal and mural diseases such as tumors, mucosal disease, and ulcerations. They are particularly useful in the small bowel, where endoscopy is technically difficult.
- US is the primary imaging modality for obstetrics and useful for detecting gallstones, renal and gynecologic disease, and abdominal aortic abnormalities.
- Abdominal CT is the method of choice for detection, localization, and characterization of tumors.
- CT diagnosis of appendicitis is very reliable, with direct visualization of the inflamed appendix in most cases.
- CTU and US are the methods of choice for most urinary tract abnormalities. EU offers less information.
- CT is the study of choice in evaluating the trauma patient.
- MRI is useful in a variety of special situations in the abdomen.

FURTHER READINGS

Brant WE, Helms CA. *The Brant and Helms Solution: Fundamentals of Diagnostic Radiology.* 3rd ed. Philadelphia, PA: Lippincott Williams & Wilkins, 2006.

Dillman JR, Caoili EM, Cohan RH. Multidetector CT urography: A one-step renal and urinary tract imaging modality. *Abdom Imaging.* 2007;32:519–529.

Gore RM, Levine MS. *Textbook of Gastrointestinal Radiology.* 3rd ed. Philadelphia, PA: WB Saunders, 2008.

Haaga JR, Lanzieri CV, Gilkeson RC, eds. *CT and MR Imaging of the Whole Body.* 5th ed. St. Louis, MO: Mosby, 2008.

QUESTIONS

1. True or false: Regarding evaluating an abdominal radiograph
   a. The stomach usually does not contain gas
   b. The long axis of the kidneys usually parallels the lateral margin of the psoas muscle
   c. Patients with adynamic ileus usually have gas in both the small and large bowel
   d. Rectal air is uncommon in normal patients

2. True or false: When using abdominal ultrasound
   a. Cysts and ascites are usually sonolucent
   b. Ultrasound waves are predominately blocked by bone
   c. Ultrasound is the modality of choice to diagnose gallstones
   d. Ascites reflects more ultrasound than normal liver

3. True or false: In patients with acute abdominal pain
   a. CT is the best imaging modality to diagnose ureterolithiasis
   b. Ultrasound is the best imaging modality to confirm a renal mass is a cyst
   c. Excretory urograms are more sensitive than CT for the diagnosis of solid renal tumors
   d. Primary liver tumors are more common than metastasis to the liver

4. True or false: Regarding imaging of solid abdominal organs
   a. An abdominal CT is a sensitive test in confirmed cases of pancreatitis
   b. An MRI is the best primary diagnostic imaging test for acute cholecystitis
   c. Hepatic cirrhosis is a disease where imaging diagnosis is specific but not sensitive
   d. MRI is very specific for distinguishing hepatic hemangioma from other hepatic tumors

5. True or false: In an abdominal trauma patient
   a. A "fast scan" is an operator skill dependent test with variable accuracy
   b. CT scan for blunt abdominal trauma should be performed with only oral contrast
   c. Screening angiography plays a major screening role in blunt abdominal trauma
   d. A positive "fast scan" is highly specific for ascetic fluid

6. True or false: In abdominal imaging
   a. The valvulae conniventes are reliable features of colonic bowel
   b. Pneumoperitoneum usually means a ruptured hollow viscous
   c. Common causes of adynamic ileus are sepsis, hypercalcemia, and narcotics
   d. The presence of pneumotosis intestinalis is a normal finding in some patients

Pediatric Imaging

Ethan A. Smith • Wilbur L. Smith

Ask any pediatrician and they will tell you: Children are not just little adults. Sure, the body parts (hearts, eyes, noses) are the same, but the fact that children are constantly growing and changing subjects them to different diseases as well as different radiographic appearances. As children evolve from young neonates to adult-sized (but not necessarily adult brained!) adolescents, the changing proportions and appearances of the various structures can be confusing.

The classic illustrative example of this is concept is the thymus, that ubiquitous but often misinterpreted anterior mediastinal "mass" seen on chest radiographs in young children (Fig. 5.1). This organ, important in the immune response, usually becomes inconspicuous by age 5 or so; however, its appearance and size are both extremely variable. It is not uncommon to find thymic tissue on chest computed tomography (CT) scans in patients up to age 20 years (Fig. 5.2). The thymus is a living piece of tissue that changes its configuration in a number of ways. In response to stress, it may shrink; after the stress has abated, it may grow (so-called "thymic rebound").

When indented by the ribs, it may form a wavy border; in pathologic conditions, such as a pneumomediastinum, it may even be displaced superiorly and laterally over the lung fields. With this variability in mind, the first rule in looking at children's radiographs is to expect change and variation and consider those factors before inventing pathology that is not real (Fig. 5.3).

In general, congenital abnormalities are much more likely to present as clinical problems in neonates and younger children than they are in adults. Basically, if a patient gets to adulthood without a congenital anomaly bothering them, it is unlikely to cause clinical problems (i.e., it may just be a normal variant as opposed to a true disease). When you deal with an abnormal abdomen in a neonate, a congenital anomaly is extremely likely; in a 4-year-old it is somewhat likely; and in a 15-year-old it is less likely. If you play the odds, in an 80-year-old you probably should not even think of a congenital abnormality as the cause of an acute abdomen. Having said this, I know that everyone will be able to find the unusual case of a

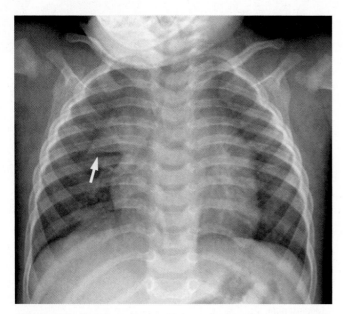

FIGURE 5.1. The triangular opacity (*arrow*) arising from the mediastinum in this healthy 3-month-old is a typical appearance of the normal thymus. The triangular shape is sometimes referred to as the "sail sign."

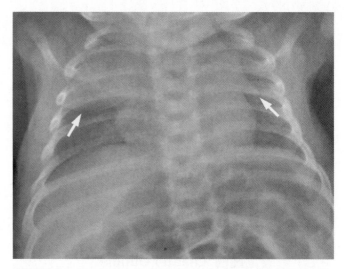

FIGURE 5.3. The large soft tissue structure (*arrows*) in the superior and anterior mediastinum of this 1-month-old is all due to normal thymus. If you call anything in the anterior superior mediastinum of a neonate normal thymus, you will be right 99% of the time.

congenital defect causing grief to an 80-year-old, but remember that it is the zebra, not the horse!

In this chapter we will discuss some of the common radiographic diagnoses of children, first neonates and infants, then the older children. The intent is not to be comprehensive, as there are 1,000-page tomes for that; rather, this is intended to show practical imaging approaches to common diagnoses.

CHEST: NEONATE AND INFANT

The newborn chest radiograph is a complex study with a substantial number of differences from that of an adult (Fig. 5.4). Along with our confusing friend the thymus

come a variety of other factors that can make newborn chest radiographs difficult to interpret. The respiratory rate of a neonate is quite fast compared to an adult, and a neonate cannot be expected to suspend respirations while we get a nice picture; therefore, radiographs are often inadvertently obtained in expiration, resulting in lower lung volumes, crowding of structures, and even patchy atelectasis. The small size of the neonatal chest also makes things more difficult because even normal structures are very close together and are often difficult to distinguish clearly from adjacent structures.

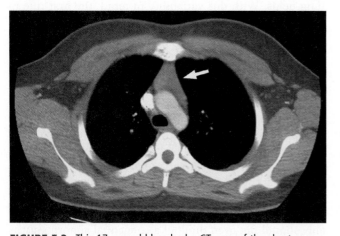

FIGURE 5.2. This 17-year-old boy had a CT scan of the chest as routine follow-up for a prior history of cancer. The triangular soft tissue in the anterior mediastinum (*arrow*) represents normal residual thymus.

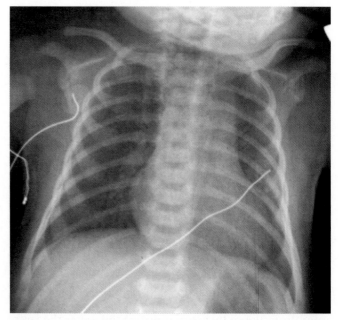

FIGURE 5.4. Normal chest radiograph of a neonate. Notice that due to the small size of the chest, the heart looks relatively prominent.

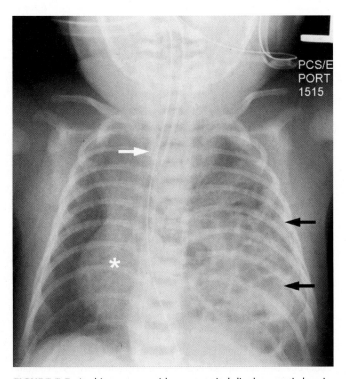

FIGURE 5.5. In this neonate with a congenital diaphragmatic hernia, the entire left hemithorax is filled with bowel loops, some of which contain bowel gas (*black arrows*). Notice how the mass effect from the bowel loops pushes the heart (*asterisk*) and mediastinal structures (*white arrow*) toward the right, away from the side of the hernia.

Neonatal and infant chest diseases can be roughly divided into two categories: Medical and surgical conditions. Medical conditions are usually diffuse processes and require medical management. Surgical diseases can be roughly defined as anything that needs prompt intervention. By this definition, for example, a tension pneumothorax needing treatment with a chest tube is a surgical disease. In assessing a newborn's chest radiograph when surgical disease is suspected, you must take two steps. First, identify which side is the more abnormal (most surgical conditions are unilateral). Second, determine the direction of shift of the mediastinum. This is best done by looking at the trachea, but the position of the heart and thymus can also be secondary clues. As a general (99%) rule, surgical conditions will displace the mediastinum *away* from the abnormal side. For example, in the instance of a diaphragmatic hernia (a condition owing to an in utero defect that allows the abdominal contents to protrude into the chest), the heart and mediastinum are clearly shifted away from the side of the hernia by the mass of the protruding bowel (Fig. 5.5).

Medical Diseases

Transient Tachypnea

All babies have to change from an intrauterine environment where their lungs are fluid filled to one where they are breathing air. This transformation, which must occur within moments of birth, involves a complex interaction of the pulmonary lymphatics, capillary vessels, and chest compression. This normal biologic process is not always smooth. In fact, many babies, if not all, have some very short-lived tachypnea in the first minute or two after being born, owing to the vagaries of clearing their normal in utero lung fluid. The physiologic phenomenon is reflected as the pleural effusions and streaky densities seen in the lungs on radiographs taken shortly after birth.

In some otherwise normal infants, the clearance of fetal fluid causes clinically significant respiratory distress and even mild hypoxia. In general, these infants are not sick enough to require an endotracheal tube, but may require supplemental oxygen or other support. This condition, called "transient tachypnea of the newborn" (TTN), improves rapidly and resolves 24 hours after birth. Radiographs obtained in an infant with TTN will show linear interstitial opacities, streaky perihilar opacities, and small (usually bilateral) pleural effusions. The lung volumes will usually be normal (Fig. 5.6). One confounding problem is that neonatal pneumonia, a much more serious condition, can also present with respiratory distress and similar radiographic findings to transient tachypnea. In this situation, the neonatologist may be forced to treat for pneumonia even if they suspect they are dealing with TTN, because the potential consequences of an untreated pneumonia can be dire. Other, less common conditions could also present with a similar radiographic picture, including congenital lymphatic abnormalities and congenital heart disease. One radiographic clue that you may

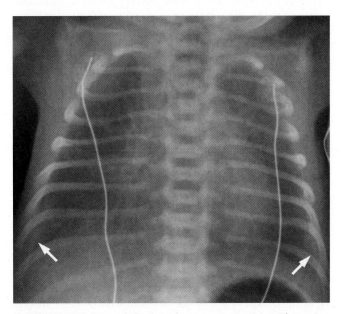

FIGURE 5.6. Full-term baby born by cesarean section with respiratory distress immediately after birth. The streaky perihilar opacities and small bilateral pleural effusions (*arrows*) are typical of transient tachypnea of the newborn. Notice that the patient is not sick enough to require an endotracheal tube.

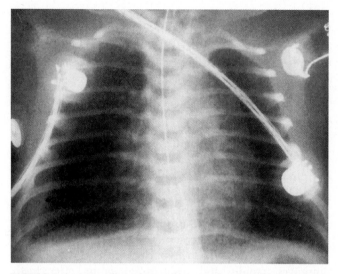

FIGURE 5.7. A very ill newborn with a streaky pattern in both lungs and a large unilateral right pleural effusion. The unilateral pleural effusion is suspicious for pneumonia. This pattern is typical of group B streptococcal infection in a neonate.

be dealing with pneumonia as opposed to TTN would be the presence of a unilateral pleural effusion (Fig. 5.7).

Respiratory Distress Syndrome (aka Surfactant Deficiency)

Previously known as "hyaline membrane disease," this process is seen almost exclusively in preterm infants (except in rare instances of congenital causes). Respiratory distress syndrome (RDS) occurs as a result of deficient surfactant, the lipid-based molecule that helps to keep alveoli open by lowering the alveolar surface tension. Surfactant is produced by the type II alveolar cells and does not begin to be made in sufficient quantities until well into the third trimester. If there is insufficient surfactant, the result is diffuse alveolar collapse leading to poor oxygen exchange and respiratory compromise. Clinical information is quite helpful in the diagnosis, as these babies will be preterm and have significant respiratory distress shortly after birth, almost uniformly requiring mechanical ventilation. The radiographic appearance of RDS is secondary to diffuse microatelectasis and has four key features: (1) Low lung volumes, (2) granular opacities, (3) air bronchograms, and (4) uniform distribution throughout both lungs (Fig. 5.8). You could argue that a fifth sign, although less specific, is the presence of an endotracheal tube indicating that the infant is experiencing severe respiratory distress. With the introduction of a synthetic surfactant, the prognosis for these babies has improved tremendously. The drug is administered as an aerosol through an endotracheal tube or at bronchoscopy. The patient is moved (rolled) around in order to distribute the surfactant throughout the lungs. Occasionally in recently treated infants you may see partial clearing with residual opacities and air bronchograms at the lung bases, representing areas where the drug has not yet distributed.

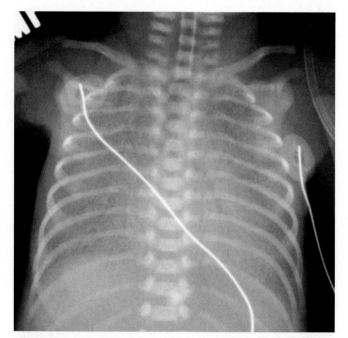

FIGURE 5.8. Extremely premature infant born at 24 weeks of gestational age. This appearance is classic for respiratory distress syndrome (i.e., RDS, surfactant deficiency, hyaline membrane disease). Note the low lung volumes, granular opacities, air bronchograms, and uniform distribution. The presence of the endotracheal tube tells you that this baby is critically ill.

Meconium Aspiration

Meconium aspiration is a disease seen in term or postterm infants and occurs if the baby passes meconium while still in the womb. The sticky, tenacious meconium can then be aspirated and cause plugging and obstruction of the small airways. Postnatally, this leads to a combination of air trapping (areas of lung where air can get in but cannot get out) and atelectasis (collapsed areas where no air can get in). These infants often also have significant respiratory distress soon after birth, often requiring intubation and mechanical ventilation. Chest radiographs will demonstrate hyperinflation, coarse and patchy bilateral airspace opacities, and even areas of relative hyperlucency secondary to air trapping (Fig. 5.9). Hyperinflation can lead to alveolar rupture and pneumothorax.

A review of the radiographic features of neonatal medical lung diseases is presented in Table 5.1.

Surgical Diseases
Pneumothorax

Although pneumothorax is rare in healthy babies, neonates and infants that require mechanical ventilation (secondary to medical processes such as RDS or meconium aspiration) are at a relatively high risk (Fig. 5.10). Remember that most neonatal chest radiographs are obtained supine, so the nice, clear apical pneumothorax and pleural edge you see in an adult may be absent. Signs of a pneumothorax

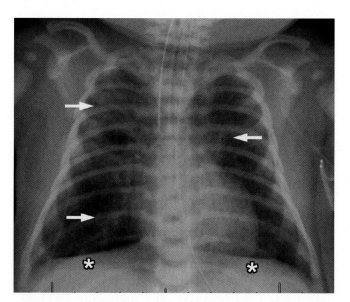

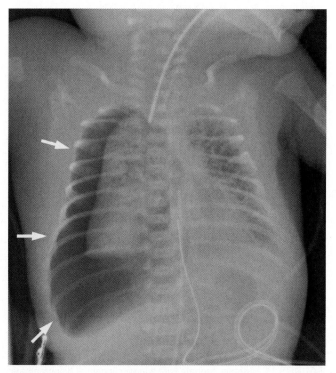

FIGURE 5.9. Neonate born at 41 weeks of gestational age with meconium aspiration. This baby is also intubated, indicated severe respiratory distress. The lungs are hyperinflated, evidenced by flattening of the diaphragm (*asterisks*). The patchy airspace opacities (*arrows*) likely represent areas of atelectasis.

in a supine baby include asymmetric hyperlucency of an entire lung, deepening of the costophrenic sulcus (the "deep sulcus sign"), and sharply defined cardiac or diaphragmatic borders (secondary to these structures being outlined by air). Remember to always look for signs of tension—if you see the mediastinal structures being shifted away, or if you see an asymmetrically flattened diaphragm, you should be concerned for a tension pneumothorax which needs prompt intervention.

Congenital Diaphragmatic Hernia

A congenital defect in the diaphragm is termed a congenital diaphragmatic hernia (CDH). If the diaphragm does not develop properly and a defect remains, bowel and abdominal contents can herniate through the hole and into the chest. The most common location for the defect is posterior and medial (a so-called "Bochdalek" hernia). CDH is also more common on the left (owing to the liver beneath the right hemidiaphragm). CDH has varying degrees of severity, depending on how big the defect in the diaphragm is and how much abdominal contents herniate

FIGURE 5.10. This premature neonate was on a ventilator due to severe respiratory distress syndrome and developed a huge right pneumothorax (*arrows*). The size of the pneumothorax should make you concerned for a tension pneumothorax, and this baby required an emergent chest tube. Notice that the right lung maintains a relatively normal shape despite the pneumothorax. This is due to the abnormal stiffness of the lung tissue because of the underlying lung disease.

through it, because the more abdominal contents there are in the chest, the less room there is for normal lung to develop. Lung hypoplasia and resultant respiratory and circulatory problems that come with it are the main cause of mortality in these patients. The radiographic appearance varies with the patient's age. In the immediate neonatal period, the bowel loops in the chest will be filled with fluid, giving the appearance of a mass. Hours to days later, as bowel gas progresses through the loops, multiple lucent gas-filled bowel loops will be present. Due to the mass effect from the herniated abdominal contents, the mediastinal structures are often displaced toward the opposite side of the chest (see Figs. 5.5 and 5.11).

Table 5.1				
Neonatal Medical Lung Diseases				
	Transient Tachypnea	**Respiratory Distress Syndrome**	**Meconium Aspiration**	**Neonatal Pneumonia**
Gestational Age	Term	Pre-term	Term or Post-term	Any
Lung Volumes	Normal	Low	High	Any
Opacities	Streaky	Diffuse, Granular	Patchy	Any
Pleural Effusions	Yes(bilateral)	No	No	+/−
Endotracheal Tube	No	Yes	Yes	+/−

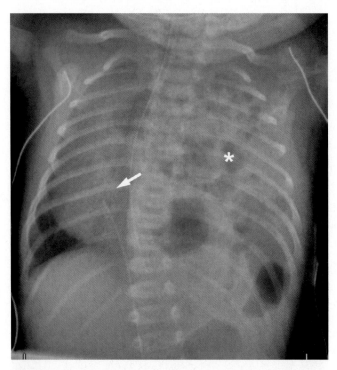

FIGURE 5.11. Another neonate with a large congenital diaphragmatic hernia. Similar to the patient in Figure 5.5, this child has a large left CDH with bowel loops filling the left hemithorax (*asterisk*) and shift of the heart and mediastinal structures to the right (*arrow*). The left lung is severely hypoplastic.

Congenital Lung Lesions

Other congenital lung masses occur infrequently, but are worth a brief mention here. The first is congenital lobar hyperinflation (CLH). This entity, formerly known as "congenital lobar emphysema," is caused by an abnormal airway that causes a one-way valve. Essentially, air can get in to the affected segment of the lung, but it cannot get back out. This causes progressive hyperinflation of a portion of the lung, most commonly the left upper lobe. On radiographs, you will see a hyperlucent area with associated mass effect. In the immediate neonatal period, the affected lung is filled with fluid and may be opaque, but as the fluid absorbs and more air gets trapped, it will soon become hyperlucent (Fig. 5.12).

The second congenital lung mass worth mentioning is the heterogeneous spectrum of lesions that includes both congenital pulmonary airway malformation (CPAM; formerly known as congenital cystic adenomatoid malformation) and sequestration. Both of these entities involve abnormal development of a section of lung, which may or may not connect with the airways and often has abnormal vascularity. In general these lesions show up as solid masses on chest radiographs, although CPAM may occasionally be predominantly made up of air-filled cysts. Many are even identified prenatally on either ultrasound or MRI (Fig. 5.13). Both of these lesions are usually surgically resected due to a risk of recurrent infections and a small risk of future malignancy.

Esophageal Atresia

Our discussion so far has focused mostly on lung disease, but of course there are other significant organs in the pediatric chest, including the heart and the esophagus. Esophageal abnormalities that are of importance in children are usually related to esophageal atresia. The most common form of esophageal atresia is a blind-ending proximal esophagus with a fistula extending from the trachea or left main stem bronchus to the distal esophagus. Inhaled air travels through the fistula and into the rest of

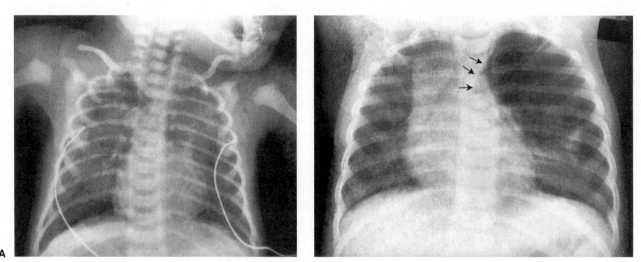

FIGURE 5.12. A: A neonatal chest film shows mediastinal shift from left to right and a partially opaque fluid density in the left upper lobe. This is a patient with congenital lobar hyperinflation and only partial emptying of amniotic fluid from the abnormal part of the lung. **B:** The same patient at the age of 11 months demonstrates findings more typical of lobar hyperinflation with a markedly hyperinflated left upper lobe herniating across the midline (*arrows*).

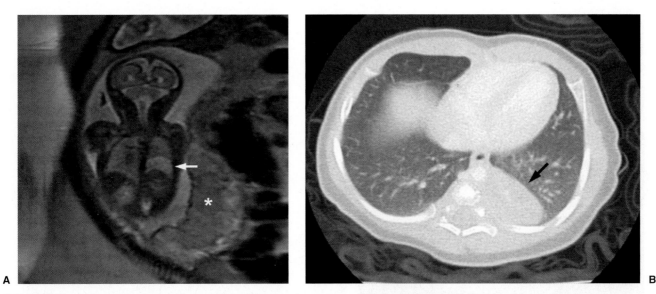

FIGURE 5.13. A: Fetal MRI obtained before birth, demonstrating an area of abnormal high signal (*light gray*) in the lower aspect of the left chest (*arrow*). Note the normal placenta (*asterisk*). **B:** A CT scan of the same patient obtained after birth demonstrates a rounded soft tissue mass in the left lower lobe (*arrow*) which proved to be a congenital pulmonary airway malformation (CPAM).

the GI tract; therefore, the initial films can look superficially normal, with a gas-filled loop of bowel. The clues are that the GI tract is more distended by air than usual and the proximal esophageal pouch is dilated. Clinicians become alert to this condition when the child chokes on feedings and the pediatrician cannot pass a nasogastric (NG) tube into the stomach. This also provides a clue on the chest radiographs as the NG tube will be seen within the pouch (Fig. 5.14).

There are two less prevalent but still frequent variants of esophageal abnormalities. The first is esophageal atresia without fistula, in which case the abdomen is gasless because the infant cannot swallow any air to displace the fluid that is in the abdomen in utero (Fig. 5.15). Such infants are usually quite ill and need emergent surgery. The second variant is tracheoesophageal fistula without esophageal atresia. This so-called H-type fistula (or sometimes termed N-type fistula because of the diagonal course of the fistula) can be a difficult diagnosis. Unlike with esophageal atresia, an NG tube can pass into the stomach, so the diagnosis is not readily apparent to the clinician. The child may present weeks later with frequent pneumonias because each time the infant eats, some of the material goes into the lung. Whenever you have an infant with frequent and recurrent pneumonia, this entity should be considered. An esophagram with careful true lateral positioning is often necessary to confirm the diagnosis (Fig. 5.16).

ABDOMEN: NEONATE AND INFANT

Abdominal radiographs of neonates are very different from those of adults, whereas radiographs of older children and teenagers begin to have a lot of similarities with adult.

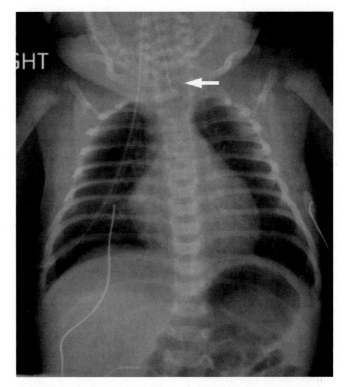

FIGURE 5.14. This baby choked on her first feeds, and the pediatrician was unable to pass a nasogastric tube. Note the tip of the nasogastric tube overlying the neck (*arrow*). The findings are consistent with esophageal atresia. There is bowel gas present, indicating the presence of a fistula between the trachea and the distal portion of the esophagus.

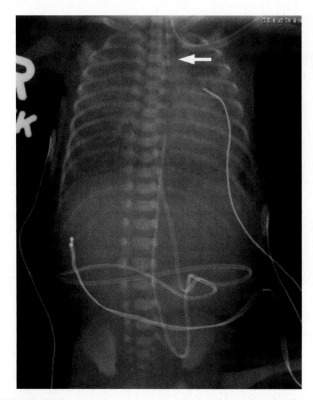

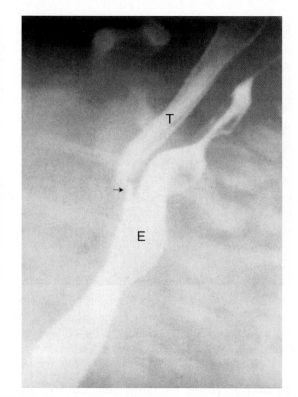

FIGURE 5.15. A premature neonate that could not tolerate feeds. The NG tube is stuck in the cervical esophagus (*arrow*). There is no bowel gas, consistent with esophageal atresia without a distal fistula. Notice that this baby also has uniform, granular opacities throughout both lungs, typical of respiratory distress syndrome secondary to prematurity.

FIGURE 5.16. A barium esophagram on a baby with recurrent pneumonia shows a connection between the esophagus (*E*) and the trachea (*T*), a so-called H-type or N-type tracheoesophageal fistula (*arrow*). This abnormality can sometimes be extremely difficult to detect.

Abdominal films of neonates are especially discrepant because of a number of physiologic factors. First and foremost, neonates swallow a tremendous amount of air during their relatively inefficient breathing and eating. It is, therefore, not at all unusual to find many loops of gas-filled small bowel on the plain film of a normal neonate (Fig. 5.17), whereas in an adult or older child it is unusual to see so much small bowel gas (Fig. 5.18). In fact, it is usually abnormal and ominous to see a gasless abdomen in a neonate (Fig. 5.19)! All of this air in the small bowel makes the interpretation of the films difficult as far as determining bowel distention. The best rule to remember is that the bowel loops of a normal neonate are thin walled and lie in close proximity to each other. The appearance of thick-walled bowel or marked separation of the bowel loops suggests an abnormal intra-abdominal process (Fig. 5.20). Comparison of Figures 6.17 and 6.20 illustrates this point.

The haustra of the colon are notoriously variable in their development and do not become prominent until about 6 months of age. For this reason, trying to differentiate large from small bowel on the plain radiographs of a neonate's abdomen is usually unreliable. Occasionally, you can get lucky and be reasonably certain in differentiation;

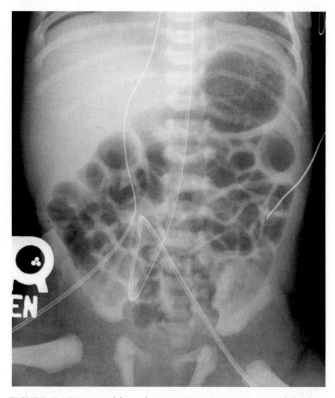

FIGURE 5.17. Normal bowel gas pattern in a neonate. While there are multiple gas-filled loops of small bowel, notice that all of the bowel loops are thin walled and are close together, not separated.

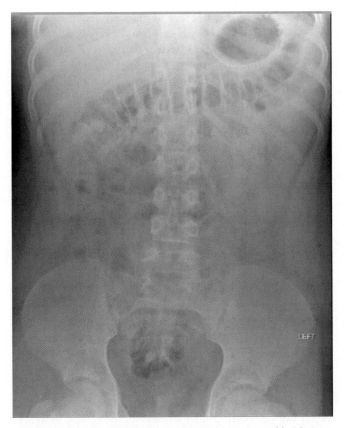

FIGURE 5.18. Normal bowel gas pattern in a 14-year-old girl. Compared to the neonate in Figure 4.17, there is much less small bowel gas. Some gas is present within the normal caliber colon, and the haustral pattern of the colon is clearly visible.

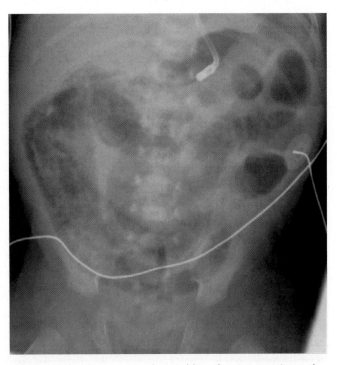

FIGURE 5.20. This is a very abnormal bowel gas pattern in another infant with necrotizing enterocolitis. Notice how the bowel loops look separated from each other. This appearance is due to thickening of the bowel walls and probably also from some free fluid within the abdomen. The linear lucencies in the bowel in the right side of the abdomen represent gas inside the bowel wall or pneumatosis, another sign that this baby is critically ill.

however, most of the time it is not even worth guessing. This makes the determination of whether there is rectal gas or not, even more critical. The vast majority of newborns will have gas all the way through their GI tract 24 hours after birth. If there is any doubt as to whether a child has bowel gas through to the rectum, the prone cross-table lateral film is invaluable in making this distinction (Fig. 5.21). Remember that on a supine image (which

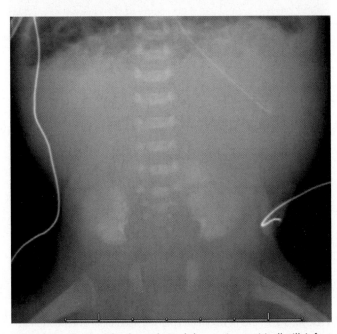

FIGURE 5.19. Completely gasless abdomen in a critically ill infant with necrotizing enterocolitis. Babies typically have at least some bowel gas, so seeing a gasless abdomen is almost always an ominous sign.

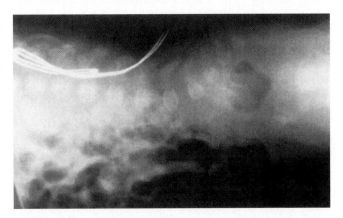

FIGURE 5.21. A prone cross-table lateral view of the abdomen can often be helpful in showing whether or not gas is present in the rectum.

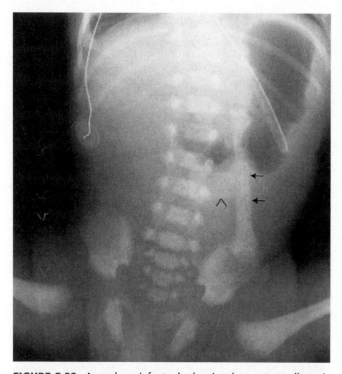

FIGURE 5.22. A newborn infant who has just begun to swallow air. Note the nasogastric tube in place in the stomach. The oblong structure to the left of the spine (*arrows*) almost looks like a bone of some sort; however, it is clearly attached to the umbilical stump (*arrowhead*) and in fact represents an umbilical cord clamp.

almost all neonatal abdominal radiographs are), the rectum is posterior (or dependent), whereas air collects in nondependent structures. By turning the patient prone, the rectum now becomes nondependent, so if bowel gas can get there (i.e., there is no obstruction), it will!

A quick mention of the belly button (umbilicus, to be proper) is in order. This necessary structure and the accessories attached to it make for sometimes confusing shadows on abdominal films of neonates. Many an unsuspecting physician has called an umbilical clamp a bone or a foreign body (Fig. 5.22). The umbilicus itself protrudes much farther in a neonate than in an adult. Any coin-shaped soft tissue density lesion in the lower midabdomen of a neonate should probably be considered the umbilical remnant until proven otherwise. A good clue is that, owing to the air surrounding the protruding umbilical stump, the edges of the umbilicus are very sharply defined, particularly the inferior edge.

Neonate

The most common indication for abdominal imaging in the immediate neonatal period is the concern for obstruction. Clinically, the child will present with feeding intolerance, often with progressive abdominal distention and sometimes with failure to pass meconium. In this setting, abdominal radiographs are commonly obtained and

demonstrate variable degrees of gaseous distention of the bowel. The savvy physician can use the appearance of the abdominal radiograph to occasionally make a definitive diagnosis, but more often as a guide as far as the next test is to be done. If there are only a few dilated loops of bowel confined to the upper abdomen, a more proximal obstruction should be suspected and an upper gastrointestinal fluoroscopy (an upper GI) should be performed. However, if there are multiple loops of dilated bowel throughout the abdomen, the higher-yield diagnostic test will be a contrast enema. Occasionally things are not this clear and both tests are done; however, as a general rule any neonatal obstruction suspected to be proximal to the ligament of Treitz should get an upper GI while anything more distal should start with a contrast enema.

Atresias

In a neonate, the most common cause of bowel obstruction is an atresia. Atresia occurs owing to a number of complex intrauterine processes, usually with the final common pathway of compromise of vascular supply to the wall of the bowel. Often, the affected segment completely disappears and all that is left is a wedge-shaped defect in the mesentery. The exception to this is duodenal atresia, which is caused by a failure of recanalization of the duodenal lumen. During normal development, the lumen of the duodenum is temporarily obliterated by an ingrowth of cells. If these cells then fail to regress, the lumen remains closed and the baby is left with an obstruction.

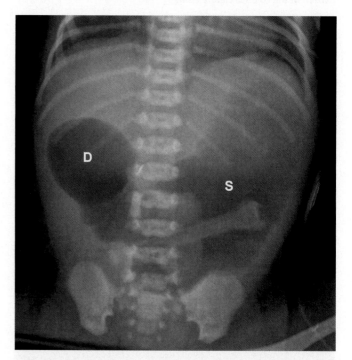

FIGURE 5.23. This newborn had marked abdominal distention shortly after birth. The abdominal radiograph demonstrates a dilated stomach (*S*) and duodenal bulb (*D*), but no distal bowel gas. This is the classic "double bubble sign" and is diagnostic of duodenal atresia.

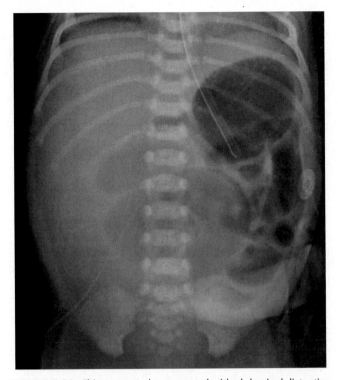

FIGURE 5.24. This neonate also presented with abdominal distention shortly after birth. Compared to the baby in Figure 4.23, there are more dilated loops of bowel, suggesting the obstruction is more distal. At surgery this baby was found to have a jejunal atresia.

Radiographs of bowel atresias vary tremendously according to the level at which the atresia occurs; however, they have common features. First, there is usually no gas distal to the level of the atresia. Second, the bowel proximal to the atresia is disproportionately dilated. Beyond that, it is just a matter of looking at the radiograph to try to guess how far down the bowel you can go before you encounter the atresia. As a general rule to help you establish the level, remember that the duodenal bulb is located in the right upper quadrant of the abdomen; therefore, if you have a dilated stomach and loop only in the right upper quadrant, duodenal atresia is likely (the so-called "double bubble sign") (Fig. 5.23). The jejunum is predominantly in the upper abdomen and predominantly on the left side, whereas the ileum is in the right lower quadrant. If you see many dilated bowel loops and particularly large loops preponderantly to the right of the spine, it is probably an ileal atresia, whereas if the loops are confined to the upper abdomen and predominantly to the left, it is probably jejunal atresia (Fig. 5.24). These are 70:30 rules, so do not get too preoccupied with them. Occasionally, an upper GI or contrast enema can be helpful to confirm the diagnosis (Fig. 5.25). Remember, the important thing is to recognize the obstruction and to think about the diagnosis of atresia—from there, it is the surgeon's job to run the bowel and find the exact location.

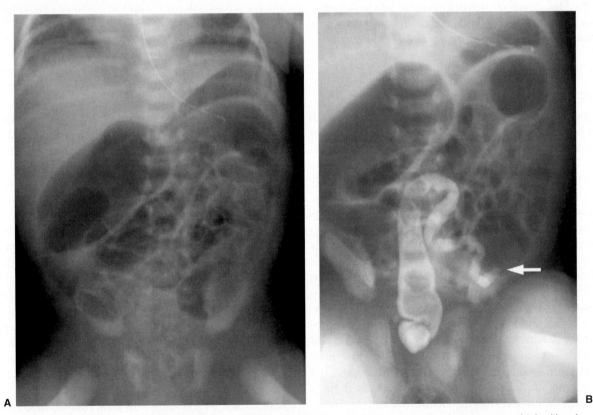

FIGURE 5.25. Another neonate with abdominal distention. **A:** Initial abdominal radiographs demonstrate multiple dilated loops of bowel. Due to the concern for a distal obstruction, a contrast enema was performed. **B:** The contrast enema shows a small caliber colon which abruptly ends (*arrow*), consistent with a colonic atresia.

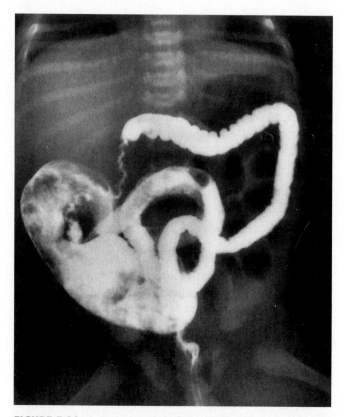

FIGURE 5.26. A contrast enema demonstrating a very small colon (microcolon) leading to a very dilated ileum distended with multiple filling defects. The filling defects are impacted meconium, which gives *meconium ileus* its name. Remember that a microcolon is a sign of a distal obstruction. The next step is to figure out the cause of the obstruction.

Microcolon

An important concept in the evaluation of a neonate with a distal bowel obstruction is the idea of a microcolon. The diagnosis of microcolon is made by doing a contrast enema. The appearance is just what you would expect, a tiny colon (Fig. 5.26). The typical microcolon is diffusely small, although there are variants where only the more distal portions of the colon are "micro." A microcolon is small because it is essentially an unused colon. This occurs because the normal secretions, mucus and cells that get excreted into the fetal GI tract (the stuff that becomes meconium), cannot get into the colon because of an obstruction, commonly in the distal or terminal ileum. The colon remains small because it does not need to grow in order to accommodate the developing bulk of meconium. This is why microcolon occurs only with a distal obstruction—the more proximal the obstruction, the more length of normal GI tract between the obstruction and the colon and therefore the more mucus and material there is to get to the colon and stimulate its normal development. The classic cause of a microcolon is meconium ileus. This condition is seen in patients with cystic fibrosis. Due to abnormal GI tract secretions, these patients have abnormally

thickened meconium which then gets stuck in the terminal ileum, causing an obstruction and resulting in a microcolon. Ileal atresia is another cause of distal obstruction that results in a microcolon. Finally, other processes such as Hirschsprung disease (absent colonic ganglion cells) can also rarely cause a microcolon, but for slightly different reasons. In summary, a microcolon is a radiographic finding that indicates an unused or diffusely abnormal colon. Further investigation is required to reveal the true diagnosis.

Infant

There are a few very important diagnoses that occur early on in life, but not necessarily in the immediate newborn period. Two examples of this type of process are malrotation with midgut volvulus and pyloric stenosis. While both occur as a result of a congenital abnormality, the presentation may (in the case of midgut volvulus) or does (in the case of pyloric stenosis) occur outside of the immediate neonatal period.

Malrotation with Midgut Volvulus

Malrotation is a congenital abnormality of fixation of the bowel and mesentery. In and of itself, having an abnormally rotated bowel is not a direct threat to the patient. However, the anatomic consequence of malrotation puts the patient at risk for midgut volvulus, a catastrophic and potentially lethal event. Remember that the fetal bowel forms about the axis of the superior mesenteric artery (I bet you never thought you would ever need that bit of embryology) and that during the first trimester the bowel herniates out of the body for a short period of time and then returns to the abdominal cavity. If, on return, the bowel does not rotate appropriately, it fixes in abnormal positions. This error in fixation of the bowel sets the scene for the bowel to twist and obstruct, causing midgut volvulus. This is truly a surgical emergency and should be considered whenever you have an abnormal film suggesting obstruction as well as the presence of bilious vomiting in a young child. Not only does this twisting cause an obstruction, but because the bowel twists about the superior mesenteric artery and vein, vascular compromise occurs. If the bowel is not untwisted, the gut will die, leaving the child a nutritional cripple. Although malrotation is discussed with the neonatal and infant abdominal diseases, be aware that it can present at any time in life. The majority of malrotation patients who develop midgut volvulus do so within the first year of life; however, older children and adults can occasionally have malrotation-related problems. The diagnostic test of choice in suspected malrotation is an emergent upper GI study (Fig. 5.27). In malrotation with midgut volvulus, this will demonstrate a duodenal obstruction, usually involving the second to third portion of the duodenum (Fig. 5.28). If there is an incomplete obstruction, the upper GI will show an abnormal

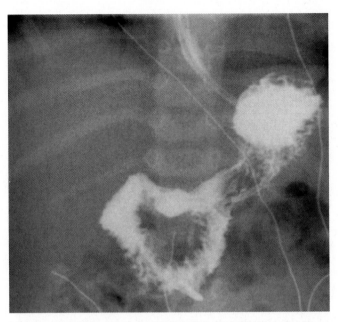

FIGURE 5.27. Contrast upper GI demonstrating the normal appearance of the duodenum, with a normal position of the ligament of Treitz. On the frontal view, the C-loop of the duodenum should descend, cross the midline, and then ascend back up to the same level of the duodenal bulb. In the setting of malrotation, the course of the duodenum will be abnormal.

course of the duodenum, occasionally with a "corkscrew"-type appearance.

Pyloric Stenosis

Pyloric stenosis is a relatively common intra-abdominal condition in babies (not brand newborns, but 4 to 6 weeks old). Pyloric stenosis is not a true congenital anomaly; instead, it is due to hypertrophy of the pyloric muscle induced by a heritable error in metabolism. Pyloric stenosis does not present right after birth because it takes some time for the abnormal chemistry to cause the pyloric muscle to hypertrophy to a sufficient degree to obstruct gastric outflow. The disease is male preponderant and classically presents with nonbilious vomiting and weight loss in a 6-week-old infant. The plain abdominal radiograph suggests a partial obstruction with a dilated stomach (Fig. 5.29). Upper GI will show elongation of the pyloric channel and the narrowing of that channel. Ultrasound has replaced upper GI in the diagnosis of pyloric stenosis for several reasons, including the lack of ionizing radiation and the anatomic detail provided that assists in surgical planning. With ultrasound, the pyloric channel appears elongated (over 14 mm) and the wall will be circumferentially thickened (over 3 mm) (Fig. 5.30). Often, the stomach will be filled with debris. Real-time imaging may demonstrate an obstruction of flow through the pylorus; however, even if some material gets through the pylorus,

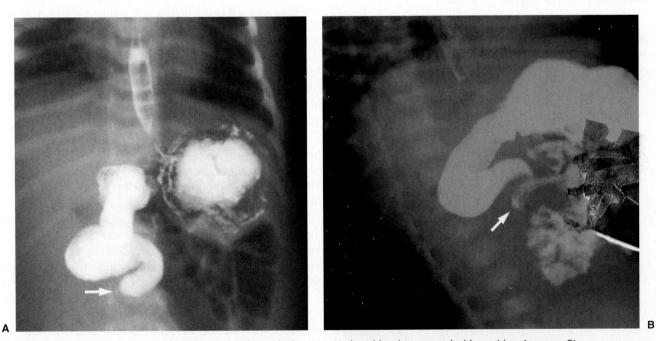

A   **B**

FIGURE 5.28. Two patients with malrotation and midgut volvulus. **A:** A 10-day-old male presented with vomiting. An upper GI was performed, demonstrating obstruction of the duodenum (*arrow*). The duodenum also appears to have a somewhat spiral or twisted appearance. **B:** This 9-day-old baby presented with bilious emesis. The upper GI demonstrates spiraling of duodenum consistent with volvulus (*arrow*). Note that some contrast does get through the twist and the bowel is not completely obstructed. Regardless, this still represents a surgical emergency due to the associated twisting of the mesenteric vasculature and risk of bowel ischemia.

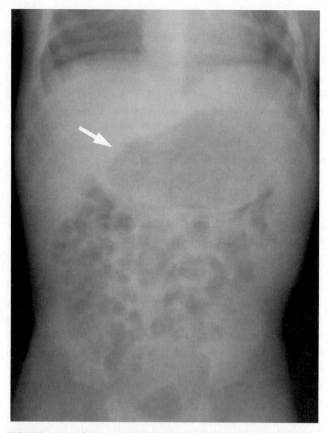

FIGURE 5.29. This 2-month-old boy presented with nonbilious emesis. The abdominal radiograph demonstrates a dilated stomach (*arrow*). The remainder of the bowel gas pattern is normal.

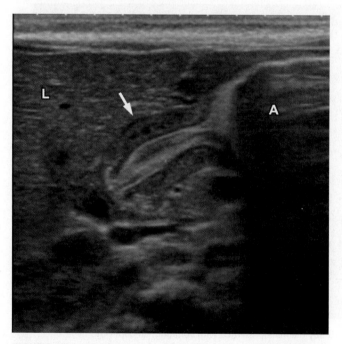

FIGURE 5.30. An ultrasound performed on the same patient as in Figure 4.29. This longitudinal image of the pylorus shows a thickened, elongated pylorus consistent with pyloric stenosis (*arrow*). The left lobe of the liver is seen in the upper left corner of the image (*L*). The gastric antrum is located immediately to the right of the abnormal pylorus (*A*).

that does not exclude pyloric stenosis. Remember, pyloric stenosis is a hypertrophy of the muscle that develops over time, so there does not have to be a complete obstruction to make the diagnosis.

CHEST: OLDER CHILDREN

As children get older, their chest radiographs gradually become more and more like adults. Older children are more able to cooperate with breath-holding instructions, so you are more likely to see a nice, inspiratory image. They are also often able to stand or sit up, so standard upright PA and lateral chest radiographs are more frequently obtained. However, there are still several important differences between children and adults, both in terms of anatomy of the chest and pathologic processes that occur. In the following section, we will look at some common conditions that occur in older children (remember: For a pediatric radiologist, older means over about 6 months of age!), focusing on processes that are more specific to children as opposed to adults.

Congenital Heart Disease

Serious congenital heart disease has a prevalence of approximately 1 per 1,000 live-born infants and, therefore, is a disease that you will likely encounter if you care for children.

Although plain film is valuable for screening for congenital heart disease, it takes a tremendous amount of experience (and luck) before you can be specific as to the type of congenital heart disease. Several principles are very important. The first is that heart size in infants and children is more difficult to estimate than that in adults. The rule of thumb of 50% cardiothoracic ratio is not valid in children. When you are looking for cardiomegaly in a child, you need to be sure *that you are not looking at thymus, that the film has been taken on a good breath, and that lateral views are used extensively.* If the heart protrudes significantly beyond the visible airway on lateral view, the heart is usually enlarged. If on an anteroposterior view the heart appears large whereas on the lateral view it is normal, then you are usually dealing with a deceiving thymus (Fig. 5.31).

The second rule is that children can have very serious heart disease and a normal-sized heart. This is particularly true in conditions in which blood flow to the lungs is insufficient because of right-to-left shunting. As a good general rule, children's hearts, being resilient, tend to dilate owing to a volume rather than a pressure overload. Conditions that cause right-to-left shunting, like tetralogy of Fallot, do not give you an enlarged heart because the volume of blood traversing the heart is actually diminished. A truly cyanotic neonate with a normal chest film (including heart size) usually has some variant of tetralogy of Fallot (Figs. 5.32 and 5.33).

Rule number three is that if you think that the pulmonary vascularity is increased in a patient suspect for

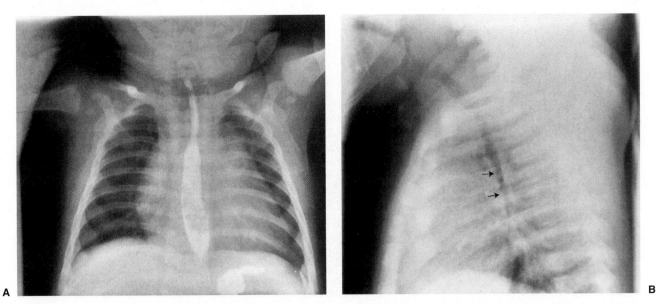

FIGURE 5.31. **A:** This child's heart measures over 60% of the transverse diameter of the chest on the radiograph. In an adult, this would be a large heart; however, this is a normal child with a large thymus simulating cardiomegaly. **B:** Note that on the lateral view, the heart does not protrude posterior to the airway (*arrows*).

congenital heart disease, you are probably right; however, if you think it is decreased, you are probably wrong. For some reason, it is much easier for humans to perceive an increase in vascularity than a decrease in vascularity in a chest film, probably because of the way our brains are wired. An enlarged heart and increased vascularity in an older child who is not cyanotic usually mean some form of left-to-right shunt such as a ventricular septal defect (Fig. 5.34).

Rule number four is applicable to neonates. We have already talked about the fact that being born is the ultimate time of transition. When you are in utero, very little blood goes through the pulmonary artery circuit. To understand this, think about physiology. In utero, the baby is not

breathing air; therefore, there is no need for blood to bring oxygen to the baby from the lungs. Immediately following birth, the baby breathes air and the situation changes dramatically. It takes some time for the pulmonary arterial flow to reach adult levels of blood flow through the lungs. All neonates, therefore, have a relative state of pulmonary hypertension. Early on, lesions that should have increased

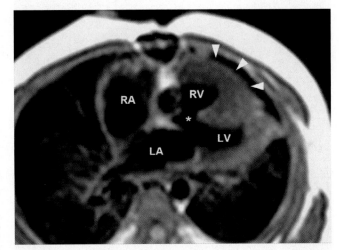

FIGURE 5.33. A different baby with tetralogy of Fallot. This is an axial image from a cardiac MR, obtained with a technique called "black blood imaging" in which the blood looks black and the soft tissues are gray. In this image, you can see the majority of the findings of TOF, including a ventricular septal defect (*asterisk*), hypertrophy of the muscle of the right ventricle (*arrowheads*), and overlap of the left ventricular outflow tract and the right ventricle. There was also stenosis of the pulmonary outflow tract and the pulmonary arteries were diminutive (not shown). LA, left atrium; LV, left ventricle; RA, right atrium; RV, right ventricle.

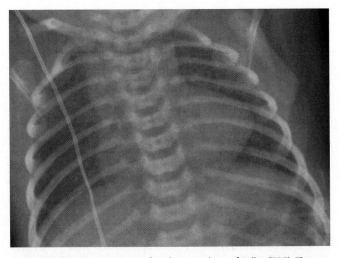

FIGURE 5.32. This cyanotic infant has tetralogy of Fallot (TOF). The cardiac size is normal, but the heart has an upturned apex, a finding that can be seen with TOF. The pulmonary vascularity is normal to decreased.

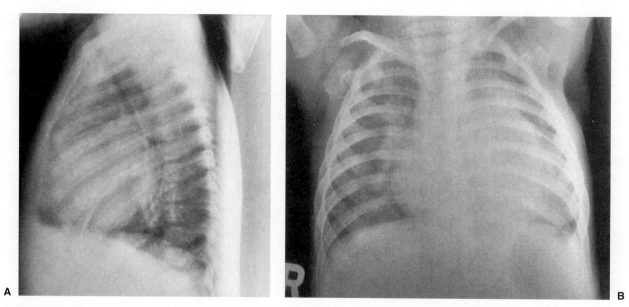

FIGURE 5.34. The anteroposterior **(A)** and lateral **(B)** radiographs of a 2-month-old infant with respiratory distress when feeding, but no evidence of cyanosis, show markedly increased pulmonary vascularity and a large heart. This combination in a child is characteristic of a congenital left-to-right shunt. The most common left-to-right shunt is a ventricular septal defect.

vascularity, such as transposition of the great vessels, are not revealed by radiograph (Fig. 5.35). The same logic explains why most left-to-right shunt lesions are not manifest until about 6 weeks of age (see rule three) when the pulmonary artery pressure has fallen significantly.

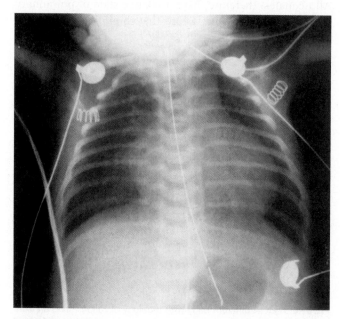

FIGURE 5.35. This very cyanotic patient has a chest radiograph showing a mildly enlarged heart, narrow superior mediastinum, and pulmonary vascularity that is slightly, but not dramatically, increased. The patient is a 3-day-old infant with transposition of the great arteries; the vascularity is going through the transition between very high vascular resistance in utero to the lower vascular resistance of an air-breathing baby. Over the course of subsequent days, the vascular resistance will drop further and the lungs will become flooded.

With those rules to consider, it is possible to set out a systematic approach to looking at the chest film of a newborn with congenital heart disease. First, see whether the heart is enlarged and whether you can determine which chamber is enlarged. Next, determine whether the vascularity is normal or increased, keeping in mind that the younger the baby, the less confident you can be to find increased vascularity. Finally, you need to talk to your clinical colleagues and find out whether the baby is truly cyanotic, as defined by arterial oxygen saturation of less than 80% with a normal arterial CO_2 saturation. With those pieces of information you can use Figures 6.36 and 6.37 and make a rough estimate as to what type of congenital heart disease the baby may have.

Infections

The most common indication for chest imaging in older children is to investigate for possible infection. Children get pneumonias just like adults and the manifestations on chest radiographs are similar in some cases. However, due to the less developed architecture of the pediatric lung, children also occasionally develop what is called a "round pneumonia," which is a bacterial pneumonia that appears round and can look like a mass on a chest radiograph (Fig. 5.38). Awareness of round pneumonia is important, because the child may only need antibiotics and possibly a follow-up chest radiograph after treatment, as opposed to a much more extensive (and invasive) work-up to evaluate a suspected mass. The small size of the pediatric airways also makes children more susceptible to viral processes such as respiratory syncytial virus (RSV). Typically, RSV and other viruses cause airway inflammation which then shows up clinically with wheezing, along with infectious

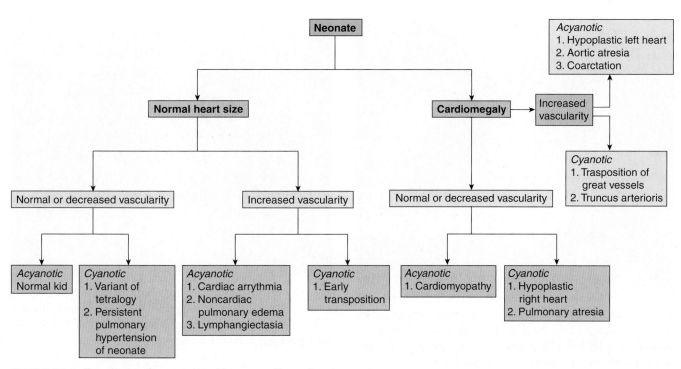

FIGURE 5.36. Flow diagram for neonates with suspected heart disease.

symptoms such as fever. Radiographs will demonstrate peribronchial thickening, streaky opacities (from subsegmental atelectasis) and hyperinflation due to mild air trapping (Fig. 5.39). Occasionally the radiographs will be normal, which is fine. The whole point of getting a chest radiograph of these children is to exclude a bacterial pneumonia that may require antibiotics for treatment. Supportive treatment is generally adequate, although rarely causes of RSV can cause critical illness.

Cystic Fibrosis

Cystic fibrosis, the most prevalent lethal genetic disease among the Caucasian population, begins with recurrent pneumonias but also has a number of features that allow a specific diagnosis from chest radiographs. The lungs are usually hyperexpanded because of the blockage of many of the smaller airways by mucous plugs. The mucus-filled bronchi manifest on radiographs as branching opacities, often in the periphery of the lungs. The hilar structures

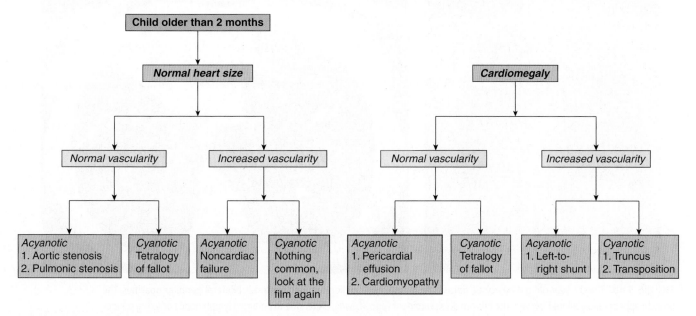

FIGURE 5.37. Flow diagram for older children with suspected heart disease.

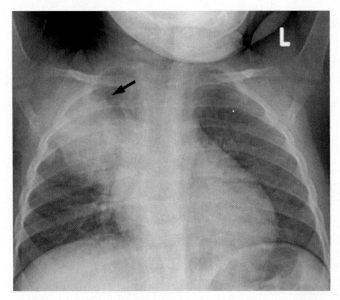

FIGURE 5.38. This 20-month-old presented to the emergency department with cough and fever. The chest radiograph shows a focal opacity in the right upper lobe with a somewhat well-defined and rounded margin (*arrow*). The radiographs and the clinical picture were consistent with a round pneumonia and the patient was treated with antibiotics. On follow-up imaging, the opacity completely resolved.

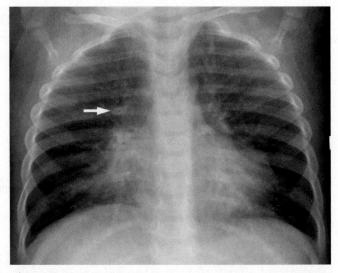

FIGURE 5.39. A 22-month-old boy who presented to the emergency room with fever and cough. This patient has typical findings of a viral process, including perihilar opacities and peribronchial thickening or cuffing (*arrow*).

may be prominent, due to the combination of the inflamed lymph nodes and pulmonary artery enlargement resulting from pulmonary hypertension (due to lung damage and chronic hypoxia). The last common finding of cystic fibrosis is that of peribronchial cuffing, or thickening of the walls of the bronchus, due to the intense inflammatory change induced by the disease (Fig. 5.40). None of these

signs are pathognomonic for cystic fibrosis; however, all of these signs taken in combination make the likelihood of this disease very high.

Foreign Bodies

Young children explore their environment with their mouths. As a child crawls around a room, they are constantly putting things in their mouth, testing which things are edible, how things feel, and how they taste. Even older children tend to still manifest this behavior, often putting

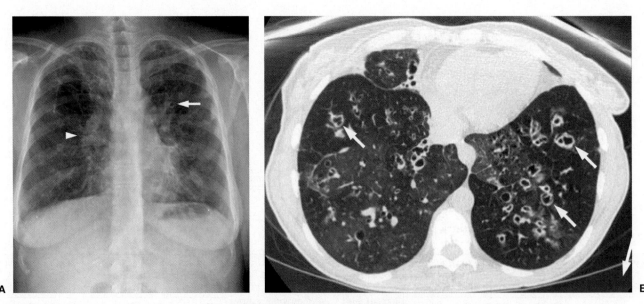

FIGURE 5.40. This 17-year-old girl has cystic fibrosis. **A:** Frontal chest radiograph demonstrates bilateral perihilar opacities. The bronchi appear mildly dilated (*arrow*). The hila are also prominent (*arrowhead*), either due to enlarged lymph nodes or to big pulmonary arteries related to pulmonary hypertension. **B:** CT image in the same patient demonstrating thickened, dilated bronchi (*arrows*).

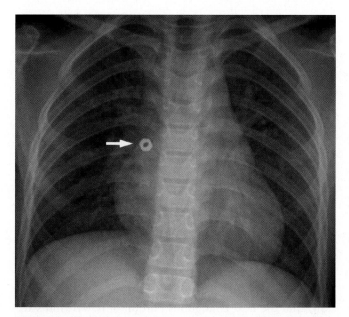

FIGURE 5.41. This 12-year-old boy had a nervous habit of putting things in his mouth. He accidentally aspirated a nut (as in "nuts and bolts") and it became lodged in his right main bronchus (*arrow*). Bronchoscopy was required to remove the foreign body.

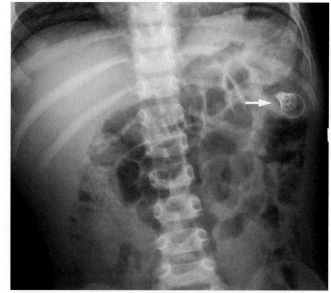

FIGURE 5.42. An abdominal radiograph from a 3-year-old girl who swallowed a small light bulb from the family Christmas tree (*arrow*).

things in their mouths as part of a nervous habit or for no reason at all. Older children with autism spectrum disorders and some development problems are particularly susceptible to this behavior. Foreign bodies can be either swallowed or aspirated, and can cause a variety of clinical manifestations and radiographic appearances (Figs. 5.41 and 5.42). Some foreign bodies (such as coins) are radiopaque and thus the diagnosis is relatively easy. Other foreign bodies, such as organic materials and plastic, do not show up on radiographs, which makes the diagnosis more challenging. In these cases, one has to look for secondary signs of a foreign body such as air trapping (for an airway foreign body) or soft tissue swelling (for an esophageal foreign body) (Fig. 5.43). There are some tricks you can do to investigate a suspected foreign body; for example, obtaining inspiratory–expiratory views or decubitus views in order to accentuate air trapping. The key to the diagnosis is to remember foreign body in your differential diagnosis and to always ask yourself; "could this be a foreign body?"

ABDOMEN: OLDER CHILDREN

Abdominal diseases in older children are less likely to be due to congenital abnormalities and more likely to be an acquired process. One of the most common causes of abdominal pain in children is viral gastroenteritis, which does not usually require imaging for diagnosis. Another relatively common cause of abdominal pain in children is constipation, which also does not usually require imaging

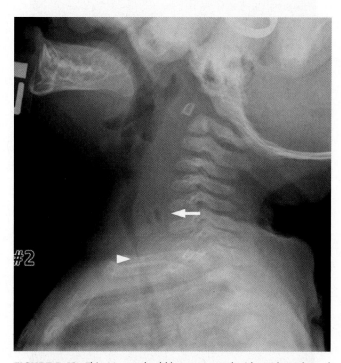

FIGURE 5.43. This 11-month-old boy presented with stridor. A lateral radiograph of the neck demonstrates soft tissue swelling and soft tissue gas (*arrow*). Notice the focal narrowing of the trachea at the same level (*arrowhead*). After further investigation, it was discovered that the patient's 4-year-old brother had been feeding the patient pistachio nuts, and one had become lodged in his esophagus, causing an inflammatory reaction. Remember to always consider a foreign body in your differential diagnosis in children.

for management. However, children do frequently have more serious causes of abdominal pain and imaging can play a critical role in the diagnosis and management of these patients. For example, there is an increasing prevalence of inflammatory bowel disease in pediatric patients, for which imaging is an important component of the diagnosis. For this section, we will focus on a few common conditions in which imaging plays a key role in the diagnosis and that may require relatively prompt intervention.

Obstruction

Bowel obstruction in children is relatively uncommon. Depending on the level of the obstruction, abdominal radiographs will generally show multiple dilated loops of bowel with air–fluid levels on upright or decubitus views (Fig. 5.44). Diagnosing an obstruction is great, but the real key is figuring out the underlying cause of the obstruction. Common causes of pediatric bowel obstruction are relatively few and can be remembered with the pneumonic "AIM" (really AAIIMM): A, adhesions, appendicitis; I, intussusception, inguinal hernia; M, malrotation, Meckel diverticulum. The differential diagnosis can be further refined based on the patient's age and clinical history. For

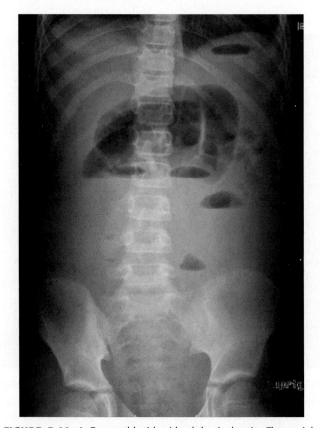

FIGURE 5.44. A 7-year-old girl with abdominal pain. The upright abdominal radiograph shows multiple dilated loops of small bowel with air–fluid levels, consistent with an obstruction. In this case, the patient turned out to have a congenital internal hernia that caused the obstruction.

example, appendicitis is relatively rare in children under age 2, so if you have a toddler with an obstruction that "A" is less likely. Intussusception would be unlikely in a 17-year-old, so you can throw out that "I." If there is no history of prior surgery, adhesions are unlikely, so there goes another "A." Using this technique, you can usually get the differential diagnosis down to a reasonable list of two or three entities.

Intussusception

Intussusception, a disease in which one segment of bowel telescopes into a more distal segment has its maximum prevalence between the ages of 6 months and 2 years. The bowel is constantly in motion because of normal peristaltic activity. If an inflamed intramural lymph node or some other structure alters this peristaltic activity, such that one segment of bowel begins to be propelled at a differential rate, this can lead to prolapse of one segment (intussusceptum) into the next contiguous portion of bowel (intussuscipiens). The prolapsed segment (intussusceptum) becomes edematous and swells because the blood supply is compromised. This compounds the problem and leads to further extension of the intussusception. The ultimate extension is protrusion of the intussusceptum from the rectum! In fact, in nineteenth century textbooks, the differential diagnosis of intussusception was rectal prolapse. The most common anatomic area involved in intussusception is the terminal ileum and most intussusceptions are ileocecal.

Radiology plays a key role in the diagnosis as the clinical presentation can vary from classic findings (abdominal pain, bloody stools) to nonspecific (somnolence, lethargy, poor feeding). Plain radiographs often show evidence of partial bowel obstruction, and the intussusceptum may be visible as a rounded soft tissue density near the point of obstruction (Fig. 5.45). The diagnosis is usually confirmed by ultrasound (Fig. 5.46). Increasingly, ultrasound is being used as the first line test in suspected intussusception. Rarely a diagnostic enema is performed. Radiology often plays both a diagnostic and a therapeutic role in intussusception. Up to 80% of intussusceptions can be nonoperatively reduced using either an air enema or a contrast enema. With an air enema, the radiologist fills the colon with air and uses the resultant pressure to "push" the intussusceptum back to its normal location, all the while closely monitoring the pressure in the colon to prevent a perforation. These techniques are very specialized and should be performed only by trained personnel. They are, however, part of the standard armamentarium of any board-certified radiologist.

Appendicitis

Appendicitis is the most common surgical condition in children. Imaging of appendicitis in children is somewhat different than in adults, as there is a greater focus placed on ultrasound. Although CT has excellent sensitivity and specificity in the diagnosis of appendicitis, the

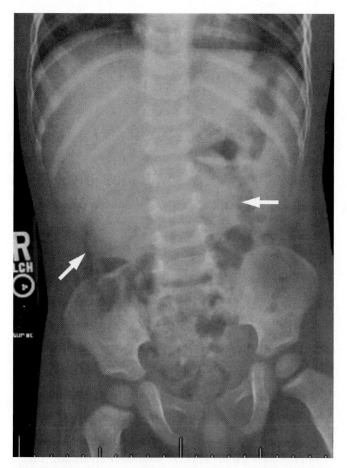

FIGURE 5.45. This 2-year-old presented to his pediatrician with intermittent abdominal pain and one episode of bloody stools. The abdominal radiograph shows a soft tissue mass in the right upper quadrant (*arrows*), suspected to represent an intussusception.

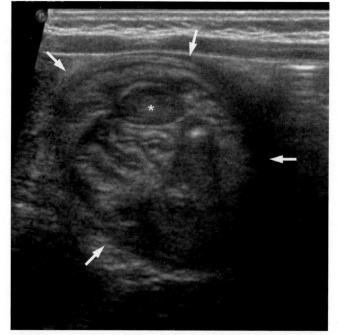

FIGURE 5.46. Abdominal ultrasound in the same patient as in Figure 4.45. There is a round structure in the right upper quadrant with concentric layers, consistent with an intussusception (*arrows*). Notice the oval-shaped gray structures (*asterisk*). These are mesenteric lymph nodes that have been pulled in with the intussusceptum. The more light gray ("hyperechoic") material centrally represents mesenteric fat which has also been pulled into the intussusception.

ONCOLOGY

Fortunately, cancer is relatively rare in children. The most common childhood malignancy is leukemia which is not usually diagnosed by imaging (although rarely the radiologist may make the diagnosis based on changes in the bones or kidneys). Solid tumors in children are also rare,

relatively high amount of ionizing radiation used, and the relatively common (but nonspecific) chief complaint of right lower quadrant pain in children, makes CT suboptimal as a first line test. Therefore, great effort has been made to optimize focused right lower quadrant ultrasound to evaluate the appendix in children. In the setting of acute appendicitis, ultrasound may show a dilated appendix (greater than 6 mm), a thickened appendiceal wall, an appendicolith, periappendiceal fluid, and, in cases of perforation, abscesses. Ultrasound is a great test if the appendix can be found, whether normal or abnormal (Fig. 5.47). However, the location of appendix is somewhat variable and sometimes you just cannot find it, while other times the appendix is obscured by bowel gas (which the ultrasound waves cannot penetrate). In these cases, you have to turn the case back over to the ED physician or surgeon—if they are concerned enough based on clinical findings, they may take the patient to the OR anyway. If there is still confusion, an additional test, usually a CT, may be needed (although MRI is sometimes being used) (Fig. 5.48).

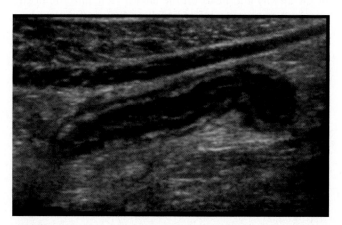

FIGURE 5.47. Focused right lower quadrant ultrasound in a 6-year-old who presented to the emergency department with fever and abdominal pain. The tubular structure in the middle of the image represents the dilated appendix, consistent with acute appendicitis.

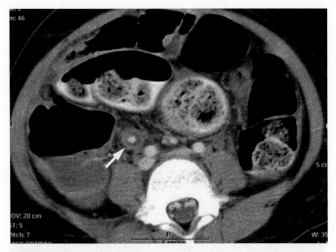

FIGURE 5.48. A different 6-year-old who also presented with abdominal pain and fever. This axial CT image demonstrates a dilated appendix in the right lower quadrant (*arrow*). The higher attenuation structure within the appendix represents an appendicolith. The findings are consistent with acute appendicitis.

although if your practice includes children you may come across one or two over the course of your career. Localizing the site of origin of the tumor is critical. Combining the location of the tumor with a few of the imaging characteristics, occasionally a relatively definitive diagnosis can be made based on the imaging alone.

Mediastinum

The differential diagnosis of mediastinal masses is kind of like real estate—the most important thing is location, location, location. The mediastinum is divided into four sections: Anterior, middle, posterior, and superior. The location of a mediastinal mass can usually be determined by what it is doing to its neighbors. The anterior mediastinum is defined as part of the mediastinum visible in front of the airway and heart on the lateral view, and the posterior mediastinum is defined as that portion of the mediastinum just posterior to the anterior edge of the vertebral bodies on the lateral view. Everything else is the middle mediastinal compartment (Fig. 5.49). The whole trick is telling these compartments apart and there are a few clues.

- *Clavicle cutoff sign:* The anterior chest is anatomically lower than the posterior chest, so if a mass stops at the inferior margin of the clavicle on the PA chest radiograph, it has to be in the anterior mediastinum (Fig. 5.50).
- *Hilum overlay sign:* Structures in the far anterior mediastinum overlie the vessels at the lung hilum; therefore, the vessels are usually seen through these structures (Fig. 5.51).
- *Posterior rib effacement:* Posterior mediastinal masses frequently spread the posterior ribs; therefore, distortion or asymmetry of the posterior ribs is a good sign that the mass is posterior (Fig. 5.52).

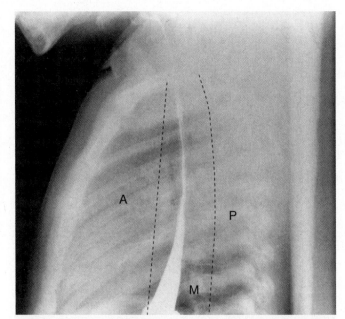

FIGURE 5.49. A normal lateral view of the chest with barium in the esophagus delineates the boundaries of the anterior (*A*), middle (*M*), and posterior (*P*) mediastinum. When you consider mediastinal masses, it is important to divide the mediastinum into these components as it will help you refine your differential diagnosis for the mass.

- *Airway distortion sign:* Masses that distort the esophagus or compress the airways are almost surely middle mediastinum (Fig. 5.53).

Once you have applied these rules and decided in which compartment to look, the pathologic processes tend to categorize themselves fairly easily. Anterior mediastinal masses are almost always lymphoma or thymus related with the occasional thyroid mass or teratoma. An Aunt Minnie applies here: If the anterior mediastinal mass contains calcium or fat, always go for teratoma. Middle mediastinal masses are generally either lymph nodes or anomalous vessels related to the aortic arch. Esophageal and bronchial duplications are less frequent but also occur in the middle mediastinum. Posterior mediastinum masses are neurogenic in origin (including neuroblastoma). When confronted with a suspected pediatric mediastinal mass, the first rule is to place it in the proper compartment; thereafter, it is a matter of pursuing the differential diagnosis.

Neuroblastoma

Neuroblastoma is one of the most common solid malignancies in young children. The tumor arises from immature neural crest cells along the path of the sympathetic nervous system. The typical location for neuroblastoma is the adrenal glands, but the tumor can arise anywhere along the sympathetic chain. On imaging, the tumor presents as a solid mass with calcifications in up to 50% of cases. Another characteristic feature is that neuroblastoma

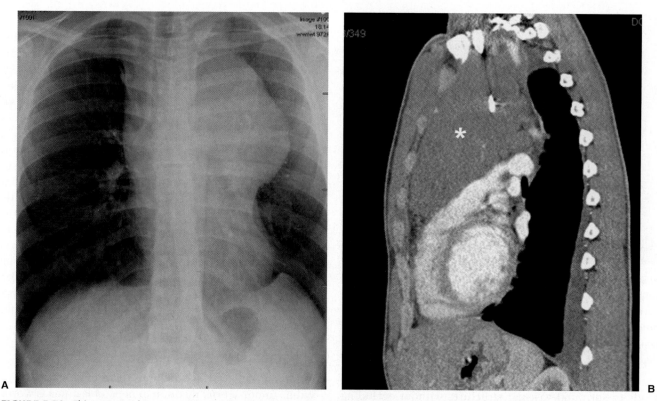

FIGURE 5.50. This teenager has an anterior mediastinal mass. **A:** The frontal radiograph demonstrates a mediastinal opacity that stops at the level of the left clavicle (the "clavicle cut-off sign"). Notice that the left lung apex can still be seen above the mass. **B:** A sagittal CT image in the same patient showing the anterior location of the mass (*asterisk*).

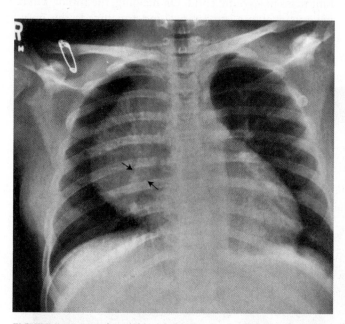

FIGURE 5.51. Another child with an anterior mediastinal mass. Note that the descending branch of the right pulmonary artery (*arrows*) is clearly visible through the mass, documenting that the tumor is not in the same plane as the vessel; otherwise, the silhouette sign would prevent the vessel from being visible. This is called the "hilum overlay sign" where masses out of the plane of the hilum allow the hilar structures to be visualized.

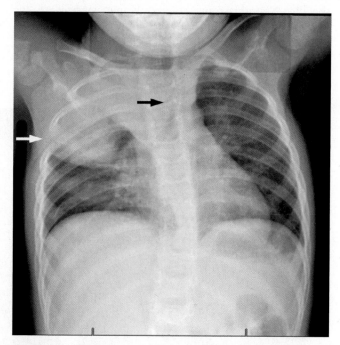

FIGURE 5.52. This 2-year-old boy presented with Horner syndrome. The chest radiograph shows a mass at the right apex. Notice how the right posterior ribs are being spread apart (*white arrow*). This tells you that the mass is located in the posterior mediastinum, in this case a posterior mediastinal neuroblastoma. The mass is so large that it also extends to the middle mediastinum and causes some displacement of the trachea (*black arrow*).

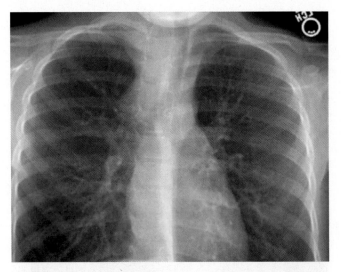

FIGURE 5.53. A 14-year-old boy with newly diagnosed lymphoma. Notice how the trachea is displaced to the left, indicating that the mass is located within the middle mediastinum. The differential diagnosis for a middle mediastinal mass includes enlarged lymph nodes, abnormal vasculature, or a congenital lesion like an esophageal duplication cyst.

tends to surround vascular structures without occluding them, whereas most other masses just push the vessels out of the way and compress them (Fig. 5.54). Lymphoma can also surround vessels, though, so this finding is not 100% specific. Neuroblastoma commonly metastasizes to the bones and to the liver, but only rarely goes to the lungs (which can help differentiate neuroblastoma from Wilms tumor in some cases).

Wilms Tumor

The most common renal mass in a young child is a Wilms tumor. Due to their retroperitoneal location, these masses can often grow quite large before they are found. The typical story will be a caregiver finding an abdominal mass in a toddler while changing the child's diaper. Imaging will show a large, heterogeneous mass arising from the kidney. One clue to the renal origin of the mass is "claw sign," a claw-shaped rim of renal tissue surrounding a portion of the mass, almost like it was holding the mass in a lobster claw (Fig. 5.55). Wilms tumors commonly metastasize to the lungs and liver, and have also been known to invade the renal vein, sometimes going all the way up into the inferior vena cava and right atrium. Metastasis to the bone is a relatively uncommon finding in Wilms tumor, which may be an important clue to differentiate it from neuroblastoma and other much more rare renal tumors. There is a differential diagnosis, but in a young child the other renal masses are so much less common, it is probably fair to say a solid renal mass is a Wilms tumor until proven otherwise.

Hepatoblastoma

Although much less common than neuroblastoma or Wilms tumor, a brief mention of hepatoblastoma is worthwhile. Hepatoblastoma is a rare tumor that arises from the liver in younger children. There is an increased incidence of this tumor in formerly premature infants. Clinically, hepatoblastoma presents as a palpable right upper quadrant mass in a young child. On imaging, the tumor will be heterogeneous in appearance and can invade the portal vein and other vascular structures (Fig. 5.56). Metastases

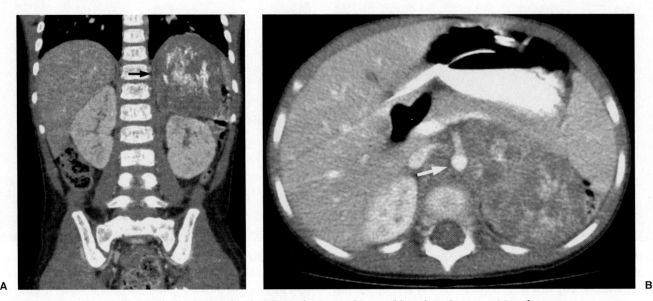

FIGURE 5.54. An 18-month-old girl who presented with abdominal pain. An ultrasound (not shown) was suspicious for a mass above the left kidney, so a CT was performed. **A:** Coronal CT image demonstrating a left suprarenal mass with multiple calcifications (*arrow*), consistent with neuroblastoma. **B:** Notice how the abnormal soft tissue surrounds the aorta (*arrow*) but does not narrow or occlude it. This is typical of either neuroblastoma (which this child had) or lymphoma.

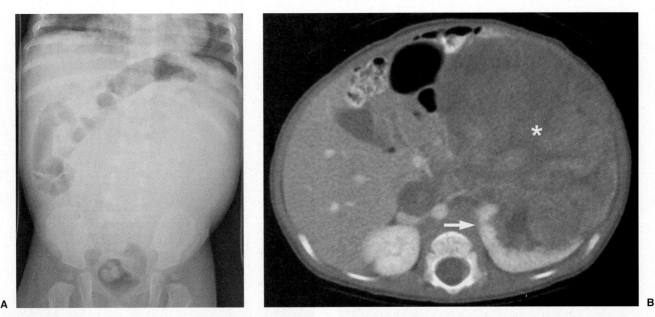

FIGURE 5.55. Wilms tumor in a 2-year-old boy. **A:** All of the bowel gas is displaced superiorly and to the right on this abdominal radiograph, indicating there is a large mass in the left side of the abdomen. If you look closely, you will see there are lung nodules at the left lung base consistent with metastasis. **B:** An axial CT image in the same patient demonstrating a large mass (*asterisk*) in the left side of the abdomen surrounded by a "claw" of residual, normally enhancing left kidney (*arrow*).

are relatively uncommon at presentation, but when they are present they are usually to the lung. One clue to the diagnosis is that the serum alpha-fetoprotein (AFP) will be elevated. The differential diagnosis includes hepatocellular carcinoma, although this is usually seen in much older children with underlying liver disease.

SKELETON

Like the rest of a child's body, the pediatric skeleton is a growing and changing entity. The child's skeleton has to be rigid enough to support the body and facilitate movement, while at the same time being flexible enough to allow for

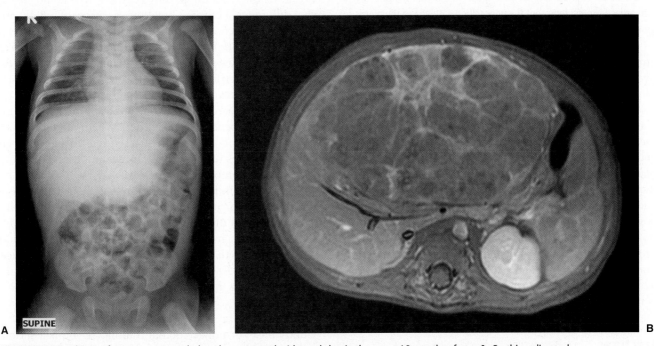

FIGURE 5.56. This is a former premature baby who presented with an abdominal mass at 18 months of age. **A:** On this radiograph, the bowel gas is pushed inferiorly and to the left, indicating a mass in the right upper quadrant. **B:** An axial contrast-enhanced MR image of the same patient showing a large, heterogeneous mass arising from the liver, consistent with hepatoblastoma.

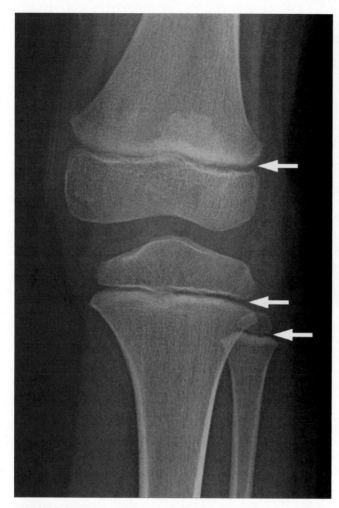

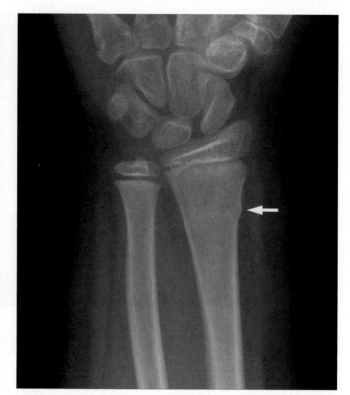

FIGURE 5.58. This child fell on an outstretched hand while playing. Notice how the cortex of the distal radius appears to be buckled (*arrow*). This is a typical buckle fracture, an injury that occurs in children due to the relative plasticity of growing bones compared to the more stiff bones of adults.

FIGURE 5.57. A normal knee radiograph in a 4-year-old girl. The lucent areas (*arrows*) represent the nonossified cartilage of the physis (or growth plate).

growth. Long bones (bones of the extremities) grow primarily through a process called "enchondral ossification," through which longitudinal growth occurs at the physis (or growth plate) (Fig. 5.57). Most long bones have two growth plates, one proximal and one distal. Some bones, such as the metacarpals, only have one growth plate. During enchondral ossification, cartilage cells within the growth plate undergo a programmed sequence of proliferation, hypertrophy, apoptosis (cell death), and mineralization, the end result of which is formation of new bone and increased bone length. A different process, call "membranous ossification," contributes to bone circumference as well as to the growth of some of the flat bones, such as those in the skull. Bone growth can be abnormal because of congenital problems (such as achondroplasia), trauma (if the growth plate is injured), or metabolic abnormalities preventing the normal mineralization of new bone (such as rickets).

Fractures

Children's bones are more pliable than those of an adult. As such, a child's bones can bend slightly before they

break, or they can break only partially. It is analogous to the difference between breaking a piece of chalk and breaking a piece of celery. If you try to bend a piece of chalk (adult bone), it will not bend, but rather it will break across its whole width; however, if you try to break a piece of celery (pediatric bone), it will bend slightly, then break partially, and only with continued force will it break all the way across. Fractures in pediatric bones are a spectrum, ranging from bending deformities (where no actual fracture is apparent) to complete fractures. In between are buckle fractures (*aka* torus fractures) and greenstick fractures (*aka* incomplete fractures) (Fig. 5.58).

Another unique consideration in pediatric fractures is the potential for involvement of the growth plate or physis. Fractures at the ends of the bones have the potential to extend into the growth plates and can have consequences on further growth (Fig. 5.59). The Salter–Harris classification is used to describe the location of the fracture in relation to the growth plate.

Child Abuse

Child abuse, or nonaccidental trauma (NAT), is a serious public health problem. Most abused children are under 1 year of age at the time of presentation, with the peak incidence being around 4 months. Certain skeletal injuries

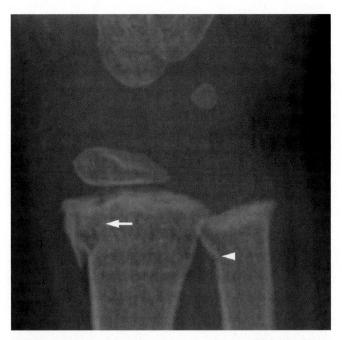

FIGURE 5.59. Another child who presented to the emergency department after a fall. There is a linear lucency that extends from the metaphysis into the growth plate, consistent with a Salter–Harris type 2 fracture (*arrow*). Note that there is also a buckle fracture of the distal ulna (*arrowhead*).

have a high specificity for abuse, including posterior rib fractures and metaphyseal corner fractures (Figs. 5.60 and 6.61). Other fractures are less specific but also occur, including long bone fractures and skull fractures. In reality, any fracture in a young child, and especially in a nonambulatory child, without an adequate explanation should

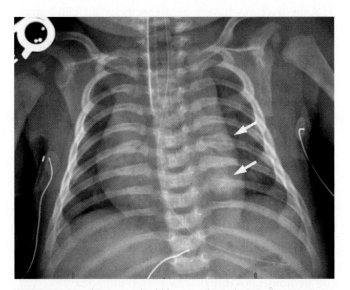

FIGURE 5.60. This 3-month-old boy was brought into the emergency department with lethargy and respiratory distress. A chest radiograph was obtained, demonstrating multiple healing posterior rib fractures (*arrow*). On further investigation, the child was found to have been abused by his mother's boyfriend.

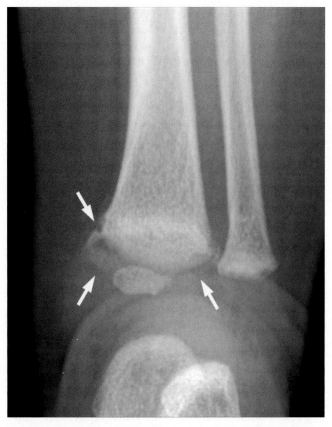

FIGURE 5.61. Metaphyseal corner fracture (or "bucket-handle fracture") (*arrow*). This type of fracture has high specificity for nonaccidental trauma (child abuse). Remember that any fracture or injury in a child without a sufficient explanation should be further investigated for possible abuse.

raise the concern for abuse and should be investigated. If abuse is suspected, a standard skeletal survey should be performed and the proper authorities (such as the local child protective services agency) should be notified. A wise pediatric radiologist once told me that every chest x-ray and plain radiograph on a child should get a second look to screen for child abuse before being put back in the film jacket (or, nowadays, before hitting the "*close*" button on the viewing monitor).

SUMMARY

In this chapter, we have discussed the radiographs of children with particular emphasis on those conditions that are common and unique to pediatrics. As in any imaging, there will always be exceptions, but a few rules are key. Always remember the thymus as a deceiver in evaluating chest films in children, particularly younger children. Any anterior mediastinal mass is thymus, thymus, and thymus! Neonatal medical and surgical chest disease can be easily differentiated by remembering the rules of mediastinal shift and unilateral abnormality. If you apply carefully the rules of looking at congenital heart disease and mediastinal masses, you should be able to get into the ballpark about 80% of the time for making an accurate diagnosis of the correct lesion.

In the abdomen, remember that it is normal for neonates to have considerable gas in their small bowel. As long as the walls are thin and the bowel loops are approximating each other, do not worry. Also remember that up to 6 months of age it is extremely difficult to tell large bowel from small bowel, and guesses as to whether a loop represents large or small bowel on plain film are exactly that—educated estimates.

The pediatric skeleton is growing and changing, and as such may respond differently to trauma, including buckle and incomplete fractures. Trauma through the growth plate can, but does not always, affect future growth. Finally, remember that child abuse does occur and treat every pediatric imaging test as a screening for abuse!

Key Points

Chest

- In some babies, in utero lung fluid takes more than a few minutes to clear, resulting in TTN. This appears on radiographs as pleural effusions and streaky densities. TTN should resolve within the first 24 hours after birth.
- TTN is indistinguishable on radiographs from early neonatal pneumonia.
- The best clue to diagnosing congestive heart failure in babies is a radiograph displaying a streaky density pattern in the lungs and cardiomegaly. If the heart protrudes significantly beyond the visible airway on a lateral radiograph, the heart is generally enlarged.
- HMD displays four characteristic radiographic features: Diffuse granularity, uniform disease, air bronchograms, and a relatively small lung volume.
- Generally, surgical conditions are unilateral and will displace the mediastinum away from the more abnormal side.

- Radiographic features of cystic fibrosis include hyperexpanded lungs, mucoid impactions, very prominent hili, and peribronchial cuffing.

Abdomen

- In summary, the rules for evaluating an infant's abdomen are different from those used for adults.
- The younger the child, the more discrepant the rules.
- Babies have a lot of air, and it is difficult to differentiate large from small bowel by plain film.
- Young children usually have congenital anomalies or atresias; slightly older children have manifestations of either congenital anomalies or heritable anomalies such as pyloric stenosis and malrotation.
- In children beyond 6 months, intussusception and appendicitis are the major clinical entities.
- In looking at abdominal films of children, remember that your odds are much better in diagnosing an unusual manifestation of a common disease (such as appendicitis) than in diagnosing a common manifestation of a rare disease.
- If you stick with the diagnosis and rules from this chapter, you will be right more often than you will be wrong.

Skeleton

- Pediatric bones are growing and changing, so normal variants are very common.
- Younger children have relatively pliable bones, so bending fractures, including buckle fractures and incomplete (greenstick) fractures happen frequently.
- Use the Salter–Harris classification when describing fractures that involve the growth plate.
- Some fractures have a high specificity for child abuse (posterior rib fractures, metaphyseal corner fractures), but all fractures without a satisfactory explanation should raise your suspicion.

QUESTIONS

1. An infant is born at 26 weeks of gestational age and rapidly develops significant respiratory distress requiring intubation. A chest radiograph is obtained, demonstrating uniform granular opacities throughout both lungs and low lung volumes. What is the most likely diagnosis?
   a. Transient tachypnea of the newborn
   b. Meconium aspiration
   c. Congenital heart disease with pulmonary edema
   d. Respiratory distress syndrome

2. True or False: The presence of small bowel gas on abdominal radiographs in a 3-day old is abnormal and indicates a bowel obstruction.

3. A 3-month-old child presents with respiratory distress and feeding difficulties. A chest radiograph demonstrates diffusely increased pulmonary vascularity and a mildly enlarged heart. Which of the following is the most likely diagnosis?
   a. Ventricular septal defect
   b. Atrial septal defect
   c. Cystic fibrosis
   d. Viral pneumonia

4. An infant presents to the emergency department with a 2-hour history of bilious emesis. What is the most appropriate radiologic test?
   a. Chest radiograph
   b. Abdominal ultrasound to evaluate for pyloric stenosis
   c. Upper gastrointestinal series
   d. Abdominal CT

5. True or False: An ultrasound is ordered on a 2-month-old male patient with projectile vomiting. During the ultrasound, the pyloric channel appears thickened (4 mm) and elongated (20 mm). These findings are consistent with pyloric stenosis.

6. A 14-month-old presents to the emergency department with wheezing, fever, and cough. A viral process is suspected clinically. What findings would you expect to see on chest radiographs?
   a. Low lung volumes, dilated bronchi, focal airspace opacities
   b. A rounded opacity with well-defined borders
   c. Hyperinflated lungs, peribronchial thickening, and streaky opacities
   d. Enlarged heart and increased pulmonary vascularity

7. A 10-month-old child presents with stridor and respiratory distress, and the parents suspect the child may have aspirated one of their sibling's small plastic toys. Unfortunately, the suspected toy is plastic, so it will not be expected to be radiopaque. What diagnostic imaging test could you perform?
   a. Airway ultrasound
   b. Decubitus chest radiographs to look for air trapping
   c. CT
   d. MRI

8. You see a focal opacity on a frontal chest radiograph of a 2-year-old. The opacity causes spreading of the adjacent ribs. What is the most likely location of the mass?
   a. Within the lung parenchyma
   b. Anterior mediastinum
   c. Middle mediastinum
   d. Posterior mediastinum

9. True or False: Calcification within a mass excludes a diagnosis of neuroblastoma.

10. A 2-month-old boy is brought in to the pediatrician's office because of leg swelling. A radiograph is obtained which demonstrates a displaced femur fracture. The patient's mother states that she does not recall any specific injury. What is the appropriate next step?
    a. Obtain a complete skeletal survey and contact the child protective agency to investigate for possible abuse
    b. Obtain a follow-up radiograph in 2 weeks to confirm the fracture
    c. Check the patient's vitamin D levels
    d. Council the patient's mother on accident prevention

Musculoskeletal System

Carol A. Boles

NORMAL DEVELOPMENT

Bones are visible on nearly all radiographs; therefore, radiologic anatomy of the musculoskeletal system is extremely important, but it can be time consuming to learn. Entire textbooks are dedicated to specific joints, but a solid knowledge of normal anatomy is a prerequisite for intelligent image evaluation. Despite many advances in imaging using other modalities such as computed tomography (CT), magnetic resonance (MR) imaging, and ultrasound, radiographs remain the mainstay of musculoskeletal imaging. Anatomy is anatomy no matter how you look at it and imaging is less confusing when thought of in this way. Let us begin with a general overview and then normal image anatomy of the hand and move systematically cephalad to the shoulder girdle. This will be followed by normal image anatomy of the lower extremity from the foot to the hip.

The bones develop in a rather systematic fashion. Bone formation is by either intramembranous (transformation of mesenchymal tissue) or endochondral (conversion of an intermediate cartilage form) formation, or by both methods.

Many flat bones, such as the skull and mandible, form by intramembranous bone formation. Both methods are found in the extremities, spine, and pelvis. With endochondral ossification, cartilage is replaced by bone initiated at specific sites called centers of ossification. These centers of ossification appear in such a predictable order that they may be used for estimation of age (Table 6.1). Understanding this aids in evaluation of fractures in the pediatric population as a small bone adjacent to a joint potentially may be assumed to be an ossification center when it is, in fact, a fracture. The area of cartilage between the centers of ossification is called the growth plate or physis. Eventually, the centers of ossification fuse across the physes.

Joints develop between the ends of bones. There are three types of joints: Synchondrosis, symphysis, and synovial joints. A synchondrosis has hyaline cartilage between the ends of bone and not movable while symphysis joints have fibrocartilage and a small amount of motion. Synovial joints, typically thought of as a "joint," have a hyaline cartilage covering and synovium, which produces fluid to lubricate these movable joints.

Table 6.1	
Average Age of Appearance of Some Major Ossification Centers	
Ossification Center	**Average Age (Girls Usually Earlier than Boys)**
Head of humerus	2 wk
Head of femur	4 mo
Distal radius	1 y
Patella	4 y
Elbow	
Capitellum	3 y
Radial head	5 y
Medial epicondyle	6 y
Trochlea	8 y
Lateral epicondyle	10 y
Olecranon	11 y
Acromion	13 y
Coracoid process of scapula	14 y
Ischial tuberosity	15 y
Inner margin clavicle	19 y

Table 6.2
Observation Checklist for Bone Radiographs
Each Bone Should Be Evaluated for
Density
Anomaly
Fracture
Destruction
New bone formation
Foreign body
Each Joint Should Be Evaluated for
Articular surface smoothness
Symmetry
Fracture
Dislocation
Arthritis
Calcification
Soft Tissues Should Be Evaluated for
Swelling
Ulcers
Calcifications
Masses
Foreign bodies

As a brief reminder of radiographic terminology, anteroposterior (AP) radiographs are named by the direction the x-ray beam travels through the body part, assuming the person is in anatomic position. For example, anatomic position has the arms at the sides with palms facing forward. The typical hand radiograph places a hand, palm down on the radiographic plate and the x-ray beam enters through the posterior (dorsal) side of the hand to reach the plate; this is a posteroanterior (PA) radiograph. The foot, however, when radiographed with the plantar surface (sole of the foot) on the radiographic plate is an AP radiograph. This is somewhat of a misnomer since the dorsal surface of the foot is really the cephalic surface of the foot in anatomic position.

Upper Extremity

People commonly injure their extremities because they actively encounter the environment with their arms and legs. Consequently, you will probably order many radiographs of the extremities in your clinical practice. Thus, we need a system to evaluate upper and lower extremity images (Table 6.2). Each bone in an image must be carefully evaluated for density, variations of normal, and fracture. Also, each joint must be evaluated for width, smoothness of the articular surfaces, dislocation, arthritis, fracture, and foreign body. The soft tissues should be evaluated for edema, hemorrhage, masses, calcifications, and foreign bodies.

The hand is so complex that it is a subspecialty in both orthopedics and plastic surgery. When you request radiographs of the hand, the standard study usually consists of PA, oblique, and lateral views (Fig. 6.1). *Remember that one of the most difficult aspects of medicine is to learn the jargon and routines, so we need to get the hand terminology correct from the beginning.* Each digit of the hand must be properly named to communicate and document information accurately. The proper terminology for each digit and the numbering system for the metacarpals are displayed in Figure 6.1A. Simply numbering the digits does not suffice, especially in situations in which digits are missing. Would you refer to the index finger as the first or second finger when the thumb is missing? So, beginning on the radial side of the hand, the thumb is always the thumb and not the first finger. Next is the index finger (not the second finger and not the first finger as some say there are four fingers and a thumb). Following are the long finger (not the third), the ring finger (not the fourth), and the small or little finger (not the fifth).

Metacarpals (Fig. 6.1A) are numbered logically with the thumb articulating with the first metacarpal, the index finger with the second metacarpal, and so on. As a general rule, each hand digit has three phalanges except the thumb, which has only two. The phalanges are named proximal, middle, and distal. The joint between the proximal phalanx and the metacarpal is called the metacarpophalangeal (MCP) joint (Fig. 6.1A). The joint between the proximal and middle phalanges is the proximal interphalangeal (PIP) joint. The joint between the distal and middle phalanges is called the distal interphalangeal (DIP) joint. The thumb, with only two phalanges, has an interphalangeal joint. The distal-most aspect of the metacarpals and the

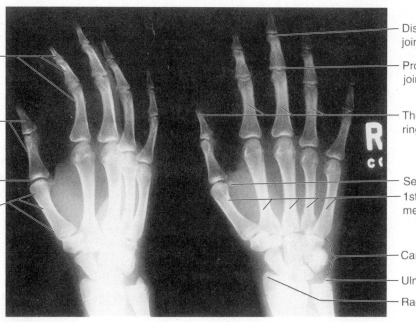

Distal, middle, and proximal phalanges

Distal and proximal phalanges of thumb

Metatacarpal phalangeal joint (MCP)

Head shaft, base 1st metacarpal

Distal interphalangeal joint (DIP)

Proximal interphalangeal joint (PIP)

Thumb, index, long, ring, and short fingers

Sesamoid bone

1st, 2nd, 3rd, 4th, 5th metacarpals

Carpals

Ulna styloid

Radius styloid

Oblique   PA

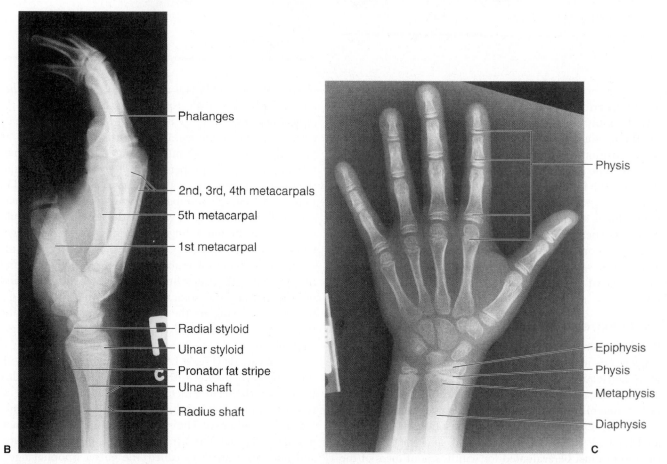

Phalanges

2nd, 3rd, 4th metacarpals

5th metacarpal

1st metacarpal

Radial styloid

Ulnar styloid

Pronator fat stripe

Ulna shaft

Radius shaft

Physis

Epiphysis

Physis

Metaphysis

Diaphysis

FIGURE 6.1. A: Right-hand oblique and posteroanterior (PA) radiographs. Normal. **B:** Right-hand lateral radiograph. Normal. **C:** Left-hand PA radiograph. Normal physis, epiphysis, metaphysis, and diaphysis. The cartilaginous physis is a lucent area on a radiograph.

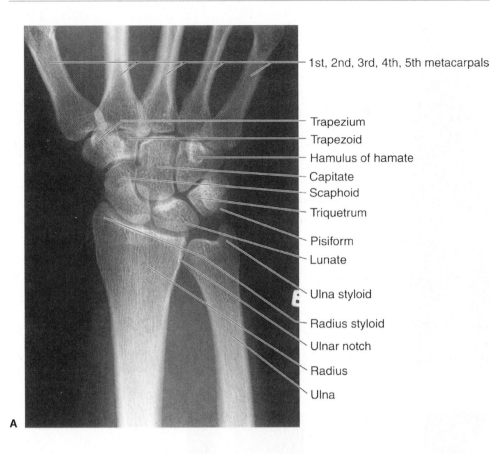

1st, 2nd, 3rd, 4th, 5th metacarpals

Trapezium
Trapezoid
Hamulus of hamate
Capitate
Scaphoid
Triquetrum

Pisiform
Lunate

Ulna styloid

Radius styloid
Ulnar notch
Radius
Ulna

A

FIGURE 6.2. Right wrist PA **(A)**, oblique **(B)**, and lateral **(C)** radiographs. Normal. Notice that the tip of the radial styloid is distal to the tip of the ulnar styloid and the radius articulates distally with the scaphoid and lunate carpals and laterally with the ulna (ulnar or sigmoid notch). The distal radial articular surface slopes toward the ulna and anteriorly (palmar). The distal ulna articulates with the radius laterally and wrist fibrocartilage distally. The ulna does not articulate directly with a carpal. (*continued*)

phalanges is the head, whereas the proximal portions are the bases. The central aspects of these bones are the shafts.

Commonly used bone terms such as physis, epiphysis, metaphysis, and diaphysis can be confusing to the novice, but actually they are very simple. The locations of these entities are demonstrated in Figure 6.1C. The physis (physeal or epiphyseal plate) is the growth plate as bone formation occurs here. The epiphysis is the end of a long bone and contains a secondary ossification center. The physis, being mostly cartilage is the lucent part of a child's bone on a radiograph and is the weakest part of a growing bone. The diaphysis (bone shaft, primary ossification center) is the long, thin center of a long bone and the metaphysis is located between the diaphysis and the physis. The term apophysis is confusing and merely refers to a secondary ossification center that does not articulate with another bone and does not contribute to bone length growth (as an epiphysis does), but, rather, to bone contour. A typical example is the greater trochanter as seen in Figure 6.23.

The wrist and forearm are common fracture sites, especially in children. If we are to understand and treat fractures in these areas, a thorough knowledge of wrist and forearm anatomy is very important. The appearance, location, and names of each carpal bone must be learned as well as their relationship to the distal radius and ulna. These relationships are well visualized on standard PA, lateral, and oblique radiographic views of the wrist (Fig. 6.2).

We generally obtain AP and lateral views of the forearm in children and adults (Fig. 6.3). Routine elbow radiographs consist of AP and lateral views (Fig. 6.4), but external rotation oblique views of the elbow may be requested on occasion (similar to the appearance in Figure 6.5A). Radiographs of the humerus usually consist of AP (Fig. 6.5A) and lateral views. Generally, an AP radiograph is obtained to evaluate the shoulder (Fig. 6.5B) and this is supplemented by either an axillary or lateral view of the shoulder depending on local practice. Musculoskeletal anatomy and disease can be nicely demonstrated by CT and MRI (Table 6.3). CT imaging is

Table 6.3
Musculoskeletal CT and MRI Indications
Computed Tomography
Bone detail
Fracture fragment evaluation
Bone tumor workup
Magnetic Resonance Imaging
Bone marrow imaging for occult fracture or metastasis
Soft tissue evaluation: Ligaments, tendons, cartilages, and vessels
Bone tumor workup

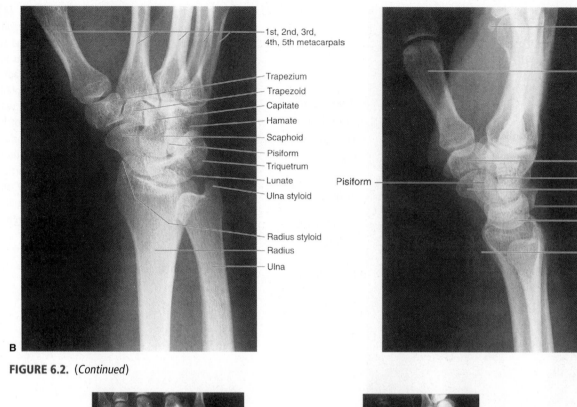

FIGURE 6.2. (*Continued*)

B

- 1st, 2nd, 3rd, 4th, 5th metacarpals
- Trapezium
- Trapezoid
- Capitate
- Hamate
- Scaphoid
- Pisiform
- Triquetrum
- Lunate
- Ulna styloid
- Radius styloid
- Radius
- Ulna

C

- Sesamoid bone
- 1st metacarpal
- Trapezium
- Capitate
- Scaphoid
- Triquetrum
- Lunate
- Anterior fat pad
- Pisiform

A

- Scaphoid
- Radial styloid
- Lunate
- Ulna styloid
- Radius shaft
- Ulna shaft
- Radial (biceps) tuberosity
- Radial neck
- Radial head
- Lateral epicondyle
- Ulna olecranon
- Medial epicondyle
- R S F

B

- 1st metacarpal
- Scaphoid
- Lunate
- Ulnar styloid
- Ulna shaft
- Radius shaft
- Radial (biceps) tuberosity
- Radial neck
- Radial head
- Humerus trochlea
- Ulna olecranon
- Humerus shaft

FIGURE 6.3. Right forearm AP **(A)** and lateral **(B)** radiographs. Normal. Note that in the correct lateral of the forearm, both the elbow and the wrist are in the lateral position. The distal radius is large and the proximal radius is small, whereas the distal ulna is small and the proximal ulna is large. The radius is far more important than the ulna in the wrist joint, whereas the ulna is more important in the elbow joint than the radius.

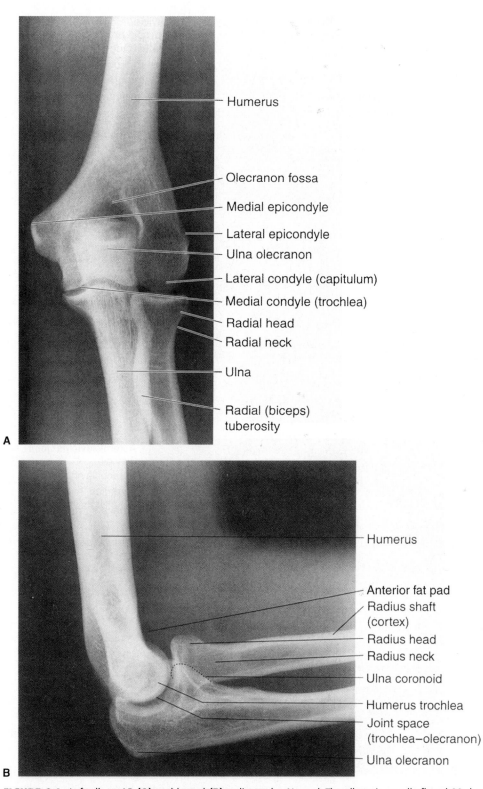

FIGURE 6.4. Left elbow AP **(A)** and lateral **(B)** radiographs. Normal. The elbow is usually flexed 90 degrees to minimize the appearance of the anterior and posterior fat pads. The *dotted line* on **B** indicates the ulna coronoid process.

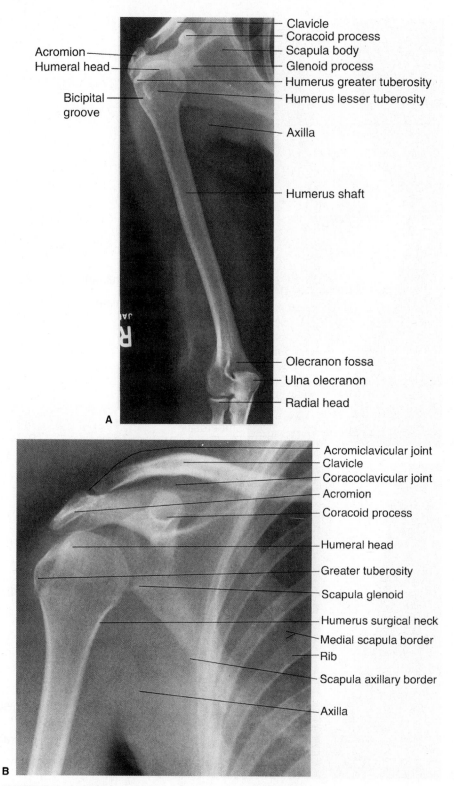

FIGURE 6.5. A: Right humerus AP radiograph with external rotation of the humerus. Normal. The right elbow is in an oblique position. **B:** Right shoulder AP radiograph with external rotation of the humerus. Normal. Note the prominence of the greater tuberosity.

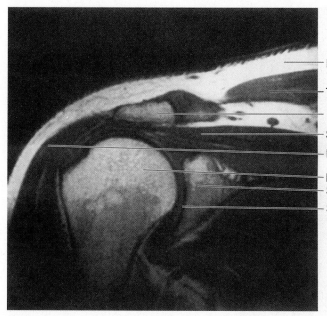

FIGURE 6.6. Right shoulder coronal T1 MR image. Normal except for mild osteoarthritis.

- Fat
- Trapezius
- Acromion
- Supraspinatus m.
- Deltoid m.
- Humeral head
- Scapula glenoid
- Shoulder joint

especially good for bone detail, whereas MRI is good for soft tissue and bone marrow imaging, revealing edema caused by bone contusions or subtle fractures not seen on the radiographs. MRI is especially helpful in displaying the soft tissue structures around joints such as shoulder rotator cuff anatomy (Fig. 6.6).

Lower Extremity

Now we approach lower extremity radiologic imaging by beginning with the foot and moving toward the hip. The standard views of the foot are AP, lateral, and oblique (Fig. 6.7). Naming of the toes is far easier than that of the

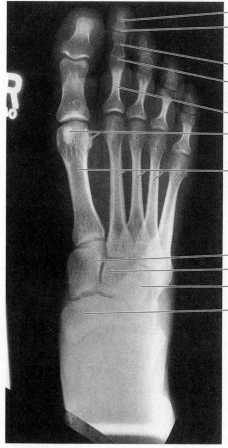

- Distal phalanx
- Distal interphalangeal joint (DIP)
- Middle phalanx
- Proximal interphalangeal joint (PIP)
- Proximal phalanx
- Sesamoid bones
- 1st, 2nd, 3rd, 4th, 5th metatarsals
- 1st (medial) cuneiform
- 2nd (intermediate) cuneiform
- 3rd (lateral) cuneiform
- Navicular

FIGURE 6.7. Right foot AP **(A)**, oblique **(B)**, and lateral **(C)** radiographs. Normal. (*continued*)

A

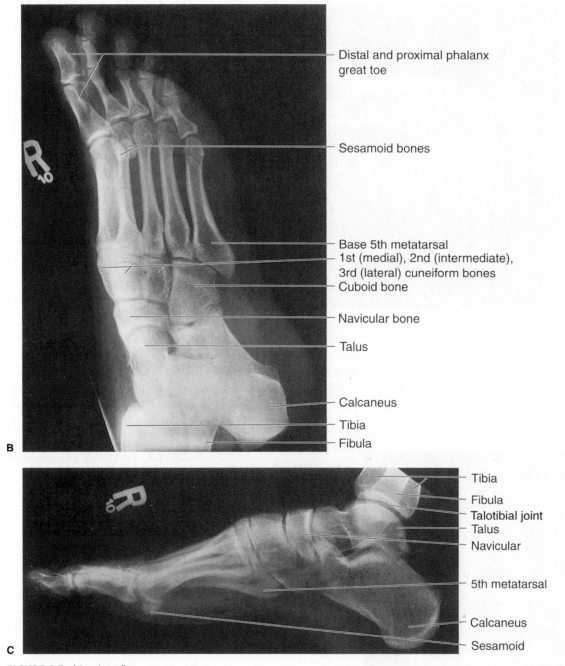

Distal and proximal phalanx great toe

Sesamoid bones

Base 5th metatarsal
1st (medial), 2nd (intermediate), 3rd (lateral) cuneiform bones
Cuboid bone

Navicular bone

Talus

Calcaneus

Tibia

Fibula

B

Tibia
Fibula
Talotibial joint
Talus
Navicular

5th metatarsal

Calcaneus

Sesamoid

C

FIGURE 6.7. *(Continued)*

fingers. The big toe or great toe may be referred to as the first toe and the remaining toes are numbered sequentially ending with the little or the fifth toe. Similarly, the metatarsals are numbered sequentially with the great toe articulating with the first metatarsal, the second toe articulating with the second metatarsal, and so forth. The ankle is usually imaged by AP-, lateral-, and, either, oblique- or mortise-view (a 10-degree internally rotated view) radiographs (Fig. 6.8). MRI may be used to image the ankle to detect soft tissue injury (Fig. 6.9).

Radiographs of the tibia and fibula usually consist of AP and lateral views (Fig. 6.10).

Routine knee radiographs consist of AP and lateral views and they may be supplemented by AP standing radiographs (Fig. 6.11) and/or oblique views. Axial, coronal, and sagittal magnetic resonance (MR) images of the knee (Fig. 6.12) are commonly requested to evaluate injuries of the knee, particularly, the nonosseous structures, including the medial and lateral menisci, articular cartilage, ligaments, tendons, and muscles. *Remember that ligaments,*

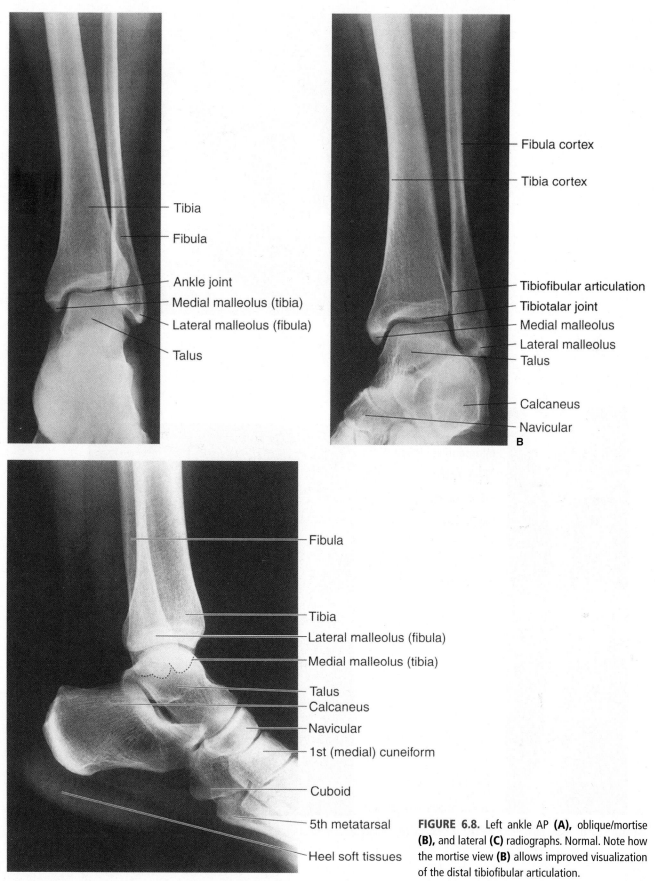

A

- Tibia
- Fibula
- Ankle joint
- Medial malleolus (tibia)
- Lateral malleolus (fibula)
- Talus

B

- Fibula cortex
- Tibia cortex
- Tibiofibular articulation
- Tibiotalar joint
- Medial malleolus
- Lateral malleolus
- Talus
- Calcaneus
- Navicular

C

- Fibula
- Tibia
- Lateral malleolus (fibula)
- Medial malleolus (tibia)
- Talus
- Calcaneus
- Navicular
- 1st (medial) cuneiform
- Cuboid
- 5th metatarsal
- Heel soft tissues

FIGURE 6.8. Left ankle AP **(A),** oblique/mortise **(B),** and lateral **(C)** radiographs. Normal. Note how the mortise view **(B)** allows improved visualization of the distal tibiofibular articulation.

FIGURE 6.9. Right ankle sagittal T1 MR image. Normal. Note that the calcaneal (Achilles) tendon has a homogeneous low-intensity (*black*) signal.

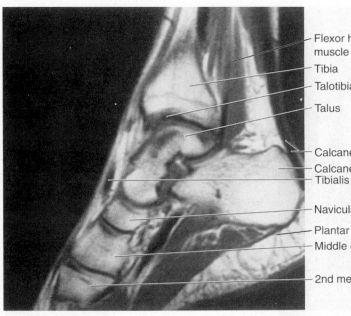

- Flexor hallucis longus muscle
- Tibia
- Talotibial joint
- Talus
- Calcaneal (Achilles) tendon
- Calcaneus
- Tibialis anterior tendon
- Navicular
- Plantar fascia
- Middle cuneiform
- 2nd metatarsal

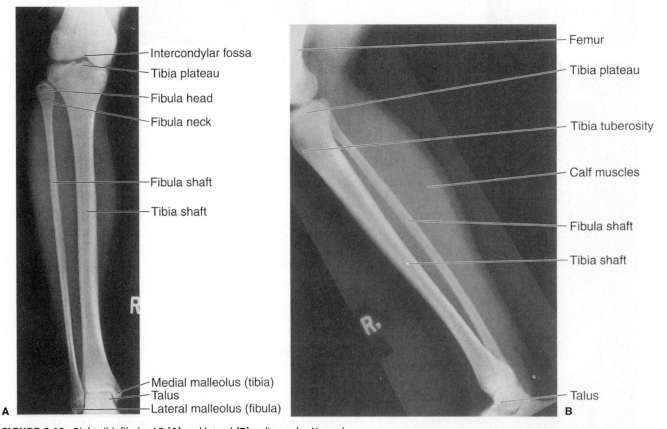

- Intercondylar fossa
- Tibia plateau
- Fibula head
- Fibula neck
- Fibula shaft
- Tibia shaft
- Medial malleolus (tibia)
- Talus
- Lateral malleolus (fibula)

- Femur
- Tibia plateau
- Tibia tuberosity
- Calf muscles
- Fibula shaft
- Tibia shaft
- Talus

FIGURE 6.10. Right tibiofibular AP **(A)** and lateral **(B)** radiographs. Normal.

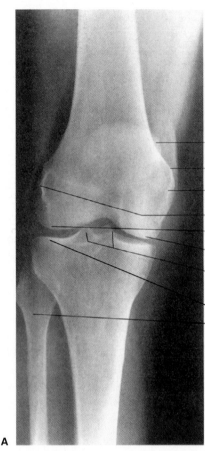

FIGURE 6.11. Right knee AP **(A)**, AP standing **(B)**, and lateral **(C)** radiographs. Normal. (*continued*)

Patella

Adductor tubercle

Medial femur epicondyle

Lateral femur epicondyle

Lateral femoral condyle

Medial femoral condyle

Lateral and medial intercondylar eminences (spines)

Lateral tibial plateau

Fibula

A

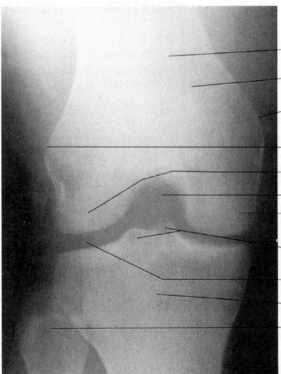

Femur

Patella

Medial femur epicondyle

Lateral femur epicondyle

Lateral femur condyle

Intercondyloid fossa

Medial femur condyle

Lateral and medial tibial intercondylar eminences

Joint space (lateral)

Tibia

Fibula head

Fibula neck

B

FIGURE 6.11. (*Continued*)

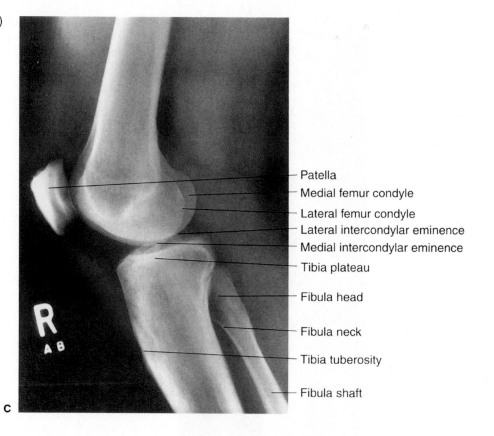

- Patella
- Medial femur condyle
- Lateral femur condyle
- Lateral intercondylar eminence
- Medial intercondylar eminence
- Tibia plateau
- Fibula head
- Fibula neck
- Tibia tuberosity
- Fibula shaft

C

tendons, and vessels have a low-intensity signal or appear black on MR images.

The femur and the hip joint are radiographed in the AP and lateral views (Fig. 6.13). A cross-table lateral view of the hip is frequently obtained in a trauma setting as seen in Figure 6.68B.

VARIATIONS OF NORMAL

There are several osseous variations of normal that can cause confusion for the novice (Table 6.4). One such variation of normal is the *sesamoid bone,* which is merely a normal extra bone, usually within a tendon. Sesamoids occur at

FIGURE 6.12. A: Right knee proton-dense sagittal MR image. Normal anterior cruciate ligament in a 36-year-old man.

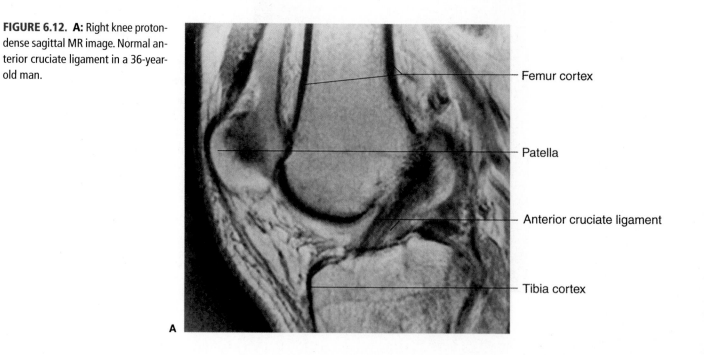

- Femur cortex
- Patella
- Anterior cruciate ligament
- Tibia cortex

A

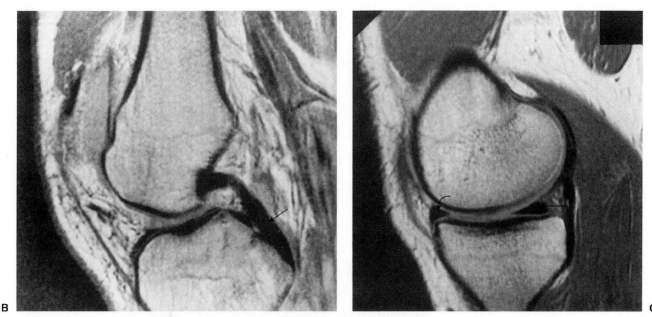

B

C

FIGURE 6.12. (*Continued*) **B:** Right knee proton-dense sagittal MR image in the same patient. Normal posterior cruciate ligament. The posterior cruciate ligament (*arrow*) is more homogeneous and has a lower-intensity signal (*blacker*) than the anterior cruciate ligament. **C:** Right knee proton-dense medial-sagittal MR image in a 32-year-old man. Normal posterior horn (*straight arrow*) and anterior horn (*curved arrow*) of the medial meniscus.

numerous sites and are commonly found in the plantar aspect of the foot near the head of the first metatarsal (see Fig. 6.7) and in the palmar aspect of the hand near the head of the first and sometimes other metacarpals (Fig. 6.14A–C; Fig 6.1A), where they are actually located in the volar plate rather than in a tendon. When you think about it, the patella is actually a sesamoid bone or a bone within a tendon. Sesamoids function to decrease the moment arm and thus, the work of a muscle. Thus, the quadriceps group of muscles becomes hypertrophied to compensate for increased work following the removal of the patella.

Ossicles are another variant of normal. They are small, supernumerary or extra bones found in a variety of places in juxtaposition to the skeletal system and usually named after the neighboring bone (Fig. 6.14D). The bipartite or multipartite patella (Fig. 6.14E–G) is another example of an accessory bone that should not be mistaken for a fracture.

Table 6.4
Normal Osseous Variations
Sesamoid bones (located within a tendon, e.g., the patella)
Ossicles (extra small bones)
Supernumerary epiphyses
Coalitions/fusions
Bone islands

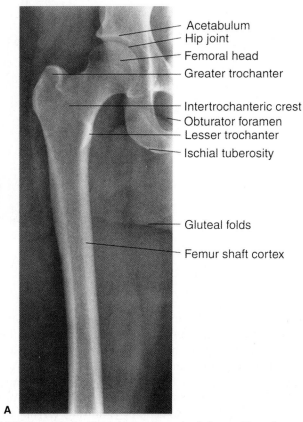

- Acetabulum
- Hip joint
- Femoral head
- Greater trochanter
- Intertrochanteric crest
- Obturator foramen
- Lesser trochanter
- Ischial tuberosity
- Gluteal folds
- Femur shaft cortex

A

FIGURE 6.13. A: Right hip and proximal femur AP radiograph. Normal. (*continued*)

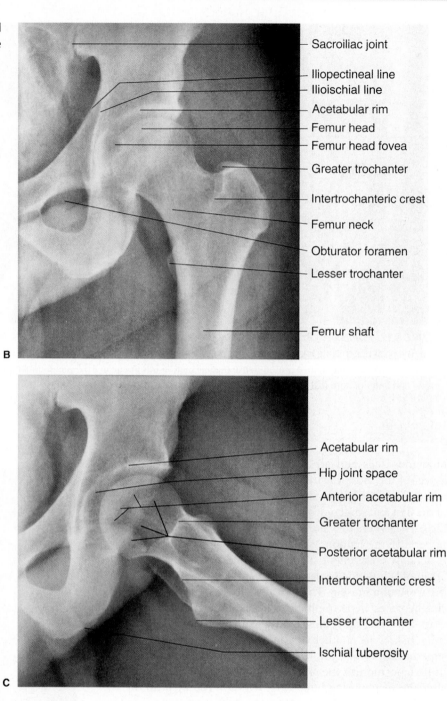

FIGURE 6.13. (*Continued*) Left hip AP **(B)** and frog-leg lateral **(C)** radiographs. Normal. See Figure 6.68B for a true lateral of the hip.

The condition results when one or more of the patellar ossification centers fail to fuse with the main patellar body. The result is that the patella has two or more sections and this male predominant variant occurs superolaterally approximately 75% of the time. Epiphyses can vary in appearance and in their number of ossification centers and still be normal (Fig. 6.14H,I). A sometimes confusing variant is a prominent scaphoid tubercle. This prominence can be mistaken for a fracture by even experienced clinicians.

CONGENITAL AND DEVELOPMENTAL ANOMALIES

Osseous congenital anomalies are not uncommon and a few of the many variations are listed in Table 6.5 and shown in Figures 6.15 to 6.20.

Coalition refers to the failure of segmentation of bones during development, resulting in a congenital fusion. This fusion may be bony or fibrous. Common locations involve

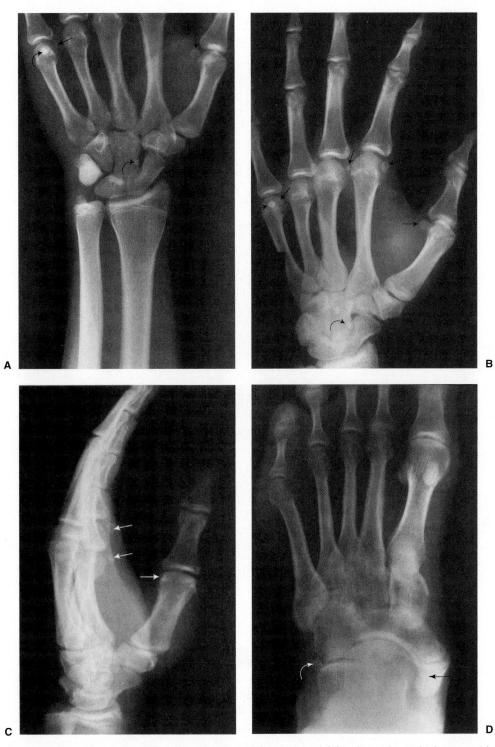

FIGURE 6.14. Left wrist PA **(A),** left-hand oblique **(B),** and lateral **(C)** radiographs. Multiple sesamoids (*straight arrows*). Bone islands (*curved arrows*) are present in the head of the fifth metacarpal and the capitate, and they have no clinical significance. **D:** Left foot AP radiograph. Os tibiale externum (*black arrow*) and os peroneum (*white arrow*). (*continued*)

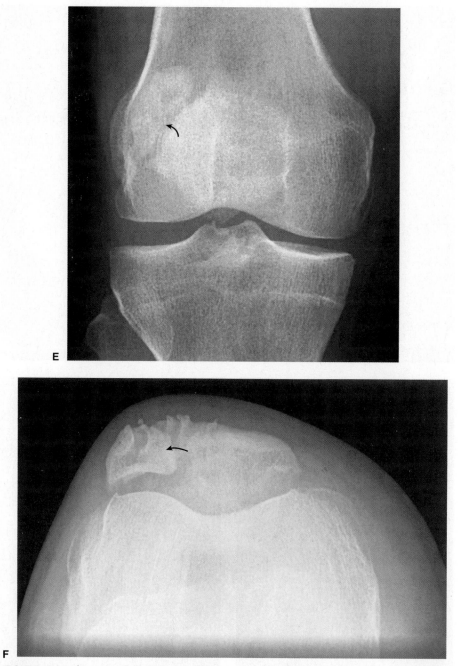

E

F

FIGURE 6.14. (*Continued*) Right knee anterior radiograph **(E),** tangential radiograph of right patella **(F),** and axial fat-suppressed MR image **(G)**. Bipartite patella. Note that the patella has two sections, and the accessory bone (*arrows*) usually lies superior and lateral to the main body of the patella.

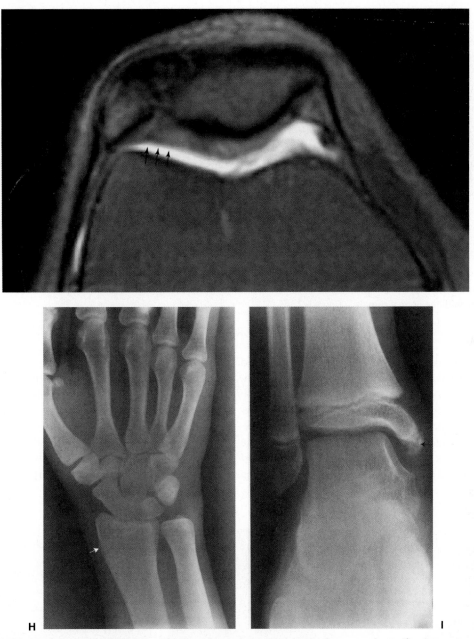

FIGURE 6.14. (*Continued*) **G:** The axial image shows the continuous cartilage over the ossification center (*arrows*) differentiating it from a fracture, which is rare in this superolateral position. **H:** Right wrist PA radiograph. Normal distal right radial epiphysis spur. This 21-year-old woman fell and had a painful wrist. This spur (*arrow*) is a variant of normal and must not be confused with a fracture. **I:** Right ankle AP radiograph. Accessory epiphysis near the tip of the distal tibia epiphysis in the region of the medial malleolus (*arrow*). This is a variant of normal.

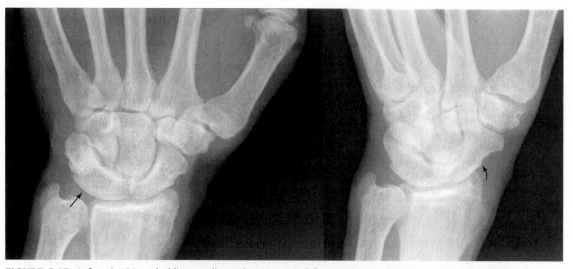

FIGURE 6.15. Left wrist PA and oblique radiographs. Congenital fusion. There is coalition of the lunate and triquetrum (*straight arrow*) and a prominent scaphoid tubercle (*curved arrow*). This tubercle should not be confused with a fracture. Compare with the normal carpals in Figure 6.2.

the lunate and triquetrum in the wrist (see Fig. 6.15) and the calcaneus and navicular or the calcaneus and talus in the foot (see Fig. 6.16).

Osteogenesis imperfecta is a congenital, nonsex-linked, hereditary abnormality with several variants of primary defects in collagen synthesis causing deficient bone matrix. These patients have bones (Fig. 6.20) that are fragile, fracture easily, and are often deformed. Achondroplasia

is a hereditary, often caused by spontaneous mutation, autosomal-dominant anomaly manifested by shortened long bones which results in this quite common form of dwarfism (Fig. 6.21).

The hip joint is the most common site of congenital dislocation and there is a strong female predominance. Developmental dysplasia of the hip (DDH), formerly known as congenital dislocation of the hip or congenital

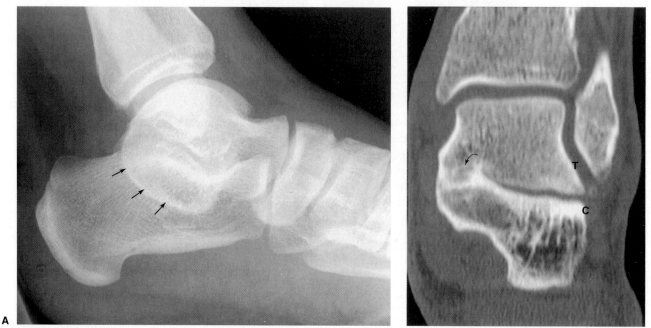

FIGURE 6.16. Lateral radiograph of the left ankle **(A)** and coronal CT image **(B)**. There is a prominent C on the radiograph (*arrows*). Compare with the normal lateral in Figure 6.8. The coronal CT clearly shows continuous bone bridging (*arrow*) between the talus (T) and calcaneus (C).

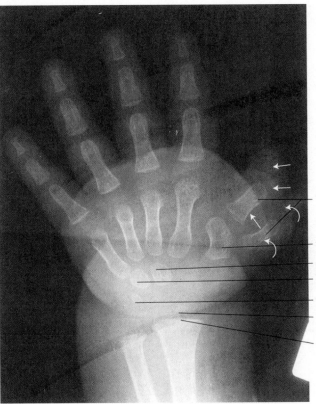

FIGURE 6.17. Left-hand PA radiograph (child). Polydactylism. There are two thumbs and one first metacarpal. One thumb has three phalanges (*straight arrows*) and the other thumb has two phalanges (*curved arrows*).

Two thumbs

1st metacarpal
Capitate
Hamate
Triquetrum
Distal radius epiphysis
Distal radius physis

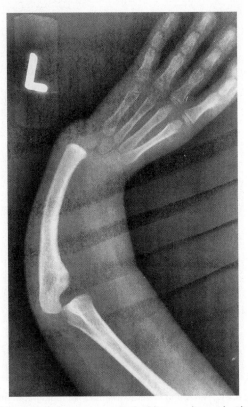

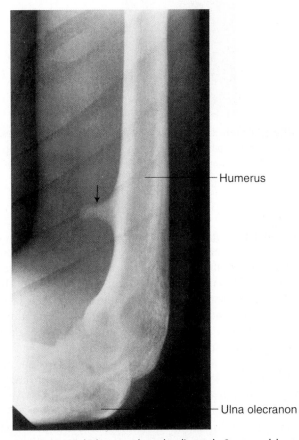

Humerus

Ulna olecranon

FIGURE 6.18. Left forearm pronated, oblique radiograph. Absence of the radius, first metacarpal, and thumb. This 6-year-old had left hand and arm deformity at birth.

FIGURE 6.19. Right humerus lateral radiograph. Supracondylar process or spur (*arrow*). It is usually located in the anteromedial aspect of the distal humerus.

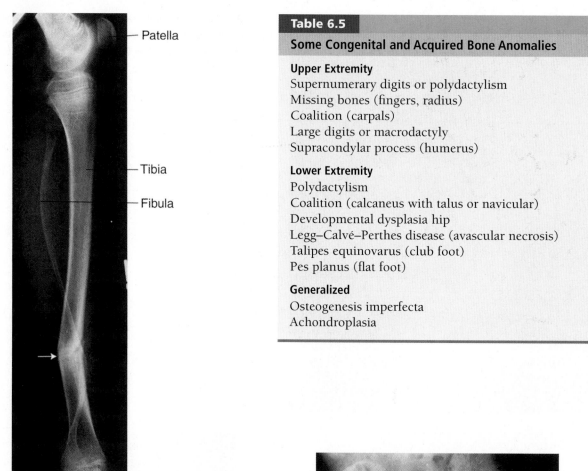

— Patella

— Tibia

— Fibula

FIGURE 6.20. Left tibia and fibula lateral radiograph. Osteogenesis imperfecta. There is a healing, apex posterior, left tibia fracture (*arrow*). Note the thin serpentine appearance of the fibula and generalized osteoporosis.

Table 6.5

Some Congenital and Acquired Bone Anomalies

Upper Extremity
Supernumerary digits or polydactylism
Missing bones (fingers, radius)
Coalition (carpals)
Large digits or macrodactyly
Supracondylar process (humerus)

Lower Extremity
Polydactylism
Coalition (calcaneus with talus or navicular)
Developmental dysplasia hip
Legg–Calvé–Perthes disease (avascular necrosis)
Talipes equinovarus (club foot)
Pes planus (flat foot)

Generalized
Osteogenesis imperfecta
Achondroplasia

hip dysplasia (Fig. 6.22) is usually diagnosed in infancy. DDH is an acquired abnormal development of the hip joint resulting in an abnormal acetabulum and femoral head owing to displacement of the femoral head deforming the acetabular cartilage. The femoral head usually displaces superiorly but can displace posteriorly. The acetabulum becomes shallow and the angle of the femoral neck between the femoral head and shaft is widened.

Two hip problems that can cause confusion are slipped capital femoral epiphysis (SCFE) and Legg–Calvé–Perthes disease (Table 6.6). SCFE (Fig. 6.23) is a hip problem that occurs during adolescence and is often associated with hip pain. The etiology is not understood, but there may be a history of trauma. It is more common in boys than girls and those who are overweight. Apparently, the physis becomes weakened during the

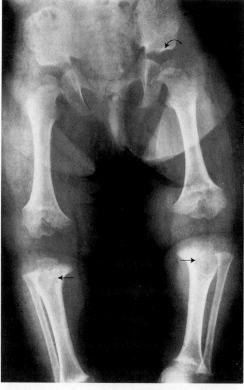

FIGURE 6.21. Pelvis and lower extremities AP radiograph. Achondroplasia. The proximal long bones are shorter and wider than normal, especially the proximal tibias (*straight arrows*). The iliac bones are rounded and the acetabula are flat (*curved arrow*).

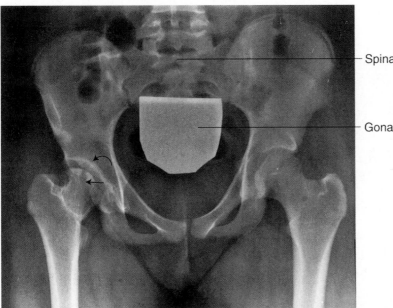

Spina bifida occulta (sacrum)

Gonadal shield

FIGURE 6.22. Pelvis AP radiograph. Developmental dysplasia of the right hip in a 14-year-old. The right hip is abnormal with a flattened femoral head (*straight arrow*) and a poorly formed acetabulum (*curved arrow*). Compare the right hip to the normal left hip and note how the femoral heads remodel to conform to the shape of their corresponding acetabulum.

rapid growth around puberty. The radiographic findings show the femoral head slipping or displacing posteriorly, medially, and inferiorly relative to the femoral neck. The proximal epiphysis becomes widened. Mild cases may go undetected and present with an earlier-than-expected onset of osteoarthritis.

Legg–Calvé–Perthes disease (Fig. 6.24A) is a form of avascular necrosis (AVN), and the etiology is unknown. It may be referred to as osteochondrosis or coxa plana. It typically occurs in a boy between 3 and 10 years of age who complains of hip pain and walks with a limp. The hip pain may be referred to the ipsilateral knee. Radiographic findings vary but may include increased density of the

femoral capital epiphysis, femoral head flattening, rarefaction (bone demineralization) of the metaphysis, and medial joint space narrowing. In general, AVN, osteonecrosis, or aseptic necrosis can occur in any joint (Fig. 6.24B,C) and can result from multiple other etiologies. Some of the other causes of AVN are listed in Table 6.7. The typical findings are sclerotic bone changes on one side of a joint that may go on to fracture, fragmentation, and eventually to collapse. MRI (Fig. 6.24C) has proved particularly useful for the diagnosis of AVN assisting in decisions for initiation of treatment prior to radiographic changes and predicting subsequent long-term complications such as early onset of arthritis.

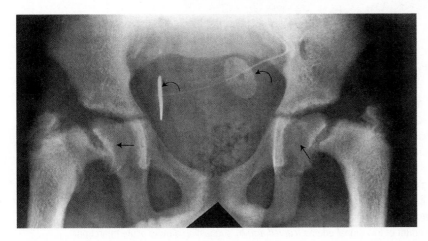

FIGURE 6.23. Pelvis AP radiograph. Bilateral slipped capital femoral epiphyses (SCFE) in a 15-year-old with chronic renal failure and on dialysis. The capital (proximal) femoral epiphyses (*straight arrows*) are displaced from their normal anatomic position. Usually, they are displaced inferiorly and posteromedially. There are monitoring electrodes projecting over the pelvis (*curved arrows*).

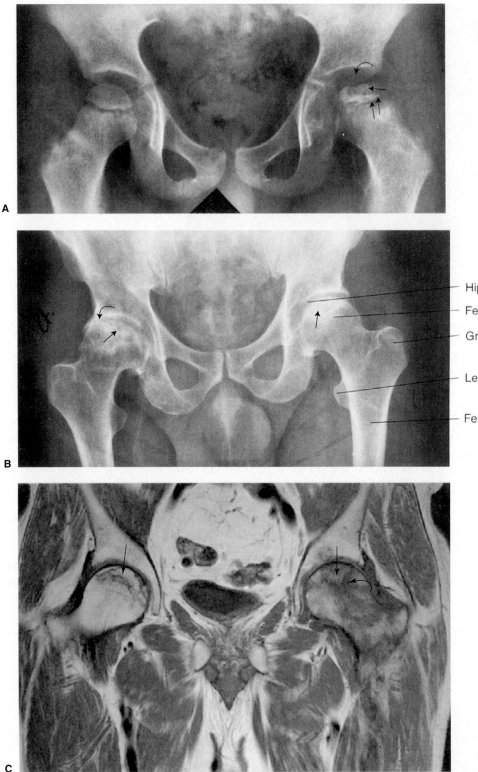

Hip joint
Femoral head
Greater trochanter
Lesser trochanter
Femur shaft

FIGURE 6.24. A: Pelvis AP radiograph. Legg–Calvé–Perthes disease. The right femoral head is normal. Note the irregular contour, flattened articular surface, and increased density of the left femoral head (*single straight arrow*). The left hip joint space is widened (*curved arrow*). The left proximal femoral epiphysis is widened (*double straight arrows*), and the metaphysis is irregular. Note that the acetabulum is normal. **B:** Pelvis AP radiograph. Bilateral femoral head avascular necrosis of unknown etiology in a 42-year-old man. Both femoral heads (*straight arrows*) are sclerotic in appearance, and the right femoral head is deformed because of mild collapse or fracture. The right hip joint is narrowed laterally (*curved arrow*). **C:** Coronal T1-weighted MRI. Femoral head osteonecrosis in a patient on chronic steroids. The crescentic area formed by low-signal lines (*straight arrows*) represents the infarcted regions. The left hip has a large amount of low-signal edema (*curved arrow*), suggesting a more acute infarction.

Table 6.6

Comparison of Slipped Capital Femoral Epiphysis (SCFE) and Legg–Calvé–Perthes Disease (LCP)

Feature	SCFE	LCP
Age	Adolescence	4–10 y
Gender	Boys more than girls (usually overweight)	Boys more than girls
Etiology	Unknown (usually during growth spurt)	Unknown
Symptoms	Hip and/or knee pain	Hip or knee pain and limping
Radiographic	Epiphysis slips posterior, medial, and inferior to the femoral neck. Early onset arthritis in adulthood	Flat and sclerotic epiphysis. Wide, slightly flattened femoral head with similarly shaped acetabulum in adulthood

TRAUMA

Fractures and Dislocations

Extremity fractures are very common, so now is the time to discuss fractures in general. The initial imaging modality to evaluate for fracture should be a radiograph. *Because a fracture or other osseous abnormality may be visible on only one of the radiographs, we obtain at least two views of a bone or joint which are 90 degrees opposed to each other.* Give yourself every opportunity to detect a fracture or other abnormality by obtaining as many views of an area as is practical. *Never accept just one radiographic view of a bone or joint.* When there is persistent concern for a fracture and the radiographs are normal, a clinical assessment is then needed. In many circumstances, the area of concern can be immobilized for a week and repeat radiographs obtained to see whether an occult fracture has now become visible. Other fractures are of such clinical importance that it is important to find out right away. The classic example is a hip fracture in an elderly patient for which an MRI should be obtained if the initial radiographs do not demonstrate a fracture. Some clinicians may get a CT scan of the hip because it is more readily available, but be wary of a negative scan in an elderly patient as these, too, may be falsely negative with a nondisplaced fracture. CT scans are, however, the screening method of choice for cervical spine fractures and are often used to better define fractures in many locations prior to treatment.

There are other rules of thumb to keep in mind. Paired bones such as the radius and ulna rarely have an isolated fracture; look closely for an associated fracture or a dislocation of the other bone at its proximal or distal joint. Structures that function as a ring, such as the pelvis, the mandible (with the facial bones), or the bones surrounding the ankle joint, also usually fracture in more than one spot. There are several fracture patterns that are typical and common, learn to look closely at the common locations for fractures.

In general, fractures can be conveniently divided into two major clinical categories.

1. Closed fracture means that there are bone fragments and the skin is intact.
2. Open fracture means the skin is not intact near the fracture. An open fracture occurs when the skin has been penetrated by one or more of the bone fragments or by a penetrating foreign body.

Many terms applied to fractures are very descriptive and quite specific (Fig. 6.25A,B). Examples of straightforward common terms for describing fractures include the following.

- Simple. Two significant fracture fragments with a single fracture plane.
- Complex or comminuted, meaning the fracture ends are smashed into multiple large pieces. Tiny bone fragments

Table 6.7

A Partial List of Avascular Necrosis Etiologies

Steroids (endogenous or exogenous) and anti-inflammatory drugs
Trauma including fractures and dislocations
Sickle-cell anemia
Hemophilia (synovitis and elevated intra-articular pressure)
Alcohol
Systemic lupus erythematosus
Renal transplant
Infection
Pancreatitis

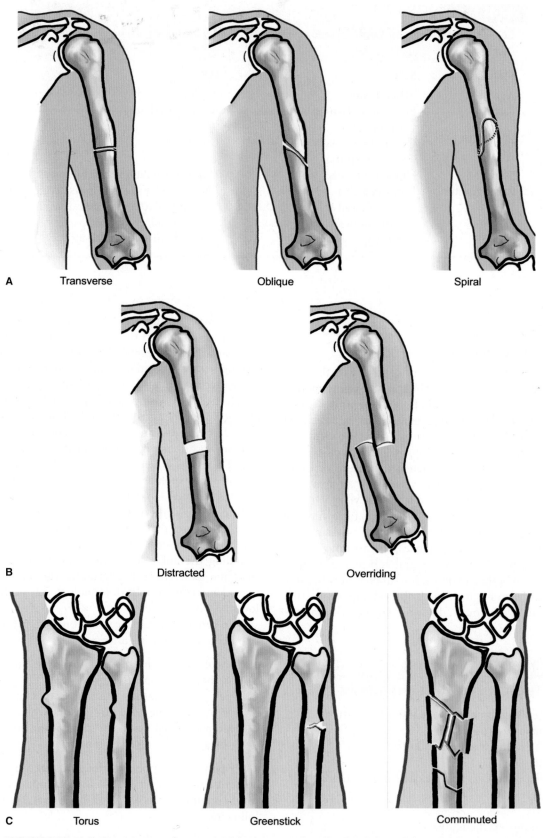

A   Transverse   Oblique   Spiral

B   Distracted   Overriding

C   Torus   Greenstick   Comminuted

FIGURE 6.25. A,B: Some common fractures and the terms used to describe them and their alignment. **C:** Common descriptive terms for fractures which are not simple. Illustration by CBoles Art.

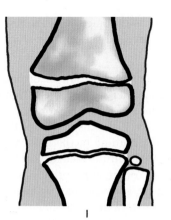

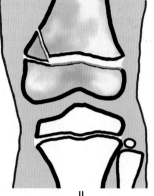

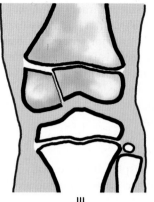

D   I
Fracture through physis

II
Fracture through
physis and metaphysis

III
Fracture through
physis and epiphysis

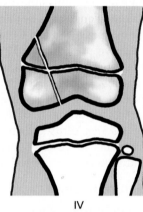

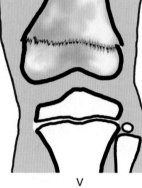

IV
Fracture through
physis, metaphysis
and metaphysis

V
Fracture with
compressions and crushing
of physis

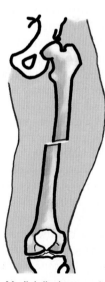

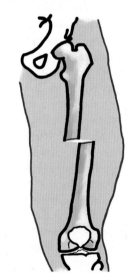

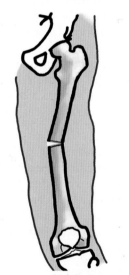

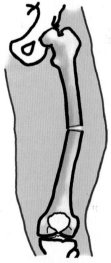

E   Medial displacement

Lateral displacement

Valgus or apex medial
angulation

Varus or apex lateral
angulation

FIGURE 6.25. (*Continued*) **D:** The Salter–Harris classification of physis fractures. **E:** Illustrations of the nomenclature used to describe fracture displacement and angulation. Illustration by CBoles Art.

are not considered fracture fragments because they are clinically irrelevant. A good way to think about this is to determine if a major tendon or ligament is attached or if the bone piece is large enough to secure with a screw, then they are comminuted fractures.

- Spiral, transverse, oblique.
- Nondisplaced.
- Overriding.
- Distracted.
- Angulated.
- Offset, or displacement, usually described by the percentage of the fracture fragments abutting or touching each other.

Some descriptive fracture terms (Fig. 6.25C) that are not quite so obvious include the following.

- Torus fracture (often involving the distal radius) looks like the bump at the base of a Greek column and has nothing to do with a bull. This is an incomplete fracture that occurs in children. The bump is created by a buckling of the flexible bone cortex without an obvious fracture line.
- Greenstick fracture describes a bone that fractures by bending like a green twig and is also incomplete.
- Pathologic fracture is one that passes through abnormal bone such as a metastasis, a primary bone tumor, or a bone cyst.
- Stress, or fatigue, fractures are secondary to unusual or excess stress, for example, tibial fractures in runners who overdo it.
- Insufficiency fractures describe fractures in bone with decreased strength, for example, caused by osteoporosis. Such a fracture may result from a normal stress such as merely walking across a room.
- An avulsion fracture is usually a fracture that occurs at the site of a tendon attachment. This fracture results when the tendon and muscle remain intact while the bone gives way (avulses) at the site of the tendon attachment to the bone.

The Salter–Harris classification of fractures (Fig. 6.25D) is helpful in describing and understanding fractures around a physis. The classification of basic five types has been expanded in recent years, but remains the standard. The higher the grade of Salter–Harris fracture, the more likely there is to be premature fusion of the growth plate. *Remember that the physis represents the weakest point in a bone.*

Type I: The fracture involves only the physis.
Type II: The fracture involves the physis and metaphysis and is the most common.
Type III: The fracture involves the physis and epiphysis.
Type IV: The fracture involves the physis, metaphysis, and epiphysis.
Type V: The fracture involves only the physis, but there is compression of the physis. This type is less common, but more serious than type 1 because there is a high risk of

the physis fusing as the fracture heals. As a result, the bone stops growing and the limb is shorter than the opposite side.

When describing the position of displaced fracture fragments, we use another set of terms. Traditionally, the distal fragment is described relative to the proximal fragment. This means that if the distal part of the fracture is displaced toward the midline of the body, it is displaced medially. One may substitute medial with volar, dorsal, radial, ulnar, or any other appropriate direction of displacement. The same concept may be used to describe angulation. Unfortunately, much confusion can be created by the nomenclatures for fracture angulation. A fracture described as medially angulated by one nomenclature (using the position of the distal fragment) may be described as laterally angulated by another nomenclature (using the fracture apex). You can see where confusion may arise! An alternative uses the word "apex" of the angle created by the fracture fragments as the key. If the apex of the fracture fragments points laterally, the fracture is described as "apex lateral." I prefer using the word apex in the description so that everyone understands which system is used (Fig. 6.25E). Varus and valgus angulation are other common terms to describe angulation (favored by many to avoid unnecessary confusion) and are also illustrated.

Fracture Healing

The rate at which a fracture heals depends on the fracture site, type of fracture, displacement, patient age, adequacy of immobilization, nutrition, and presence or absence of infection. When a fracture occurs, there usually is an associated hemorrhage into the fracture site with subsequent hematoma formation around and between the fracture fragments. The fibrin in a hematoma serves as a framework for fibroblasts, osteoblasts, and a general inflammatory reaction. Bone matrix or osteoid appears in the repair process after a few days, and this is called soft callus or provisional callus. The soft callus is not visible on a radiograph. As calcium salts precipitate in the soft callus and new bone grows, this is called callus. As the callus gradually becomes denser, it becomes visible on a radiograph. Eventually, the callus becomes solid and bone union is established between the fracture fragments.

In a few days following a fracture, some absorption or removal of bone occurs as a part of the repair process near the ends of the fracture fragments. Because of this bone resorption, the fracture line becomes more visible on subsequent radiographs. This explains why some subtle fractures may not be visible on radiographs obtained immediately following injury but become visible approximately 7 to 10 days following injury.

Self-explanatory terms used to describe problems in the fracture healing process include the following.

- Nonunion—although this term can be somewhat confusing since nonunion implies that there is continued

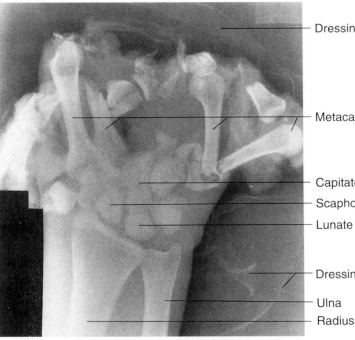

— Dressing

— Metacarpals

— Capitate
— Scaphoid
— Lunate

— Dressing

— Ulna
— Radius

FIGURE 6.26. Left-hand AP radiograph. Obvious severe hand injuries secondary to a corn-picking accident. The phalanges are essentially missing and there are fractures of the metacarpals and carpals.

motion between fracture fragments. A bone may not have well-formed bone across the fracture, but the non-bone or fibrous union may prevent motion. You may see the phrase "no radiographic union" as a fracture may be clinically healed (no pain, no motion across the fracture).

- Delayed union.
- Malunion.

Upper Extremity

Fractures of the hands result from a wide variety of activities. Some fractures and injuries are so obvious that the average person could readily spot them on a radiograph (Fig. 6.26). Subtle fractures can involve any bone and are common in the phalanges of the hand (Figs. 6.27 and 6.28). Joint dislocations may occur in almost all joints, and the hand phalangeal joints are common dislocation sites, often related to sports (Fig. 6.29). Metacarpal fractures are also common, and fractures of the fifth metacarpal often result from punching a solid object (Fig. 6.30). These fractures are appropriately called boxer fractures although they clearly demonstrate an amateur status because professionals would strike using the second and third metacarpals. We will review some other frequently encountered fractures of the upper extremity.

The most commonly fractured carpal is the scaphoid (Fig. 6.31). The carpal scaphoid is occasionally referred to as the navicular (an archaic term) by clinicians, but it is correctly termed the scaphoid. "Scaphoid" avoids confusion

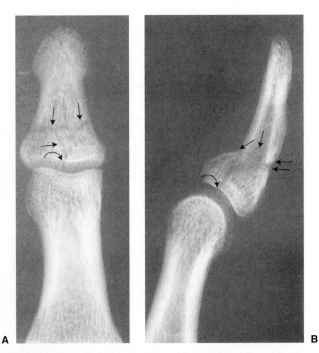

A   B

FIGURE 6.27. Left thumb PA **(A)** and lateral **(B)** radiographs. Comminuted fracture (*straight arrows*) that extends to the articular surface of the interphalangeal joint (*curved arrow*). There is mild apex palmar angulation at the fracture site (*double arrows*).

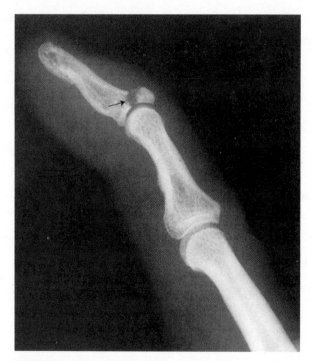

FIGURE 6.28. Right index finger lateral radiograph. Mallet finger. The distal phalanx demonstrates a slightly flexed attitude due to fracture (*arrow*) at site of the insertion of the extensor digitorum mechanism. The loss of the extensor mechanism continuity with the distal phalanx allows the distal phalanx to assume a flexed position or a mallet finger.

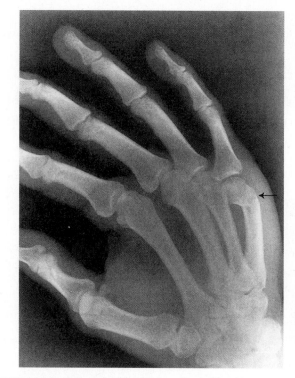

FIGURE 6.30. Right-hand PA oblique radiograph. Boxer or Saturday night fracture. The apex dorsal angulated fracture (*arrow*) is through the neck of the right fifth metacarpal.

with the tarsal navicular in the foot. Scaphoid fractures result from the injury lines of force being transmitted along the long axis of the thumb, and the majority of these fractures are located in the scaphoid waist. Because of the location of its blood supply and variable arterial branches,

scaphoid fractures may develop complications such as nonunion and AVN, which may result in secondary development of arthritis. These complications are more apt to occur when there is delayed diagnosis and delayed or inadequate treatment. If a scaphoid fracture is suspected but the

FIGURE 6.29. Left-hand PA radiograph. Dislocation at the proximal interphalangeal (PIP) joint of the left long finger. The middle and distal phalanges are completely dislocated relative to the proximal phalanx. There are no fractures.

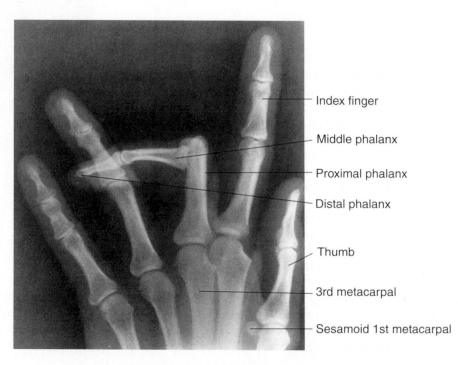

Index finger

Middle phalanx

Proximal phalanx

Distal phalanx

Thumb

3rd metacarpal

Sesamoid 1st metacarpal

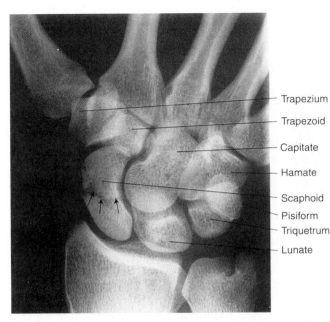

Trapezium
Trapezoid
Capitate
Hamate
Scaphoid
Pisiform
Triquetrum
Lunate

FIGURE 6.31. Right wrist PA radiograph. Essentially nondisplaced fracture (*arrows*) of the scaphoid waist.

initial radiographs are negative, additional radiography, CT, or MRI is indicated if casting and repeat radiograph in 1 week is not practical (Fig. 6.32).

Using arms and outstretched hands to cushion falls often results in fractures about the wrist. Whereas young adults typically fracture the scaphoid, children and older adults are more likely to fracture the distal radius and ulna. One such common fracture is called the Colles fracture (Fig. 6.33). It is imperative to reduce these fractured bones as close to their normal anatomic alignment as possible. Anything less than anatomic realignment may result in a painful and/or poorly functioning wrist. Therefore, it is important to know that the radial styloid tip is 1 to 1.5 cm distal to the ulnar styloid tip and the distal radial articular surface slopes 15 to 25 degrees toward the ulna and 10 to 25 degrees volar or anteriorly. Anatomic reduction may not be necessary in the nondominant hand of a person, where "less than anatomic" may still lead to a functional outcome. Children, of course, have a remarkable ability to remodel and anatomic realignment is not usually needed, depending on the age of the child. In fact, to avoid future limb length discrepancy, anatomic realignment may be purposely avoided.

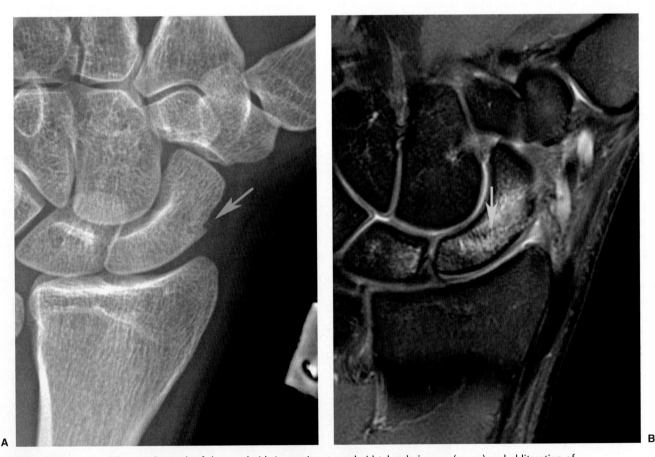

A   B

FIGURE 6.32. A: PA oblique radiograph of the scaphoid. A prominent scaphoid tubercle is seen (*arrow*) and obliteration of normal fat next to the bone, but no definite fracture is seen. **B:** Fat-suppressed T2-weighted MR image of the scaphoid reveals edema and a fracture line (*arrow*), which does not extend through the medial margin consistent with an incomplete fracture.

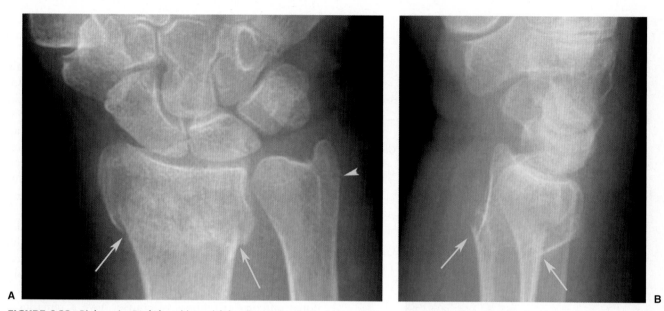

FIGURE 6.33. Right wrist PA **(A)** and lateral **(B)** radiographs. Colles fracture. There are fractures of the distal radius (*arrows*) and the ulna styloid (*arrowhead*) with dorsal tilting of the distal radius fracture fragment. The pronator fat stripe is obliterated when compared with Figure 6.1B. The ulna styloid is not displaced. Note that the radius is slightly impacted with its articular surface proximal to the ulnar head. Reduction will try to bring to neutral or restore the volar (anterior) tilt.

A subtle fracture in the distal forearm of children is the torus fracture (Fig. 6.34). As mentioned previously, torus does not refer to a bull but rather the convex molding/projection (torus) located at the base of a classical column. The torus fracture on a radiograph usually appears as a minimal bump on the bone without a visible fracture line. It represents a buckling of the bone cortex since a child's bones are more elastic and able to bend. On occasion,

the force may create an incomplete or greenstick fracture (Fig. 6.35A,B), so named because a "green" or freshly cut stick will not break through and through when bent as a dried one will. However, most fractures of the radius and ulna that are encountered in practice are much more obvious (Fig. 6.35C–E).

Elbow fractures (Figs. 6.36–6.38) and dislocations (Fig. 6.39A–D) can occur when children and adults fall

FIGURE 6.34. A: Left wrist PA, oblique, and lateral radiographs. Torus fracture (*arrows*) or a nondisplaced fracture of the distal left radius. Left wrist PA **(B)** and lateral **(C)** radiographs. Healing left radius torus fracture 6 weeks following the radiograph shown in **A**. The dense white zone (*arrows*) is the typical appearance of a healing fracture. **D:** Right wrist lateral radiograph in a younger child demonstrates a more obvious torus fracture (*arrow*).

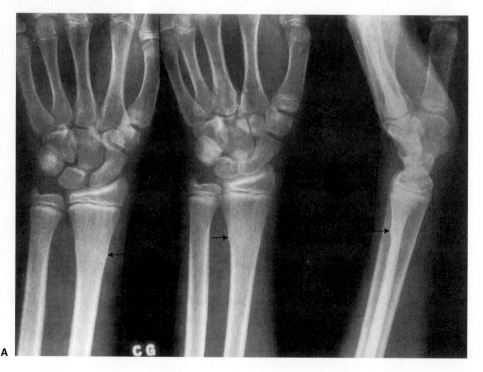

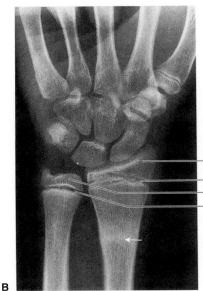

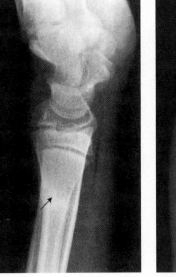

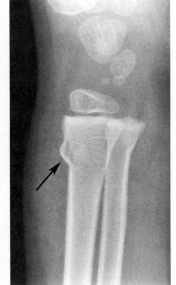

Radius epiphysis
Radius physis
Ulna epiphysis
Ulna physis

B

C

D

FIGURE 6.34. (*Continued*)

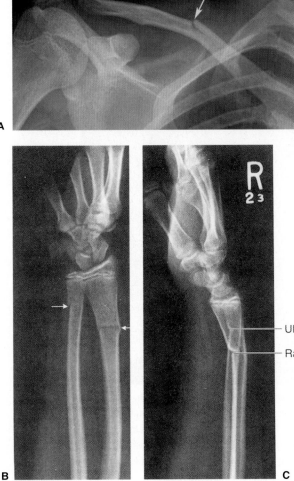

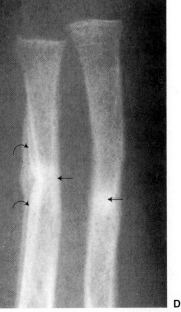

A

B

C

D

R
2 3

Ulna fracture
Radius fracture

FIGURE 6.35. **A:** AP view of the right clavicle shows a greenstick fracture of the superior cortex of the clavicle (*arrow*). Note the open physis of the humerus indicating the young age of the patient. Right forearm AP **(B)** and lateral **(C)** radiographs. Complete transverse fractures (*arrows*) of the distal shafts of the radius and ulna in a 15-year-old. There is mild apex volar, or apex anterior, angulation at the radius fracture site. The fracture fragments in the ulna are mildly offset. **D:** Right forearm AP radiograph. Healing fractures (*straight arrows*) of the radius and ulna in a young child. The fractures are remodeling to near-anatomic alignment and the *curved arrows* indicate periosteal reaction and new bone formation. The fracture lines are not visible, suggesting early bone union.

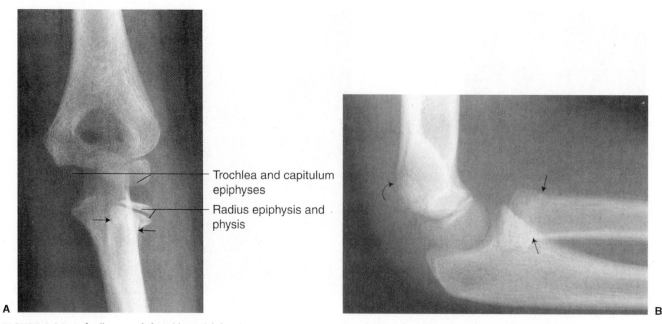

A   B

FIGURE 6.36. Left elbow AP **(A)** and lateral **(B)** radiographs. Radial neck fracture. The *straight arrows* indicate the site of the fracture and the radial head is tilted laterally on the AP view. The fracture is very difficult to see on the lateral view (*straight arrows*). A positive fat pad sign is faintly visible posterior to the distal humerus (*curved arrow*) on the lateral view and this always means that one should carefully evaluate for a fracture. A visible fat pad anterior to the distal humerus is normal so long as it is not overly prominent (see Fig. 6.4).

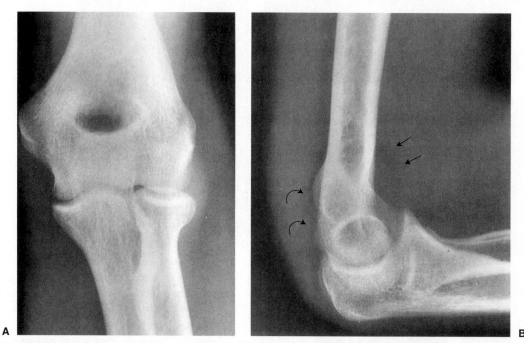

A   B

FIGURE 6.37. Left elbow AP **(A),** lateral **(B),** and oblique **(C)** radiographs. Fracture of the radius neck. The patient fell from a bicycle and complained of a painful elbow. A fracture is not definitely visible on the AP and lateral radiographs; however, it should be strongly suspected because the anterior fat pad (*straight arrows in* **B**) is more prominent than normal and a posterior fat pad (*curved arrows*) is present. The fracture (*arrow in* **C**) can be clearly visualized on the oblique radiograph. This demonstrates the importance of obtaining multiple views of a suspected fracture site and reiterates the significance of a positive posterior fat pad sign and a prominent anterior fat pad.

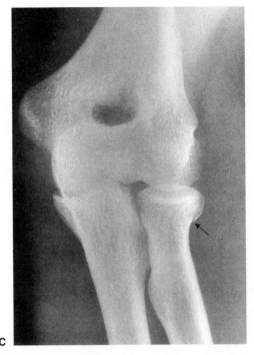

FIGURE 6.37. (*Continued*)

The radiographic anatomy of the elbow is complicated. This is especially true in children because of the presence or absence of multiple ossification centers. *When in doubt about an elbow fracture or dislocation, the noninvolved elbow may occasionally be useful for comparative purposes* (see Fig. 6.38). This principle of comparative views applies to all areas of difficult anatomy. However, knowledge of the anatomy and ordered development of the ossification and subsequent fusion of the physes are fundamentally more important. Note that fractures and dislocations of the elbow can be a threat to the brachial artery because of its proximity to the distal humerus (see Fig. 6.39E).

Soft tissue injuries to the elbow may be more difficult to assess on radiographs. Although a biceps tendon tear may be obvious clinically due to the bulge of a retracted muscle (Fig. 6.40A), an MR study can demonstrate how far the tendon is retracted and some degree of the structural integrity of the torn tendon (Fig. 6.40B). MRI is also frequently used to assess tendons and the ulnar collateral ligament of the elbow, particularly in throwing athletes, such as baseball pitchers (Fig. 6.41).

A very common injury to the shoulder occurs when a senior trips on the rug or stairs. If they land on their extended hand and do not fracture their wrist, they may sustain a fracture of the surgical neck of the humerus (Fig. 6.42). Generally, this is very easily treated with a sling or a light, hanging cast but may require an extended time for healing due to the patient's age and the fewer stresses compared to a weight-bearing bone. A similar fracture can occur through the physis of the proximal humerus in children (Fig. 6.43).

directly on their elbow or on an extended arm or hand. In general, children are more likely to have a supracondylar fracture of the distal humerus and adults a radial head fracture. Dislocations of the elbow are named for the direction the radius and ulna dislocate relative to the humerus. When the radius and ulna dislocate posterior to the humerus, it is a posterior dislocation.

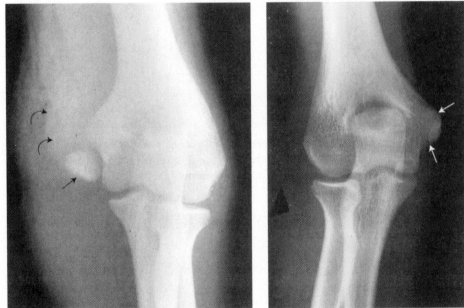

FIGURE 6.38. A: Left elbow AP radiograph. Avulsion fracture of the medial epicondyle epiphysis (*straight arrow*) in a 13-year-old. There is considerable soft tissue prominence (*curved arrows*), probably due to edema and hemorrhage secondary to the avulsion fracture. Remember that the pronators and flexors of the forearm attach to the medial epicondyle and the extensors and supinators to the lateral epicondyle. **B:** Right elbow AP radiograph for comparison. Normal. The medial epicondyle epiphysis (*straight arrows*) is normal. (*continued*)

FIGURE 6.38. (*Continued*) **C:** Right elbow oblique radiograph. Bucket-handle fracture of the distal humerus (*curved arrow*) in a 14-month-old child. Bucket-handle–type fractures can be found in child abuse situations. The *straight arrows* indicate periosteal reaction that occurs as a part of the healing process.

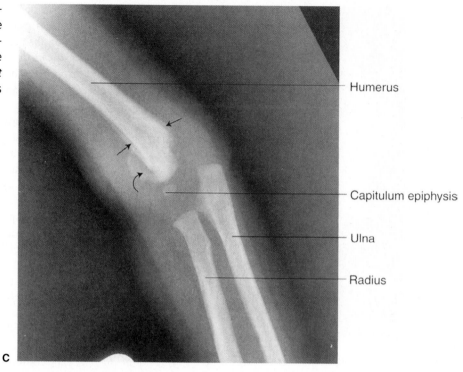

Humerus

Capitulum epiphysis

Ulna

Radius

C

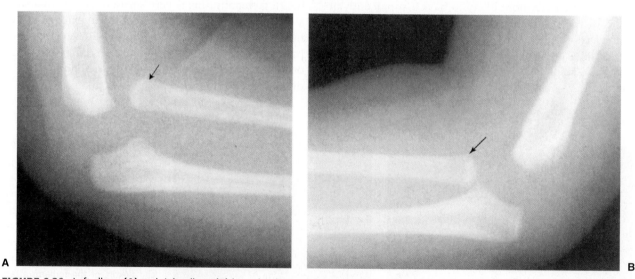

A   B

FIGURE 6.39. Left elbow **(A)** and right elbow **(B)** lateral radiographs. Anterior dislocation of the left (*arrows*). The right elbow lateral radiograph is normal and was obtained for comparative purposes as elbow anatomy may be especially difficult in children. Note the significant difference in position of the proximal left radius relative to the left humerus compared to the normal right proximal radius relative to the right humerus.

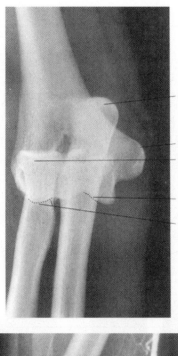

C

Ulna olecranon

Medial epicondyle
Radial head

Trochlea

Capitulum

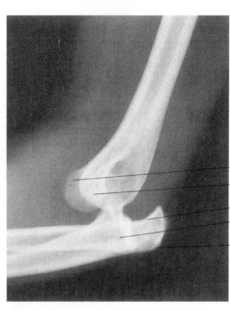

D

Capitulum
Trochlea

Trochlear notch
Radial head

Ulna olecranon

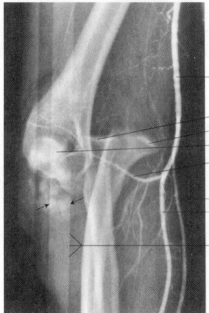

E

Brachial artery

Radial head
Ulna coronoid
Ulna olecranon
Recurrent ulnar artery

Radial artery
Ulnar artery

Artifact

FIGURE 6.39. (*Continued*) Right elbow AP **(C)** and lateral **(D)** radiographs. Posterior dislocation of the elbow in a 23-year-old. The proximal ulna and the radial head are posterior to their normal articulations with the distal humerus and this is best appreciated on the lateral view. There are no fractures. **E:** Left elbow lateral angiogram. Fracture–anterior dislocation of the left elbow in a different patient. The radius and ulna are dislocated anteriorly relative to the humerus and there is a comminuted fracture of the ulna olecranon (*arrows*). The brachial artery is displaced anteriorly by the dislocation and the associated soft tissue edema and hemorrhage.

FIGURE 6.40. Biceps tendon tear. **A:** Lateral radiograph of the right distal humerus reveals a prominent soft tissue bump (*arrow*). **B:** Sagittal T2-weighted MR image demonstrates the retracted, torn biceps tendon (*arrow*). The level of its normal attachment on the radial tuberosity is marked by an *asterisk* and the amount of retraction can be measured.

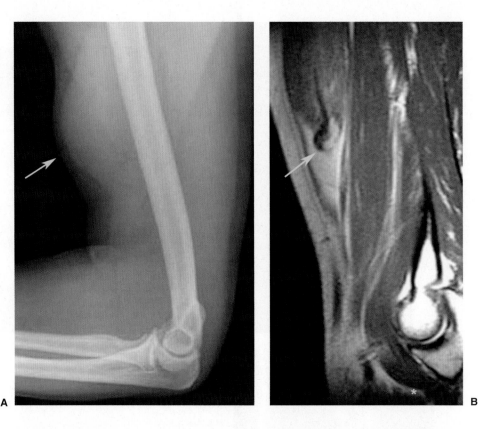

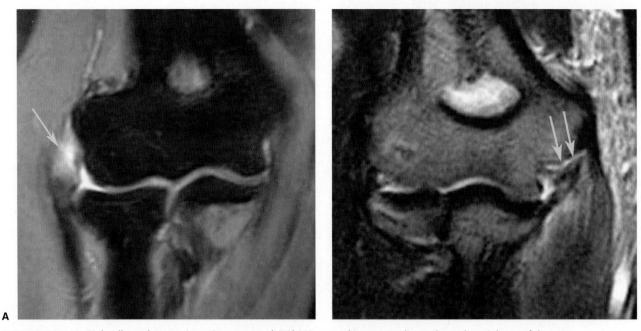

FIGURE 6.41. A: Right elbow short tau inversion recovery (STIR) MR coronal image. Tendinopathy and partial tear of the common extensor tendon (*arrow*). This is sometimes mistakenly called lateral epicondylitis. **B:** Right elbow coronal fat-suppressed T2-weighted MR image of a tear of the humeral attachment of the ulnar collateral ligament (*arrows*).

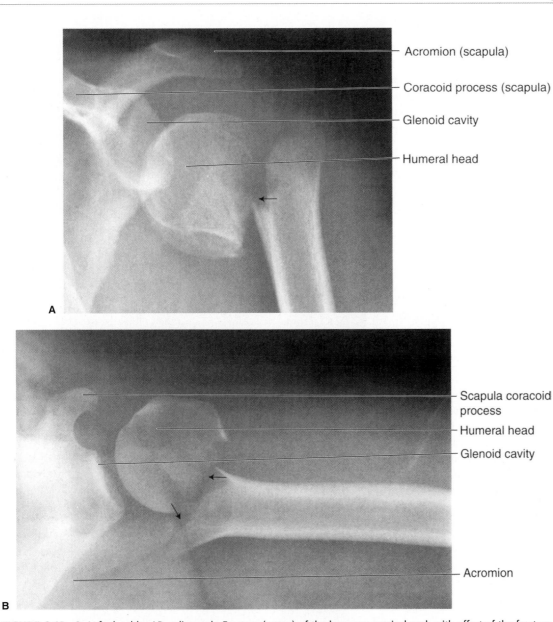

- Acromion (scapula)
- Coracoid process (scapula)
- Glenoid cavity
- Humeral head

A

- Scapula coracoid process
- Humeral head
- Glenoid cavity

- Acromion

B

FIGURE 6.42. A: Left shoulder AP radiograph. Fracture (*arrow*) of the humerus surgical neck with offset of the fracture fragments in a 19-year-old patient. The humeral head is rotated and subluxated medially on the AP view resulting in an abnormal relationship between the humerus head and the scapula glenoid cavity. **B:** Left shoulder axillary radiograph of the same patient as in **A.** The central x-ray beam travels through the axilla to demonstrate nicely the offset fracture fragments (*arrows*). Note that the humeral head now is in a normal relationship with the scapula. The scapula coracoid process projects anteriorly and the base of the scapula acromion projects posterior to the glenoid cavity on this view. Surgical internal fixation was required.

Dislocation of the shoulder is another common injury that can occur in all age groups. In the much more common anterior dislocation of the shoulder, the humeral head displaces medial and inferior to the glenoid cavity on an AP radiograph and an impaction fracture of the greater tuberosity, a Hill–Sach deformity, may result (Fig. 6.44A–C), or the greater tuberosity may fracture completely (Fig. 6.44D). A dislocation is often very difficult to diagnose on a single anterior view and an axillary or scapular Y view should be obtained (Fig. 6.44E). In a posterior dislocation, the glenohumeral joint often appears slightly widened on an AP view (Fig. 6.45A) while overlap of the humerus and glenoid is seen on the oblique, or Grashey, view (Fig. 6.45B). CT can assess for fractures and occasionally discover an unanticipated dislocation (Fig. 6.45C). Anterior dislocation of the shoulder is much

FIGURE 6.43. Left shoulder AP radiograph. Salter I fracture (*arrows*) through the proximal physis of the left humerus in a 15-year-old patient. The patient fell on an outstretched arm. The major clue to the presence of a fracture is that the physis width is greater than normal. Be careful not to overcall the normal physis a fracture (see Figs. 6.44E and 6.49).

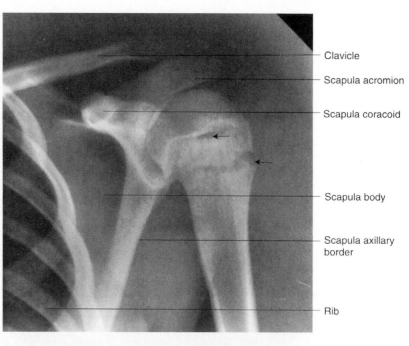

Clavicle

Scapula acromion

Scapula coracoid

Scapula body

Scapula axillary border

Rib

FIGURE 6.44. A: Left shoulder AP radiograph. Anterior dislocation of the shoulder without fracture. The humeral head is inferior to the glenoid cavity and not rotated; this is the classic position of the humeral head in an anterior dislocation. The intertubercular (bicipital) groove is well visualized and within it rests the tendon of the long head of the biceps brachii. **B:** Left shoulder axial CT of an anterior dislocation. Note how the humeral head (H) may impact the glenoid (G).

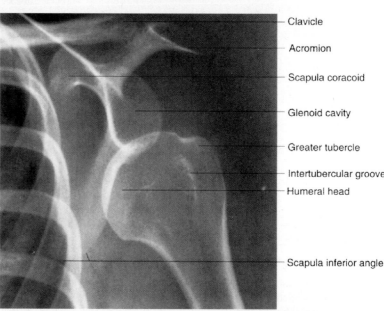
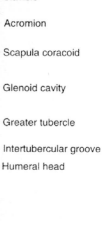

Clavicle

Acromion

Scapula coracoid

Glenoid cavity

Greater tubercle

Intertubercular groove

Humeral head

Scapula inferior angle

A

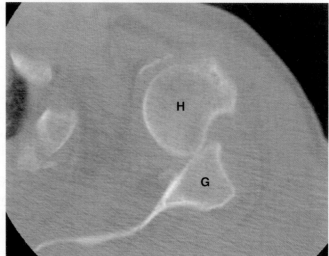

B

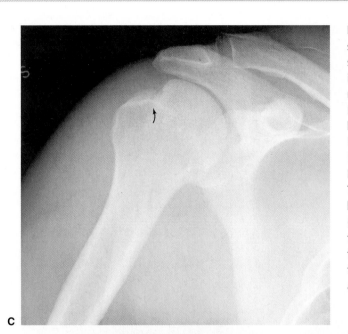

FIGURE 6.44. (*Continued*) **C:** Right shoulder AP radiograph. Postreduction study demonstrates a Hill–Sach deformity (*arrow*) from impaction fracture. **D:** AP radiograph of left shoulder. Anterior dislocation with fracture of the greater tuberosity (*straight arrow*). Note a fat–fluid level (*curved arrow*) on this upright study. Fat from the marrow floats in blood. **E:** Scapular Y-view. Anterior dislocation. The coracoid, acromion, and scapular body form the limbs of the Y. The glenoid (*dashed circle*) is located at the intersection. The humeral head should contact this intersection. Note the open physis in this 17-year-old, not to be mistaken for a fracture.

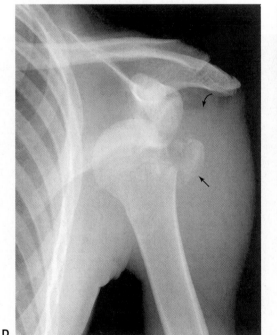

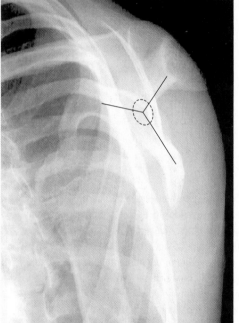

more common than a posterior dislocation. Associated fractures of the humerus or scapula and rotator cuff tears may occur, however, neural and vascular injuries are much less frequent.

Occasionally, a severe humeral head fracture or other disease process of the proximal humerus necessitates shoulder prosthesis (Fig. 6.46). Fractures of the scapula are not common and usually result from a high-force injury as in motor vehicle accidents. These are frequently evaluated by CT to determine whether the fracture involves the glenoid or the suprascapular notch where the nerve to the supraspinatus and infraspinatus muscle travels (Fig. 6.47). Fractures of the clavicle are very common, especially in children who fall (Fig. 6.48). The most common site for clavicle fractures is at the junction of the middle and distal thirds.

MRI is a powerful tool for evaluating shoulder rotator cuff and the glenoid labrum (Figs. 6.49 and 6.50). An arthrogram is performed by distending a joint, usually with fluid that will provide contrast to the structures of

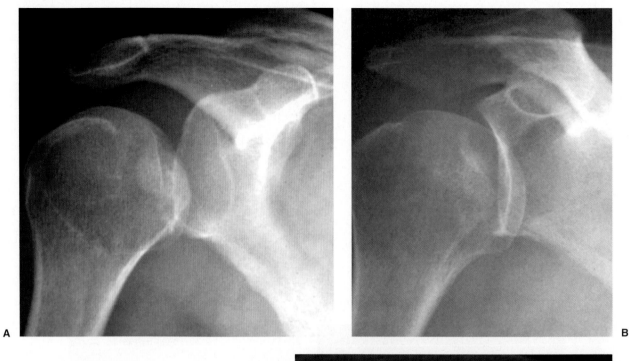

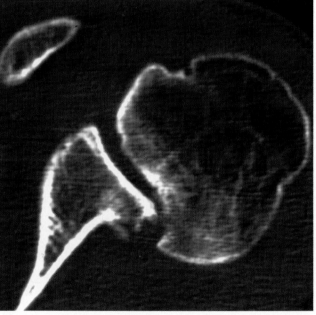

FIGURE 6.45. A: Right shoulder AP radiograph. Posterior dislocation may be overlooked as the shoulder joint may appear normal or slightly widened. **B:** Oblique, or Grashey, view of the right shoulder views the glenoid cavity in tangent. There is clear overlap of the humeral head and glenoid. Normally, there should be a distinct joint space on this view. **C:** Axial CT image of a left shoulder in a patient with a posterior dislocation with impaction. Note that, unlike an anterior dislocation, it is rare for the entire humeral head to be posterior to the glenoid.

interest. MR arthrograms are especially helpful for evaluating tears of the glenoid labrum (Fig. 6.51). Ultrasound can also be used to assess the rotator cuff, but requires an experienced sonographer and interpreter (Fig. 6.52). Remember that MRI is also useful for bone marrow and can identify occult fractures (Fig. 6.53).

Lower Extremity

Injuries to the feet are very common, as this is where our body meets the ground. See Figures 6.54 to 6.58 for a

gallery of common foot injuries. When evaluating the foot in young patients, remember that there is an apophysis at the base (proximal end) of the fifth metatarsal. An apophysis is a growth center (like the epiphysis) that does not contribute to bone length. It alters bone contour and usually is not located in a joint but typically has tendons attached to it. A lateral radiolucent line near the base of the fifth metatarsal that runs parallel to the long axis of the metatarsal represents a normal apophysis (see Fig. 6.54C), whereas *a transverse lucent line at the base of*

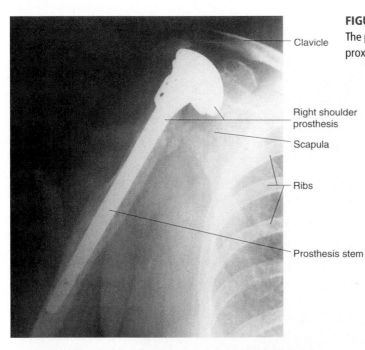

Clavicle

Right shoulder prosthesis

Scapula

Ribs

Prosthesis stem

FIGURE 6.46. Right shoulder AP radiograph. Right shoulder prosthesis. The prosthesis was necessitated by a severe old fracture deformity of the proximal humerus.

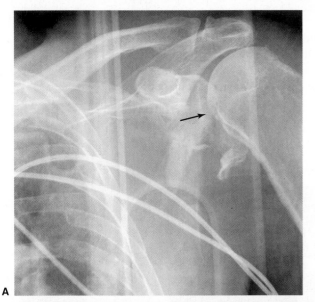

A

FIGURE 6.47. Left shoulder AP radiograph **(A)** and axial CT **(B)**. Scapular fracture. The most important finding is involvement of the glenoid (*arrows*), which can lead to arthritis.

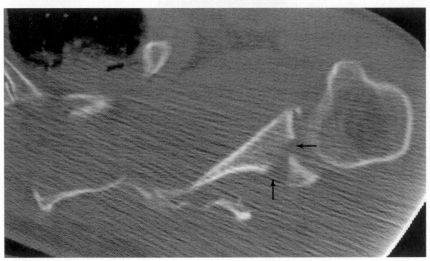

B

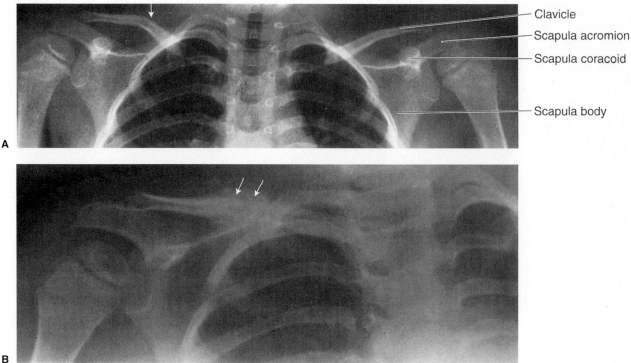

A

B

FIGURE 6.48. **A:** Right and left clavicles AP radiograph. Subtle greenstick fracture of the middle-third of the right clavicle (*arrow*) in a 3-year-old child. There is minimal apex cephalad angulation at the fracture site. The fracture is more apparent when compared to the normal left clavicle. **B:** Right clavicle AP radiograph in the same patient 4 weeks later. Healing fracture. The white material surrounding the fracture site in the middle-third of the right clavicle (*arrows*) is callus. The bone has remodeled the angulation and the clavicle alignment is normal.

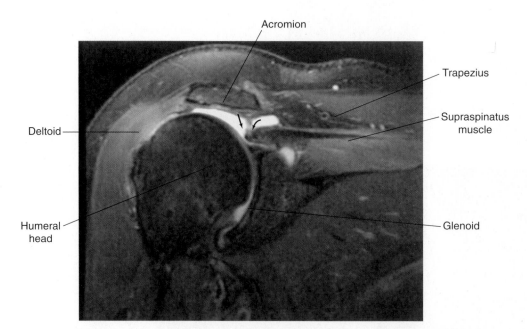

FIGURE 6.49. Right shoulder fat-suppressed T2 coronal MR image. Rotator cuff complete tear in a 55-year-old man. The area of high-intensity or white signal (*straight arrow*) represents blood, edema, and joint fluid in the laceration of the supraspinatus tendon. The free margin of the torn supraspinatus tendon is indicated by the *curved arrow*. Note that the bone cortex is black on the MR image. Note the edema (*brighter signal*) in the supraspinatus muscle.

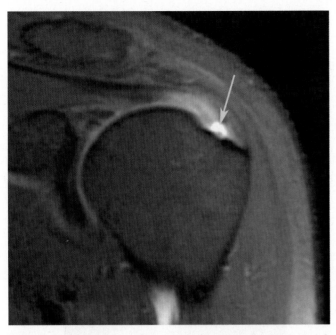

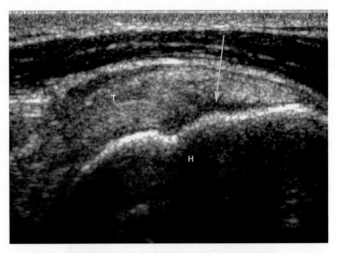

FIGURE 6.52. Ultrasound of the supraspinatus tendon insertion in oblique coronal plane. Partial tear. The curved white line with dark adjacent to it is the cortex of the humerus. Focal area of lower echogenicity at the tendon attachment (*arrow*) is partial tear. This is similar to the tear in Figure 6.50. Humerus (H), supraspinatus tendon (T).

FIGURE 6.50. Oblique coronal, fat-suppressed, T1-weighted MR left shoulder arthrogram. Partial tear of the articular surface of the supraspinatus tendon (*arrow*) at its insertion on the greater tuberosity.

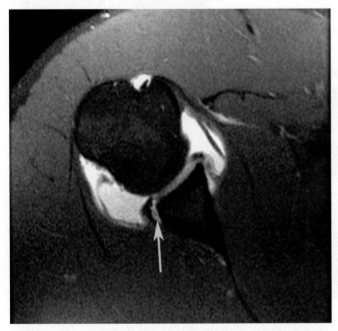

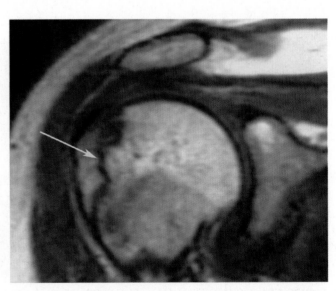

FIGURE 6.51. Axial fat-suppressed T1-weighted MR right shoulder arthrogram. Posterior labral tear. Contrast is seen between the labrum and its posterior glenoid attachment (*arrow*).

FIGURE 6.53. Right shoulder, oblique-coronal T1-wieghted MR obtained for persistent pain following a fall onto the shoulder and normal radiographs. A non-displaced fracture of the greater tuberosity (*arrow*) is demonstrated as a low signal line through the brighter marrow fat.

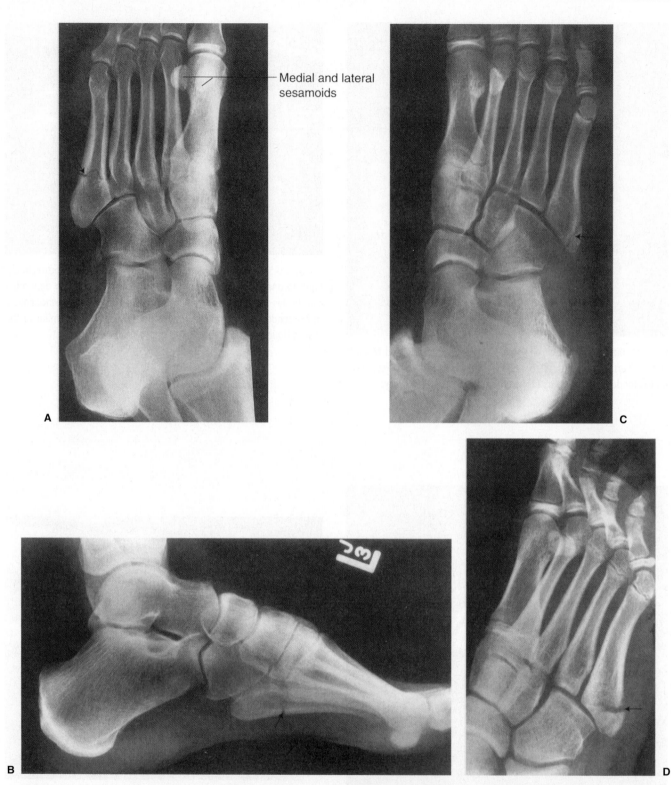

Medial and lateral
sesamoids

FIGURE 6.54. Left foot oblique **(A)** and lateral **(B)** radiographs. Nondisplaced transverse fracture of the proximal left fifth metatarsal shaft (*arrows*). **C:** Right foot AP radiograph. Normal in a 14-year-old boy. The normal apophysis (*arrow*) at the base of the fifth metatarsal appears as a longitudinal radiolucent or black line and should not be confused with a fracture. **D:** Right foot oblique radiograph. Transverse nondisplaced fracture (*straight arrow*) involving the fifth metatarsal base. This injury usually results from an inversion stress on the peroneus brevis that attaches to the base of the fifth metatarsal.

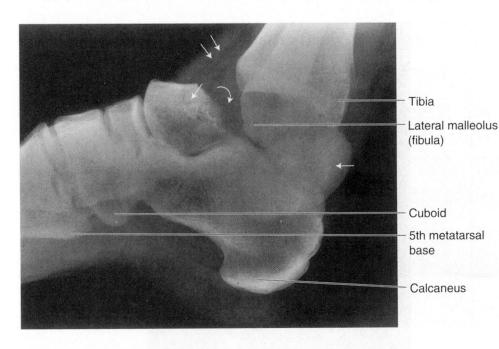

FIGURE 6.55. Right ankle lateral radiograph. Midtalus distracted fracture (*curved arrow*). The fracture fragments (*single straight arrows*) are markedly distracted and the soft tissue edema and/or blood is indicated by the *double straight arrows*. The fracture resulted from a dorsiflexion injury.

the fifth metatarsal always represents a fracture (see Fig. 6.54D).

The ankle injuries vary from minor sprains to severe trimalleolar fracture dislocations (Figs. 6.59–6.61). CT is often used to evaluate ankle fractures (Figs. 6.62 and 6.63); ultrasound and MRI may be used to evaluate soft tissue injuries (Fig. 6.64). Fractures of the shafts of the tibia and fibula are common in sports, especially contact sports and skiing. A fracture that fails to heal over 4 months and has persistent motion about it, often with pain, is called a nonunion fracture. Nonunion fractures have a variety of causes, some of which are listed in Table 6.8. Nonunions and delayed unions are frequently found in the mid- and distal tibia where adequate blood supply can be a problem (Fig. 6.65). Severe fractures of the tibia may require internal fixation to facilitate immobiliza-

tion and healing (Fig. 6.66). The tibia is also the site of stress fractures in all age groups, especially in runners (Fig. 6.67).

A wide variety of fractures occur in and around the knee, and examples are demonstrated in Figures 6.68 to 6.71. These figures demonstrate that not all fractures are visible on the initial radiographs around the time of injury. Whenever symptoms persist following an injury and the original radiographs were negative, you must consider follow-up imaging that might include radiographs, MRI, CT, or radionuclide scans. CT scans are often used for obvious tibial plateau fractures (see Fig. 6.69) to better demonstrate the number and position of fragments and depth of depression of articular surface. For tibial plateau fractures, this imaging data is important to determine whether open reduction is needed or casting will be adequate.

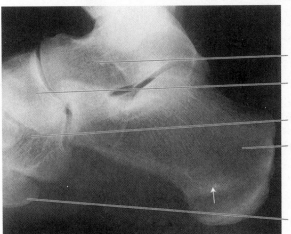

FIGURE 6.56. Right calcaneus lateral radiograph. Calcaneus insufficiency fracture in a 53-year-old woman. The white line (*arrow*) indicates a healing mildly impacted fracture that was not visible on radiographs 2 months prior to this study. The shape and height of the calcaneus are fairly well maintained. She had been on steroids for inflammatory bowel disease and the steroids caused osteoporosis. As a consequence of the osteoporosis, the bone was not strong enough to prevent fracture.

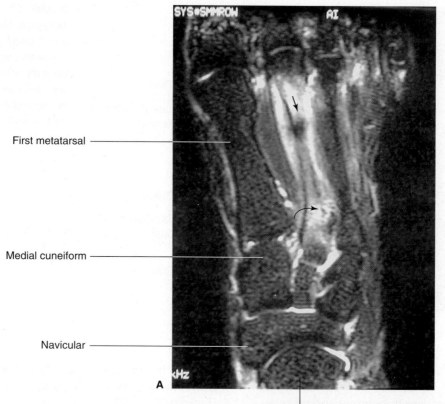

First metatarsal

Medial cuneiform

Navicular

Talus

A

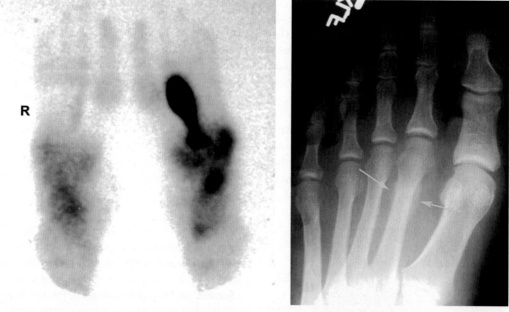

R

B

C

FIGURE 6.57. Metatarsal stress fracture. **A:** Long-axis fat-suppressed T2-weighted MR of the right foot in a runner. Second metatarsal stress fracture has some callus, which is black (*straight arrow*), and a large amount of edema in the bone and soft tissues, which is white (*curved arrows*). Bone scan **(B)** and AP left foot radiograph **(C)** in a similar patient. Callus (*arrows*) is white on the radiograph. Note the bone scan image is obtained as if looking at the bottom of the patient's feet so the left foot appears opposite to that of the radiograph.

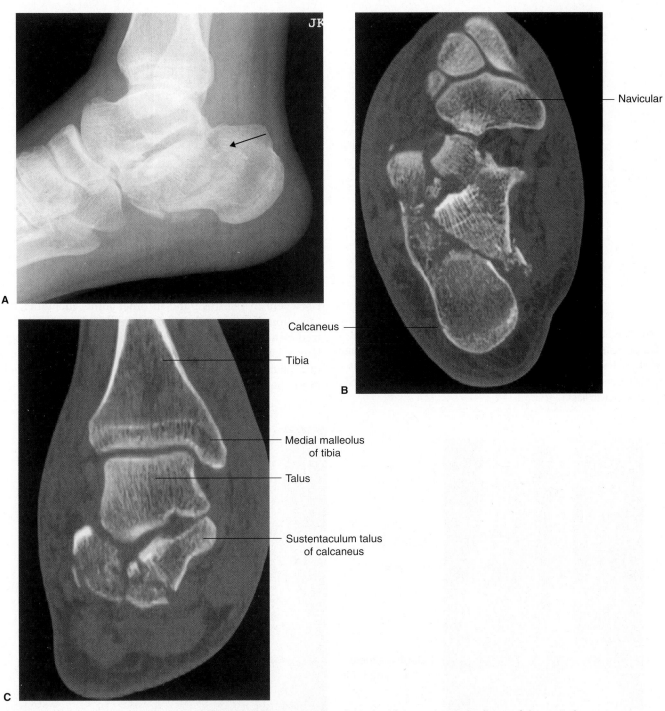

Navicular

Calcaneus

Tibia

Medial malleolus
of tibia

Talus

Sustentaculum talus
of calcaneus

FIGURE 6.58. A: Right calcaneus lateral radiograph. Calcaneus fracture (*arrow*) with impaction and collapse of the vertical height of the calcaneus. Compare the shape of the calcaneus in this patient to the calcaneus in Figure 6.55. Axial **(B)** and coronal reformatted **(C)** CT images better demonstrate the extent and comminution of the fracture.

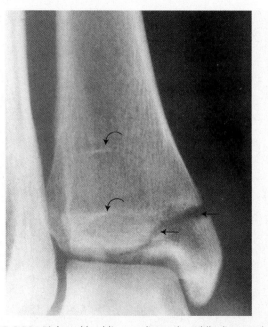

FIGURE 6.59. Right ankle oblique radiograph. Mildly distracted fracture (*straight arrow*) through the base of the medial malleolus in an adult. The fracture extends onto the articular surface of the distal tibia. The white lines (*curved arrows*) represent previous physis location and arrested growth lines.

Table 6.8
Causes of Fracture Nonunion
Infection and osteomyelitis
Inadequate immobilization
Poor blood supply
Interposition of muscle or other structure between the fracture fragments
Combinations of the above

The patella is a large, superficial sesamoid bone. It may fracture due to falls and blunt trauma (see Fig. 6.71). Osteochondritis dissecans (Fig. 6.72A,B) is a fairly common abnormality involving the knee in adolescents and young adults. It occurs most frequently along the lateral aspect of the medial femoral condyle, but it can be found elsewhere in the knee and in other joints including the hip, shoulder, ankle, and elbow. It is thought to be a localized ischemic or AVN that often occurs after injury, perhaps related to a subchondral stress fracture, which results in a piece of necrotic bone that may or may not detach from the donor site. If this necrotic fragment becomes

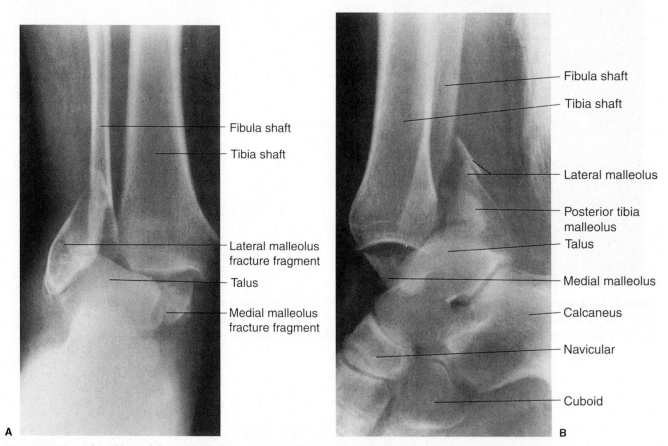

FIGURE 6.60. Right ankle AP (**A**) and lateral (**B**) radiographs. Displaced trimalleolar fractures and talotibial dislocation. The medial and posterior tibial malleoli fracture fragments and the fibula lateral malleolus fracture fragments are all displaced. The talus is severely displaced laterally and posteriorly relative to the tibia. This is an eversion injury.

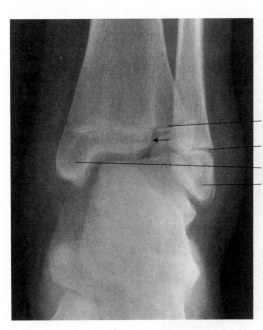

FIGURE 6.61. Left ankle AP radiograph. Salter III fracture of the left distal tibia in a 12-year-old. The fracture line (*arrow*) extends from the physis through the distal tibial epiphysis to the articular surface.

— Tibia physis
— Fibula physis
— Distal tibia epiphysis
— Distal fibula epiphysis

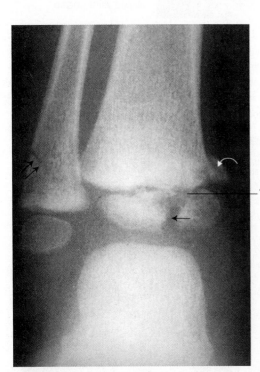

— Tibia physis

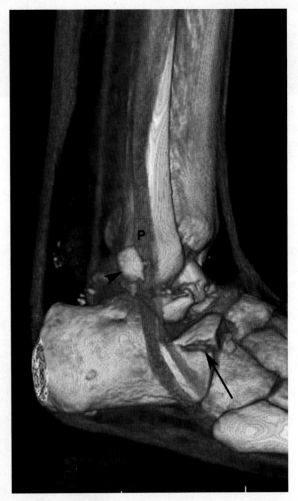

FIGURE 6.62. Right ankle AP radiograph. Salter IV fracture of the distal tibia. The fracture line (*single straight arrow*) extends from the distal tibial physis through the epiphysis to the tibial articular surface. The fracture also involves the medial tibia metaphysis (*curved arrow*). There is an associated fracture of the distal fibula (*double straight arrows*).

FIGURE 6.63. Lateral view from a three-dimensional CT reconstruction. Fractures with dislocated peroneal tendons. Fractures of the anterior process of the calcaneus (*arrow*) and distal fibula (*arrowhead*) are seen on this view. The peroneal tendons (P) should be posterior to the fibula, but are displaced anteriorly and are likely trapped by the fibular fracture fragment.

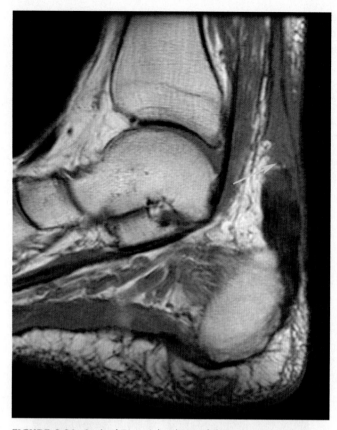

FIGURE 6.64. Sagittal T1-weighted MR of the ankle. Achilles tendon tear. There is thickening disruption (*arrow*) of the normally uniformly black Achilles tendon.

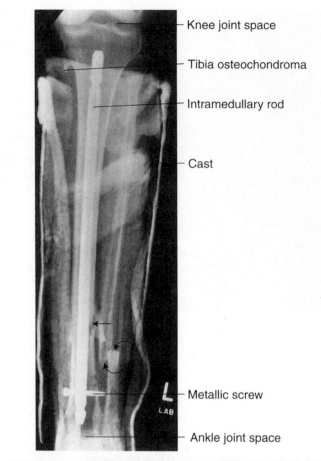

- Knee joint space
- Tibia osteochondroma
- Intramedullary rod
- Cast
- Metallic screw
- Ankle joint space

FIGURE 6.66. Left tibia and fibula AP radiograph. Intramedullary rod internally fixating a transverse fracture in the distal one-third of the left tibia (*straight arrow*). There is an offset overriding transverse fracture in the distal one-third of the fibula (*curved arrows*). The fibula is non–weight-bearing, so the displacement is not important to a good functional outcome.

FIGURE 6.65. Left tibia and fibula AP **(A)** and lateral **(B)** radiographs. Osteomyelitis and nonunion of a tibia fracture. The fracture line (*arrows*) is clearly visible 3 months following the injury and this indicates a delayed union or nonhealing fracture. Infection at the fracture site caused the delayed union.

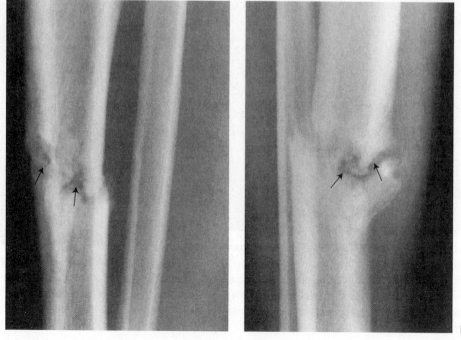

A

B

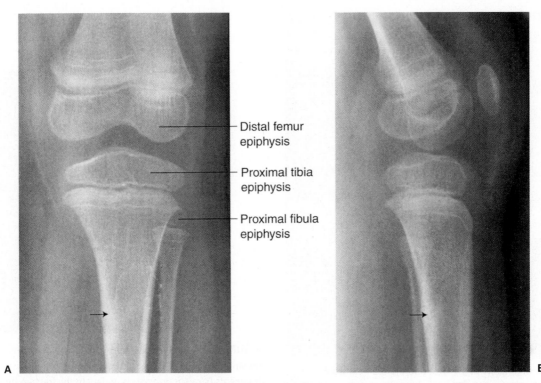

FIGURE 6.67. Left knee AP **(A)** and lateral **(B)** radiographs. A healing stress fracture in this 5-year-old is indicated by the zone of increased density in the posteromedial proximal tibia (*arrows*). The fracture resulted from excessive usage or stress.

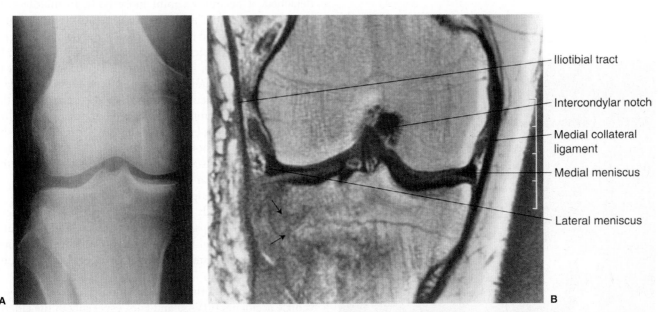

FIGURE 6.68. A: Right knee AP radiograph. This AP radiograph and a lateral (*not shown*) radiograph were interpreted as normal. The radiographs were obtained because of right knee pain immediately following knee trauma in a 31-year-old man. **B:** Right knee coronal T1 MR image. Lateral tibial plateau fracture. This study was obtained 2 weeks following the initial radiograph in **A** because of persistent knee pain and a clinical suspicion of an anterior cruciate ligament injury. The *arrows* indicate an area of low-intensity signal (*dark*) caused by blood and edema replacing the bone marrow fat (*white*) in the tibial plateau fracture site. The anterior cruciate ligament was intact. The fracture eventually became apparent on subsequent radiographs.

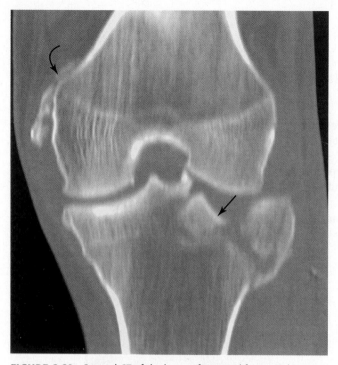

FIGURE 6.69. Coronal CT of the knee reformatted from axial images. Lateral tibial plateau fracture. CT is often used to better evaluate the amount of depression of the articular surface (*straight arrow*) and number and location of fragments. The irregular bone formation along the medial femur (*curved arrow*) is the result of a prior medial collateral ligament injury.

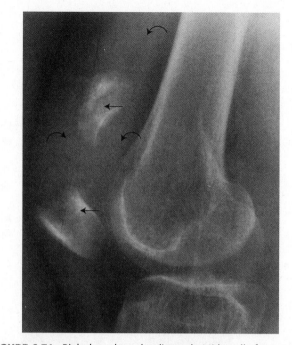

FIGURE 6.71. Right knee lateral radiograph. Midpatella fracture secondary to a motor vehicle accident. There are two distracted fracture fragments (*straight arrows*) secondary to the fracture through the mid-patella. The *curved arrows* indicate blood and increased synovial fluid in the supra-, pre-, and retropatellar spaces of the knee.

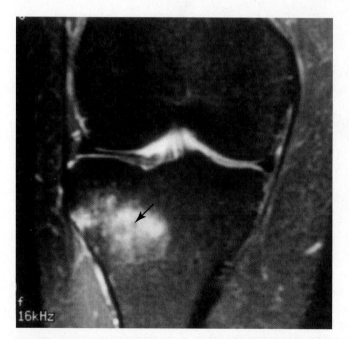

FIGURE 6.70. Coronal inversion recovery MRI of the right knee. Insufficiency fracture of the medial tibia in an elderly patient with pain. The incomplete fracture line (*arrow*) is white on this sequence from blood and edema.

detached, it becomes a joint loose body. In middle-aged to older adults, the abnormality is typically the weight-bearing aspect of the medial femoral condyle and the term spontaneous osteonecrosis is often used (Fig. 6.72C,D). In the older age group, in particular, these lesions are felt to be due to subchondral insufficiency fractures. AVN (osteonecrosis) may occur in any region of the bone and is the result of bone ischemia and localized bone death. The clinical presentations of bone ischemia vary with the bone site and size as well as bone age (see Fig. 6.24). Osteonecrosis has a variety of causes. The term infarct is used when the dead bone is not near a joint.

As a general rule, femoral shaft fractures are easy to detect both clinically and radiographically, as the patient experiences severe pain at the fracture site and is usually unable to bear weight (Fig. 6.73). This is an uncommon area for stress fractures, but they may occur here in young athletes.

The hip is another area commonly injured in motor vehicle accidents (MVAs) and falls, especially in the elderly (Fig. 6.74). MRI has become the standard in evaluating for hip fracture with seemingly normal radiographs (Fig. 6.75). Stress fractures may develop in the hip as well, most typically in runners (Fig. 6.76). Dislocations of the hip are not common and require violent trauma as in MVAs (Fig. 6.77). However, patients with a hip prosthesis may on occasion dislocate the prosthetic head with a minimal amount of stress (Fig. 6.78). As opposed to the shoulder, posterior

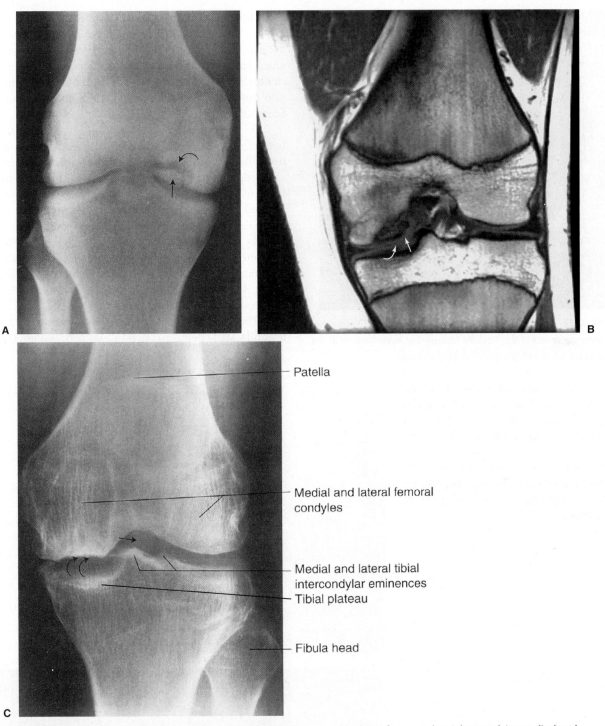

Patella

Medial and lateral femoral
condyles

Medial and lateral tibial
intercondylar eminences
Tibial plateau

Fibula head

FIGURE 6.72. A: Right knee AP radiograph. Osteochondritis dissecans. The bone fragment (*straight arrow*) is not displaced from the donor site (*curved arrow*) on the lateral aspect of the medial femoral condyle. **B:** Coronal T1-weighted MR right knee in a different patient. The fragment (*straight arrow*) is clearly seen and cartilage covers it (*curved arrow*). **C:** Left knee AP radiograph in a different patient. Spontaneous osteonecrosis. There is a displaced bone fragment or loose body (*straight arrow*) in the joint space. The radiolucent defect surrounded by the sclerotic zone (*curved arrows*) in the weight-bearing portion of the medial femoral condyle is the donor site of the loose body. (*continued*)

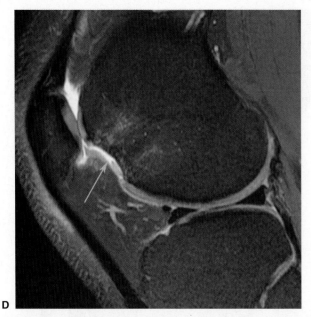

D

FIGURE 6.72. (*Continued*) **D:** Sagittal fat-suppressed T2-weighted MRI. Note the defect in the trochlea (*arrow*). The loose body is in the suprapatellar bursa and not included on this image.

FIGURE 6.73. Left femur frog-leg **(A)** and true **(B)** lateral radiographs. Transverse fracture of the femur in a 26-year-old automobile accident victim. There is apex anterior angulation. Note how the fracture fragments can change when the patient is moved. Displacement is posterior in the frog-leg lateral but was anterior on the true lateral. The patient is supine and the x-ray beam horizontal on the true lateral.

dislocations of the hip are much more frequent than anterior. Occasionally, dislocations are not visible on a single anterior radiographs and CT becomes rather important since prompt reduction of hip dislocation is imperative to minimize the likelihood of AVN of the femoral head. CT is also quite useful in the assessment of complex pelvic and acetabular fractures.

In the United States, 3.3 million reports of abuse involving 6 million children are made each year and 5 children die per day as a result of abuse. Boys and girls are affected equally. Injury to the bones is the most common form of injury with physical abuse with fractures documented in 11% to 55% of cases. Although 80% of child abuse deaths are secondary to head injuries, nonaccidental trauma can involve all parts of the skeletal system. An appropriate workup for suspected abuse includes a radiographic survey of the long bones, pelvis, spine, ribs, and skull. Bone scanning may also be useful if clinical suspicion remains high with normal radiographs.

The metaphyseal fractures (classical metaphyseal lesion [CML]) demonstrated in Figure 6.79A are typical of

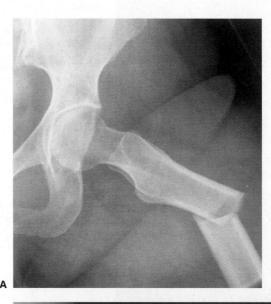

A

B

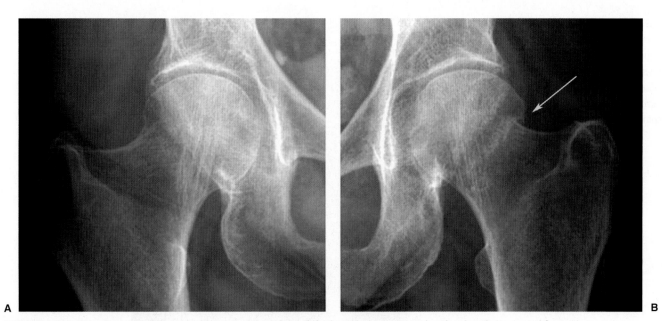

FIGURE 6.74. AP radiograph of the right **(A)** and of the left hip **(B)**. The right hip is normal and makes the impacted femoral neck fracture on the left (*arrow*) more readily apparent.

the findings in some child abuse cases and these metaphyseal fractures are probably due to a twisting mechanism. Subperiosteal hemorrhage on a radiograph is another twisting type of injury that should make you highly suspicious of nonaccidental trauma (Fig. 6.79B). Bucket-handle fractures (see Fig. 6.38C) are also associated with abuse. Skeletal injuries and fractures that should make the

observer highly suspicious for nonaccidental trauma are summarized in Table 6.9, and the common child abuse fracture sites outside the skull are shown in Table 6.10. Suspicious findings must be differentiated from normal periostitis found in infancy, osteogenesis imperfecta, congenital insensitivity to pain, and metabolic and vitamin deficiency disorders.

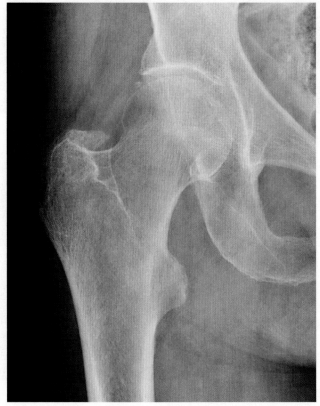

FIGURE 6.75. **A:** Right hip radiograph was interpreted as normal. With persistent clinical suspicion for fracture MR was obtained. **B:** Coronal T1-weighted MR of the pelvis reveals the nondisplaced right intertrochanteric fracture. The entire pelvis is imaged because the hip pain may be due to occult hip fracture, sacral or pubic rami fractures, or a soft tissue injury.

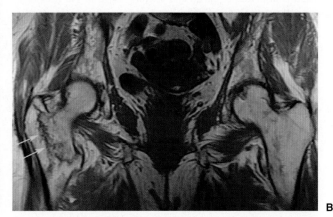

FIGURE 6.76. AP radiograph **(A)** of the left hip was interpreted as normal. This avid runner complained of persistent pain and an MR was obtained. Coronal fat-suppressed T2-weighted image **(B)** demonstrates edema (*white*) around the developing stress fracture (*arrow*). Left untreated, this might well progress to a complete fracture.

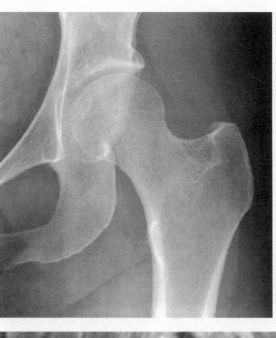

A

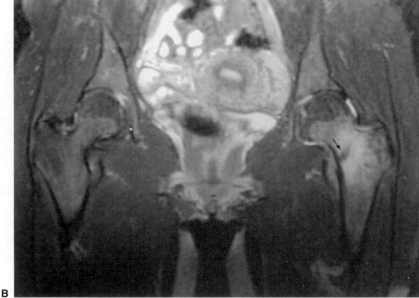

B

FIGURE 6.77. Pelvis AP radiograph. Posterior dislocation of the left hip without fracture secondary to a motor vehicle accident. The left femoral head is displaced cephalad and lateral relative to the acetabulum (*arrows*). The right hip is normal and makes an excellent comparison.

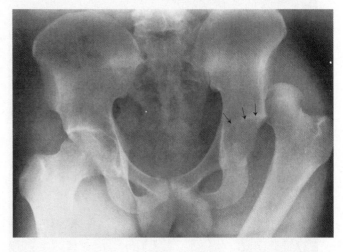

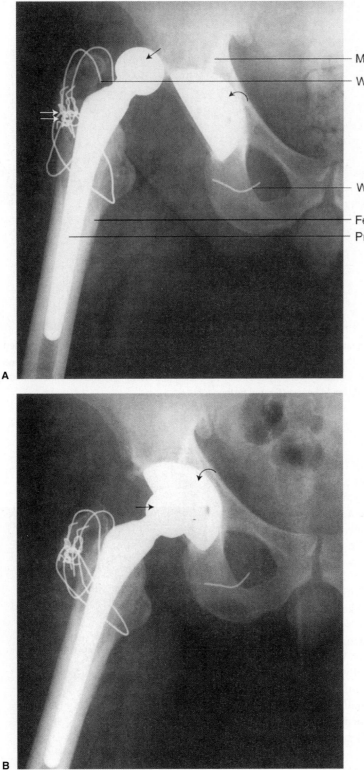

— Metallic screw
— Wire fracture

— Wire fragment

— Femur shaft
— Prosthesis stem

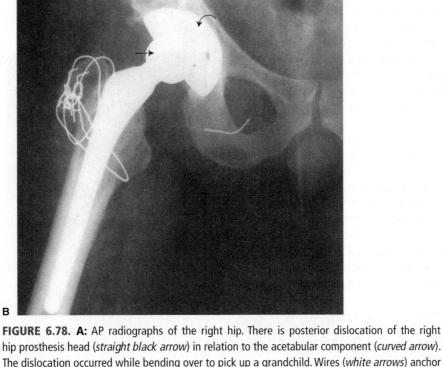

FIGURE 6.78. **A:** AP radiographs of the right hip. There is posterior dislocation of the right hip prosthesis head (*straight black arrow*) in relation to the acetabular component (*curved arrow*). The dislocation occurred while bending over to pick up a grandchild. Wires (*white arrows*) anchor the greater trochanter to the femur and at least one of the wires is fractured. A fragment of loose wire lies inferior to the prosthesis acetabular component. **B:** Following closed reduction (no surgery) under general anesthesia, the prosthetic head has been returned to its proper position relative to the acetabular prosthetic component.

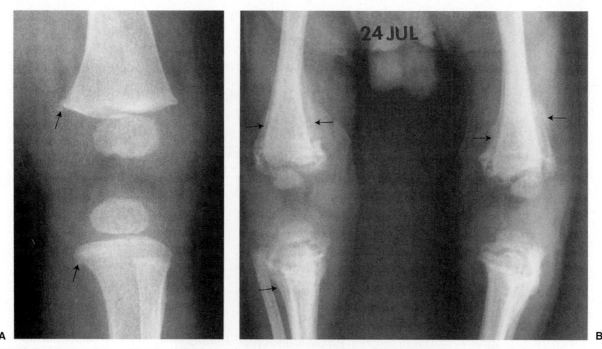

A   B

FIGURE 6.79. **A:** Left knee AP radiograph. Metaphyseal corner fractures (*arrows*). This battered child complained of knee pain and had an obvious limp. **B:** Right and left lower extremities radiograph. Subperiosteal hemorrhage. The *arrows* indicate the appearance of blood beneath the periosteum secondary to severe squeezing and twisting of the extremities. This appearance is highly suspicious for child abuse and should be investigated further.

Soft Tissue Injury

One of the most common injuries of the lower extremity is the sprained ankle. A sprain is simply an injury to a ligament around the ankle (or any other joint) and it varies in severity from a stretching of the ligament to a partial tear to a complete disruption. Ankle sprains usually result from a turning or twisting of the ankle joint while walking or running. When the foot turns outward, there is an eversion or abduction injury. When the foot turns inward, there is an inversion or adduction injury. Sprains occur with and without associated fractures. Note the tiny chip-like fracture at the ligamentous attachment is considered a "sprain equivalent" and treated more like a sprain than a fracture. A dramatic example of a severe sprain is demonstrated in Figure 6.80.

Because ankle sprains are usually treated by casting in the United States, MRI is not commonly used to image ankle sprains, and the imaging usually is limited to radiographs; an exception is high-performance athletes as the time off from his or her sport may be determined by the

Table 6.9
Osseous Injuries Suspicious for Child Abuse

Corner fractures
Periosteal hemorrhage
Bucket-handle fractures
Multiple fractures of varying ages

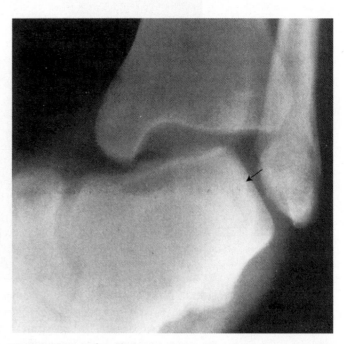

FIGURE 6.80. Left ankle inversion stress AP radiograph. Severe ankle sprain. The talus dome is tilted laterally (*arrow*) secondary to disruption of the lateral collateral ligament in an inversion or adduction injury. There are no fractures.

Table 6.10

Common Fracture Sites in Abused Children

Lower extremity: Femur (most common), tibia
Elbow
Shoulder
Ribs

severity of injury. However, in the general population, MRI of the ankle is used for specific problems such as Achilles tendon tears and confusing clinical presentations of ankle pain. The Achilles tendon or calcaneal tendon is a common injury site (Fig. 6.81). This injury can result from violent sport activities or simply stepping in a hole, and the diagnosis usually is made by the history of acute, sharp pain in the Achilles tendon. When there is a complete tear or disruption of the Achilles tendon, physical examination often shows pinpoint tenderness at the site of injury and inability to plantarflex the foot. An MRI is often requested to confirm a clinical diagnosis or suspicion and evaluate the degree of separation or gap in the tendon. This will aid in the decision for casting versus surgical intervention. Alternatively, ultrasound has also been used to evaluate the Achilles tendon (Fig. 6.82).

Injuries to muscles are often diagnosed clinically. Some muscular injuries may require further evaluation—frequently using MRI, typical of these are muscle avulsions or tears of the hamstring (Fig. 6.83) or pectoralis muscles. A muscle may also tear in its body. The extent of this intramuscular tear and hematoma is particularly important to the elite athlete since length of rehabilitation

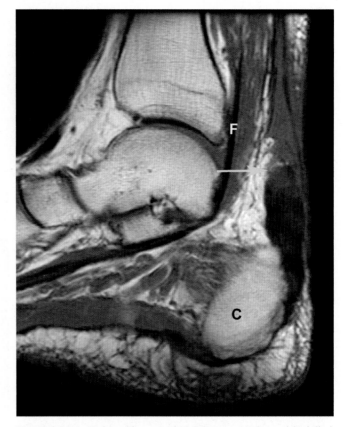

FIGURE 6.81. Right ankle sagittal T1 MR image. Calcaneal (Achilles) tendon tear (*arrow*). Note the disruption and balling up of the distal portion of the tendon. The tear is about 2 cm proximal to the calcaneal attachment—a typical location. C, calcaneus; F, flexor hallucis longus.

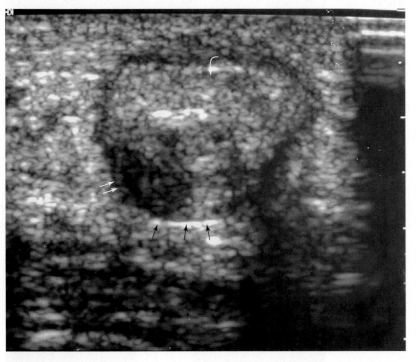

FIGURE 6.82. Transverse ultrasound image of an Achilles tendon. Partial tear. Posterior is at the top of the image. The normal portion of the tendon is echogenic (*curved arrow*). The anterior portion, which is normally flat or concave, is rounded (*straight black arrows*) and has low echogenicity (*white arrows*) due to edema and blood.

FIGURE 6.83. A: AP radiograph of the pelvis shows a partial avulsion at the hamstring origin on the right ischium (*arrow*). Note the asymmetry from the other side. **B:** Coronal plane fat-suppressed T2-weighted MR image at the plane of the ischial tuberosities in a different patient. The bright signal in the left posterior thigh is edema and blood surrounding the tear of the biceps femoris muscle of the hamstrings (*arrow*).

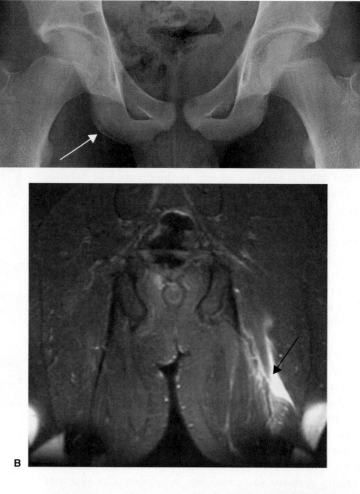

FIGURE 6.84. AP radiograph of the left hip. Following placement of an intramedullary nail for the developing fracture in the lateral shaft of the proximal femur, bone has developed in the soft tissues in the surgical bed termed heterotopic ossification (*arrows*).

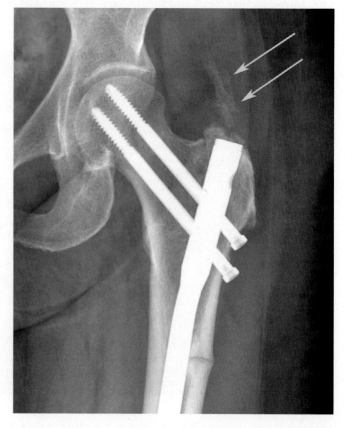

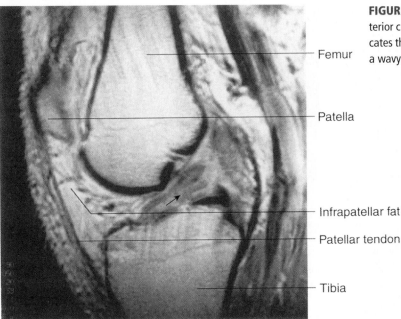

Femur

Patella

Infrapatellar fat

Patellar tendon

Tibia

FIGURE 6.85. Right knee sagittal proton-density MR image. Anterior cruciate ligament tear in a 41-year-old man. The arrow indicates the site of the anterior cruciate ligament tear manifested by a wavy high-intensity (*white*) signal.

and long-term prognosis are affected by the severity of the muscular injury. Following injury to muscles there may be subsequent calcification and/or ossification at the injury site called *myositis ossificans*, now more commonly termed *heterotopic ossification*. Common locations include the quadriceps and brachialis muscles and near the hip following hip surgery (Fig. 6.84).

MRI is a wonderful imaging tool for evaluating cartilage, menisci, tendons, and ligaments in and around the knee and other joints. Usually the radiographs are negative in such injuries, but based on the physical findings and the patient's symptoms, an MR image is requested for a more definitive evaluation of these soft tissue structures (Figs. 6.85–6.90).

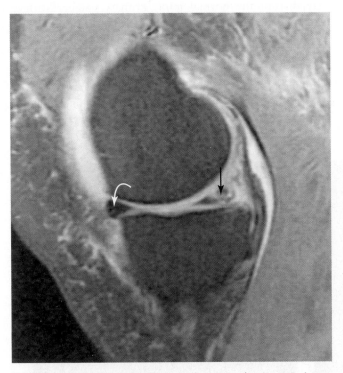

FIGURE 6.86. Sagittal fat-suppressed, proton-density MR image through medial meniscus. Tear of the posterior horn in a 45-year-old woman. The high-intensity signal (*straight arrow*) likely represents edema and synovial fluid within the tear. The anterior horn of the meniscus (*curved arrow*) is normal.

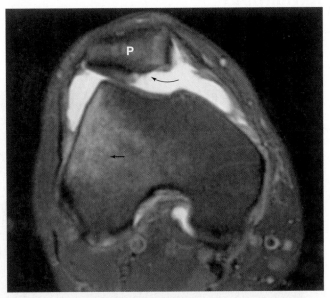

FIGURE 6.87. Axial fat-suppressed T2 MR right knee following patellar dislocation. The patella (P) is laterally subluxated: It should closely articulate with the trochlea of the femur. There is edema of the lateral femur (*straight arrow*) where the patella impacted. A cartilage defect (*curved arrow*) was created in the patella during the dislocation or relocation.

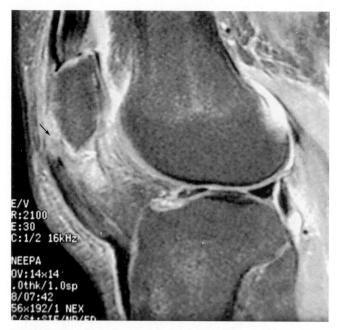

FIGURE 6.88. Sagittal proton-density MR right knee. Patellar tendon tear. There is disruption of the patellar tendon (ligament) at its patellar attachment (*arrow*).

Many foreign bodies in soft tissue and bone are radiopaque and readily identified on radiographs (Fig. 6.91A,B). Occasionally, a nonopaque foreign body in an extremity is suspected. If a foreign body is not visible on a radiograph, an ultrasound, CT, or MR study can be requested to assist in the detection and location of the foreign body (Fig. 6.91C).

ARTHRITIDES

Osteoarthritis

Osteoarthritis (degenerative arthritis) is the most common form of arthritis. You can categorize osteoarthritis into two

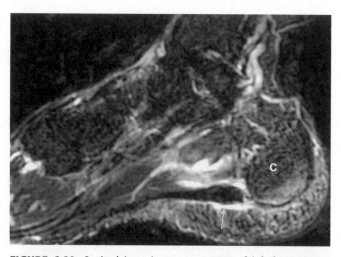

FIGURE 6.89. Sagittal inversion recovery MRI of left foot. Plantar fasciitis. The plantar fascia is thickened (*arrow*) and has surrounding edema (*white*). Mild edema is also seen in the adjacent calcaneus (*C*).

types. Secondary osteoarthritis, or degenerative joint disease, can occur at all ages but tends to appear with increasing age as a result of wearing-out processes. It may involve almost all of the joints of the extremities and spine (Figs. 6.92–6.94) but favors the DIP joints and thumb–carpometacarpal joint in the hands, hips, and knees. In younger individuals, secondary arthritis may result from trauma, infection, or any other process that may disrupt the normal joint. Primary osteoarthritis is probably familial and involves the DIP joints of the hands, the first metacarpal–carpal joint, and the hips. Another frequent location of arthritis is the great toe (metatarsophalangeal [MTP]) joint. A bunion may develop from a familial predisposition or related to shoe wear, particularly high heels. The apex at the MTP joint is displaced medial and becomes a prominent bulge along the medial side of the foot. Overlying soft tissue irritation may develop or

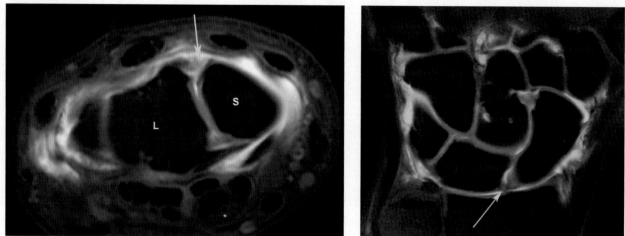

FIGURE 6.90. MR arthrogram. Axial **(A)** and coronal **(B)** fat-suppressed T1-weighted MRI of the right wrist after the injection of MR contrast into the radiocarpal joint. There is a partial tear of the dorsal (posterior) aspect of the scapholunate ligament (*arrow*) allowing contrast (*white*) to enter the midcarpal joint. *S,* scaphoid; *L,* lunate; *,* median nerve.

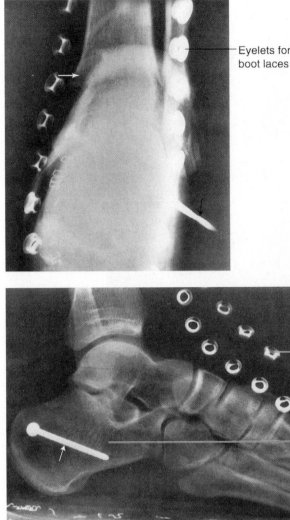

Eyelets for
boot laces

FIGURE 6.91. Left foot AP **(A)** and lateral **(B)** radiographs taken through the boot. Metallic nail (*arrows*) piercing the boot and lodged in the calcaneus. The nail was driven into its present location by a power tool. **C:** Left foot axial T2 MR image. Foreign body (*straight arrow*) in a different patient. The site of the foreign body entry wound (*curved arrow*) is marked by the white pill containing oil. The foreign body tract (*double arrows*) is white, probably because it is filled with edema, blood, granulation tissue, or inflammatory cells.

Eyelet for boot laces

Calcaneus

Boot sole

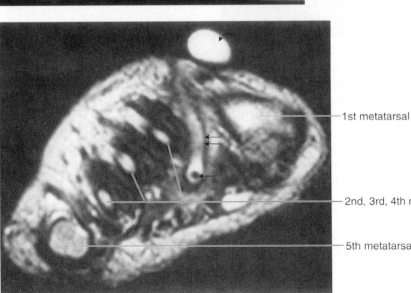

1st metatarsal

2nd, 3rd, 4th metatarsals

5th metatarsal

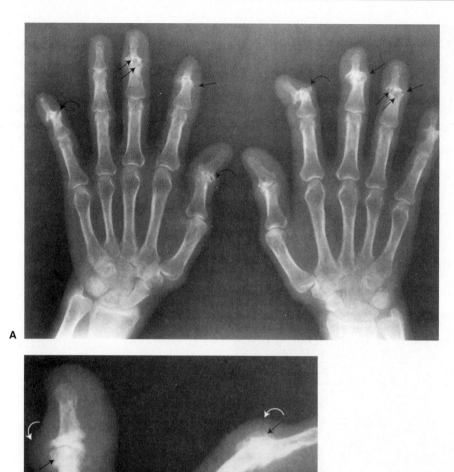

FIGURE 6.92. A: Right- and left-hand PA radiograph. Osteoarthritis or erosive osteoarthritis. This 63-year-old woman worked as a typist for 20 years. Note the advanced osteoarthritic changes (*single straight arrows*) involving the distal interphalangeal (DIP) joints of both hands. The DIP joints are markedly narrowed and osteophytes (*curved arrows*) are present. Erosions are also present (*double straight arrows*). **B:** Left index and long finger lateral radiograph. Osteoarthritis DIP joints. For many years this 60-year-old woman operated an adding machine with her left hand. There is narrowing of the DIP joint spaces due to articular cartilage destruction. There are soft tissue prominences (*white arrows*) overlying bone excrescences near the DIP joints. These bone excrescences or protuberances are called Heberden nodes (*black arrows*).

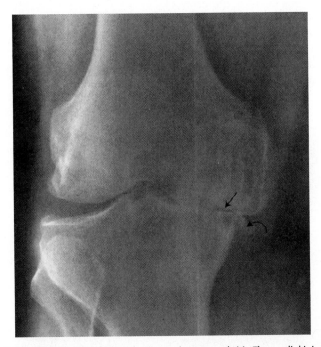

FIGURE 6.93. Right knee AP radiograph. Osteoarthritis. The medial joint space or medial knee compartment is markedly narrowed, the articular surfaces are irregular (*straight arrow*), osteophyte formation (*curved arrow*) is present, and there is varus deformity. Note that the medial joint space has all but disappeared compared to the lateral joint space.

osteoarthritis may result from the now incongruent joint (Fig. 6.95).

The radiograph is the primary tool for evaluating osteoarthritis as well as all other arthritides. Some important facts and radiographic findings of osteoarthritis are listed in Table 6.11 and include asymmetric, irregular joint narrowing because of articular cartilage destruction, osteosclerosis, and osteophyte formation. When advanced osteoarthritis involves the medial knee compartment, a genu varus deformity or bowed leg usually results. Advanced osteoarthritis in the lateral knee compartment often results in a genu valgus deformity or knock-knee appearance. When advanced osteoarthritis involves the hip, the femoral head migrates cephalad because of asymmetric cartilage destruction, whereas in rheumatoid arthritis the femoral head tends to drift centrally from uniform cartilage loss. Acetabular protrusion may result from softening of the bones due to osteoporosis.

Rheumatoid Arthritis

Rheumatoid is another type of arthritis that is frequently encountered in the everyday practice of medicine. It is an inflammatory arthritis of unknown etiology that involves synovial joints and is characterized by symmetric joint narrowing secondary to articular cartilage destruction by pannus, which is a granulation tissue derived from the

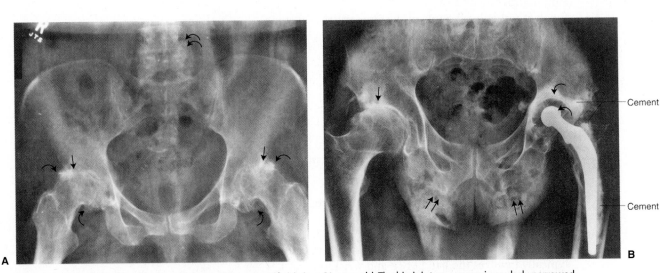

FIGURE 6.94. **A:** Pelvis AP radiograph. Bilateral hip osteoarthritis in a 61-year-old. The hip joint spaces are irregularly narrowed and the femoral heads are typically migrating in a cephalad direction (*straight arrows*). The femoral heads are cystic and sclerotic in appearance. Osteophyte formation is present along the periphery of the joints (*single curved arrows*). Osteophyte formation is also present in the lower lumbar spine (*double curved arrows*). **B:** Pelvis AP radiograph. Osteoarthritis of the right hip, left hip prosthesis, and bilateral inguinal hernias. There is irregular narrowing of the right hip joint and cephalad migration of the femoral head (*single straight arrow*). A left hip prosthesis is in place. The *curved arrows* indicate the prosthetic femoral head and acetabular components. Large bilateral inguinal hernias contain air-filled loops of bowel (*double straight arrows*).

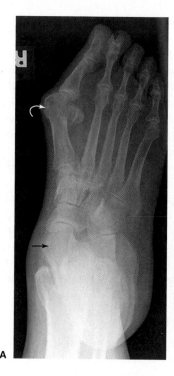

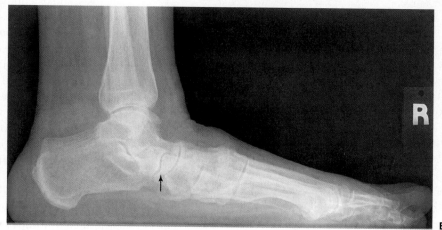

FIGURE 6.95. Anterior **(A)** and lateral **(B)** radiographs of the right foot in a 64-year-old woman. Hallux valgus. The head of the first metatarsal is uncovered as the great toe is directed laterally (*white arrow*). The great toe is also pronated and the sesamoids of the first metatarsal are subluxated laterally. This person also has a flat foot deformity (pes planus). The head of the talus is directed medially and plantar (*black arrows*).

A

B

Table 6.11

Typical Symptoms and Radiographic Findings in Osteoarthritis and Rheumatoid Arthritis

Osteoarthritis

Pain, deformity, and limitation of joint motion

Pain improves with rest

Involves virtually all joints of the extremities and spine

Typically involves the hand distal interphalangeal (DIP) joints and the first carpometacarpal (CMC) joint

Asymmetric joint narrowing

Sclerotic bone changes

Cysts or pseudocysts

Osteophyte formation

Usually absence of osteoporosis

Genu valgus and varus deformities (knees)

Cephalad and sometimes lateral migration of the femoral head

Rheumatoid Arthritis

Pain, stiffness, and limitation of motion, especially in the hands and feet, worse in the morning

Pain improves with activity

Involves all synovial joints of the extremities and spine

Typically involves the hand MCP and wrist joints

Symmetric joint narrowing (both within a joint and side-to-side)

Periarticular osteoporosis (prominent feature)

Periarticular soft tissue thickening and swelling

Marginal osseous erosions

MCP joint subluxation and ulnar deviation

Medial migration of the femoral head and acetabular protrusio

Pencil tip appearance of the distal clavicle

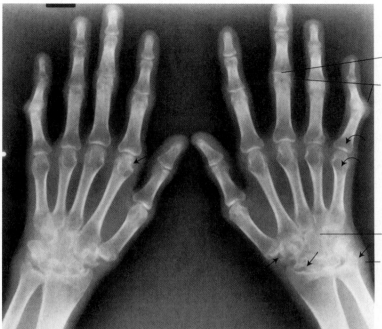

— Narrowed PIP joints

— Fusiform soft tissue changes

— Narrowed carpal joints

— Ulnar soft tissue prominence

FIGURE 6.96. Right- and left-hand PA radiograph. Rheumatoid arthritis. The radiographic findings include peri-articular osteoporosis (*curved arrows*), swan neck deformities of the little fingers, narrowing of the proximal interphalangeal (PIP) joints with associated fusiform soft tissue swelling, narrowing of the carpal and PIP joints, and soft tissue thickening or prominence around the distal ulna. Also, there are erosions involving the carpals, ulnar styloids, and metacarpal heads (*straight arrows*). The fusiform soft tissue swelling surrounding the joints represents edema and effusion. The soft tissue prominence around the distal ulna is secondary to edema and thickening around the external carpi ulnaris.

synovium. Some important facts and radiographic findings associated with rheumatoid arthritis are listed in Table 6.11. As in osteoarthritis, any or all of the joints in the extremities and spine can be involved. The most commonly affected joints, in decreasing frequency, are the MCP, wrist, PIP, knee, MTP, shoulder, ankle, cervical spine, hip, elbow, and temporomandibular joints. Often the initial symptoms of rheumatoid arthritis are stiffness, pain, limitation of movement, and swelling in the hands and/or feet. Usually, the first joints involved are the metacarpal and metatarsal phalangeal joints and this tends to be symmetric right to left. Radiographs are the standard modality in its evaluation and monitoring of progression, however, MRI can assess soft tissue changes before any radiographic abnormality (Figs. 6.96–6.100). Potentially, the earliest abnormality detectable on a radiograph is periarticular soft tissue thickening. Additional radiographic findings include periarticular osteoporosis due to hyperemia, symmetric joint narrowing, and marginal erosions. As the disease progresses, joint deformity may develop due to subluxation and ulnar deviation of the fingers at the MCP joints. This later finding is quite characteristic of rheumatoid arthritis. Despite far advanced cartilage destruction, true bone ankylosis is uncommon.

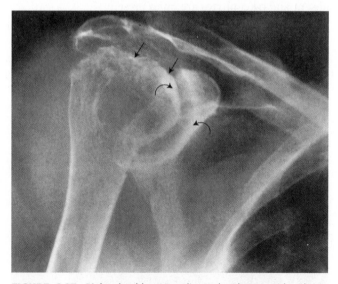

FIGURE 6.97. Right shoulder AP radiograph. Rheumatoid arthritis. There is characteristic osteoporosis, a pointed distal clavicle, and mild cephalad drift of the humeral head. The cephalad drift of the humeral head suggests rotator cuff damage that is common in this disease. There are articular bone erosions (*straight arrows*) and sclerosis (*curved arrows*). The sclerosis may be from some secondary osteoarthritis that may develop after cartilage loss when the inflammation from rheumatoid arthritis is quiescent.

FIGURE 6.98. Right and left knee AP radiograph. Rheumatoid arthritis in a 27-year-old. There are symmetric narrowing of the knee joints (*straight arrows*), periarticular cysts (*curved arrows*), erosions (*double arrows*), and osteoporosis.

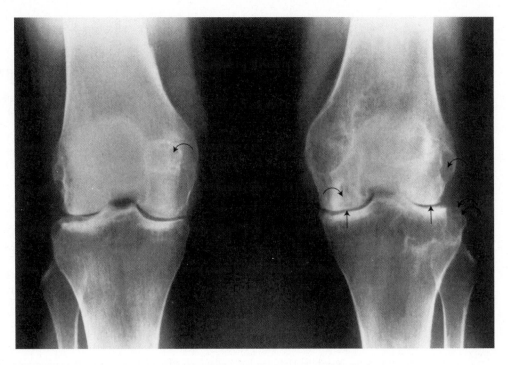

The differential diagnosis of rheumatoid arthritis as shown in Table 6.12 includes gout and infection. In gout, osteoporosis is usually absent, and articular and juxta-articular erosions are more sharply defined. In osteomyelitis and infectious arthritis, the osteoporosis is greatest near the infection site. In osteoarthritis, osteoporosis is usually absent and osteophytes are often present.

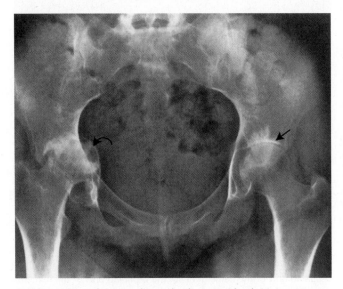

FIGURE 6.99. Pelvis AP radiograph. Rheumatoid arthritis in a 27-year-old. There is generalized osteoporosis. The entire left hip joint space is symmetrically narrowed (*straight arrow*). There is characteristic medial drift of the right femoral head and acetabular protrusio (*curved arrow*). Note that the sacroiliac joints are not involved in this patient.

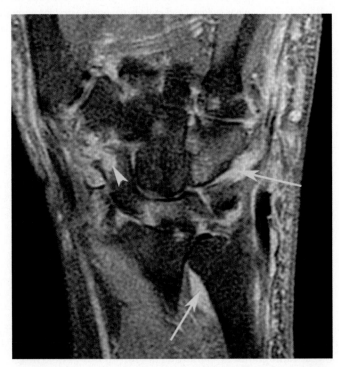

FIGURE 6.100. Coronal fat-suppressed T2-weighted MR of the wrist in a patient with rheumatoid arthritis. The wrist joints are distended, but the higher signal is not the bright white of fluid (see Figs. 6.86 and 6.87). This is synovial thickening/pannus formation *(arrows)* and may lead to erosions *(arrowhead)*. Also compare the cartilage loss in this patient with the normal cartilage in the wrist in Figure 6.90. The bones, particularly the hamate and the lunate have higher signal, likely due to edema.

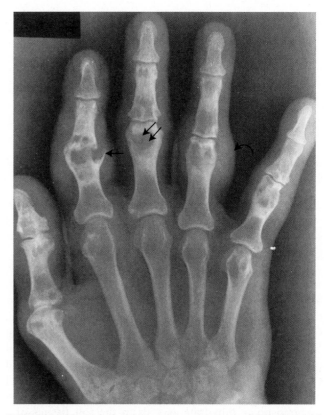

FIGURE 6.102. Right-hand PA radiograph. Gout arthritis. The proximal interphalangeal (PIP) joint spaces are at least partially preserved and the lucent areas (*double arrows*) are typical of the sharply marginated periarticular erosions. Erosions that extend into the joint often have an overhanging edge (*single straight arrow*). Note the classic appearance of a tophus (*curved arrow*). A tophus is an asymmetric swelling about the joint that may or may not be calcified.

Table 6.12

The Differential Diagnosis of Rheumatoid Arthritis

Gouty arthritis
Infectious arthritis
Sudeck atrophy
Psoriatic arthritis
Osteoarthritis
Ankylosing spondylitis
Scleroderma
Systemic lupus erythematosus

Psoriatic Arthritis

Psoriatic arthritis is found in 2% to 6% of patients with skin manifestations of psoriasis although the vast majority of those with psoriatic arthritis have had a long history of psoriatic skin disease and particularly associated with psoriatic nail changes. There are five clinical spectra of the arthritis: (1) Polyarthritis with DIP joint involvement; (2) a markedly deforming condition (arthritis mutilans) with widespread joint destruction and ankylosis (fusion across joints); (3) symmetric arthritis resembling rheumatoid arthritis; (4) single or asymmetric, few joint involvement (pauciarticular); and (5) sacroiliitis and spondylitis, which may resemble ankylosing spondylitis. The arthritis is characterized by involvement of small joints with asymmetric distribution. There are bone erosions, but, unlike rheumatoid arthritis, there is more frequent ankylosis. Bony proliferation adjacent to joints and at muscle and tendon attachment sites is characteristic (Fig. 6.101).

Gout, Pseudogout, and Hemophilic Arthritis

Some arthritides that are associated with metabolic diseases and blood dyscrasias are listed in Table 6.13. Gout arthritis (Fig. 6.102) is secondary to hyperuricemia or elevated serum uric acid levels. The patients classically present with podagra or pain and inflammatory changes near the medial aspect of the first MTP joint. While the

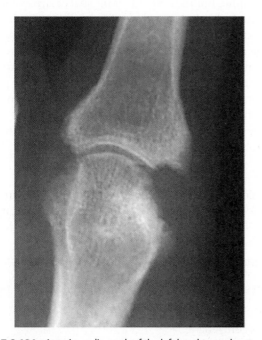

FIGURE 6.101. Anterior radiograph of the left hand second metacarpal–phalangeal joint. There are joint space narrowing and small erosions with a fluffy proliferation of new bone at the joint margins typical of psoriatic arthritis.

Table 6.13

Arthritides Associated with Metabolic Diseases and Blood Dyscrasias

Gout
Calcium pyrophosphate deposition (CPPD) disease
Hemophilia

Table 6.14

Radiographic Features of Gout

Sharply marginated and sometimes sclerotic-bordered erosions with overhanging edges near a joint
Tophus formation (paste-like calcium urate within the soft tissues) or soft tissue nodules
Normal bone mineralization
Occasionally joint deformity

Table 6.15

Causes of Chondrocalcinosis

Calcium pyrophosphate deposition (CPPD)
Hemochromatosis
Aging
Hyperparathyroidism and hypercalcemia

disease is characterized by numerous exacerbations and remissions, the disease usually is present for a number of years before it is detectable on a radiograph; the radiographic findings of gout are listed in Table 6.14.

Chondrocalcinosis means calcification of cartilage and it is most often noted in the knee. It can affect both fibro- and hyaline cartilage, with calcification in fibrocartilage more frequently related to aging and degeneration. Chondrocalcinosis can be associated with a number of conditions that are listed in Table 6.15. The arthritis of calcium pyrophosphate deposition (CPPD), or the clinical exacerbation termed pseudogout, is found in middle-aged or older people and is caused by the deposition of calcium pyrophosphate dihydrate crystals in the soft tissues of a joint, including menisci, ligaments, articular cartilage, and the joint capsule (Fig. 6.103).

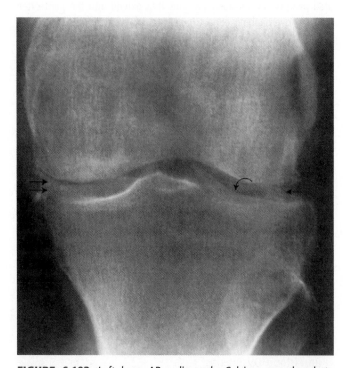

FIGURE 6.103. Left knee AP radiograph. Calcium pyrophosphate deposition (CPPD) disease or pseudogout. There are calcifications in the lateral meniscus (*single straight arrow*) and the medial meniscus (*double straight arrows*). There is also calcification of the articular cartilage (*curved arrow*).

The joints in patients with hemophilia are gradually injured by repeated bleeding into the joints. Cystic changes develop in the bones neighboring the injured joints and osteoporosis is a common feature (Fig. 6.104). During childhood and adolescence, there may be overgrowth of bones near joints related to hyperemia. In general, osteoporosis is a common feature in rheumatoid arthritis, blood dyscrasias, and osteomyelitis but not in osteoarthritis and gout. But remember that osteoporosis is common by itself and may be present in addition to, though not related to osteoarthritis and gout.

Neuropathic Joints

Chronic trauma to a joint that has lost pain sensation can result in a neuropathic or Charcot joint (Fig. 6.105). Some common causes are shown in Table 6.16. Diabetic neuropathic joints are most common in the lower extremity, whereas syringomyelia-related neuropathic joints are usually found in the shoulders and upper extremities. The radiographic findings include joint space narrowing, fragmentation of sclerotic subchondral bone, articular bone cortex destruction, joint loose bodies, and bone mass formation at the articular margins. Some of the neuropathic joint findings are similar to those found in osteoarthritis. It is generally not true that patients do not feel pain in their neuropathic joints; rather, the degree of pain is disproportionate to the amount of damage. In other words, just because a patient complains of joint pain, the underlying problem may be a neuropathic joint.

Other

Periarticular calcifications can result from acute and chronic trauma (Fig. 6.106). Although they do not involve joints, bone spurs are sometimes considered a form of

Table 6.16

Causes of Neuropathic or Charcot Joints

Diabetes mellitus
Syringomyelia
Meningomyelocele
Peripheral nerve injury
Congenital indifference to pain

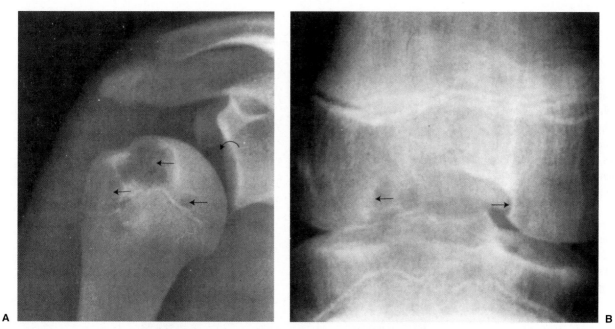

A   B

FIGURE 6.104. A: Right shoulder AP radiograph. Hemophilia in a 15-year-old boy. There are cystic changes (*straight arrows*) in the humeral head secondary to repeated bleeds and there is widening of the shoulder joint (*curved arrow*) due to hemarthrosis. **B:** Knee AP radiograph. Hemophilia in the same patient as in **A**. He has a widened intercondylar notch (*arrows*) secondary to repeated episodes of hemarthrosis. There is osteoporosis.

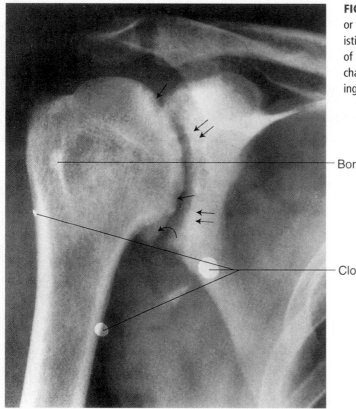

Bone island

Clothing artifacts

A

FIGURE 6.105. A: Right shoulder AP radiograph. Neuropathic joint or Charcot joint in a patient with syringomyelia. There is characteristic irregularity of the articular surfaces secondary to destruction of the bone and joint cartilage (*single arrows*). There are sclerotic changes or increased density (*double arrows*) of the bone surrounding the joint and an osteophyte (*curved arrow*). (*continued*)

FIGURE 6.105. (*Continued*) **B:** Oblique radiograph of the left foot in a diabetic person. Neuropathic joints. There are healed fracture deformities of the meta-tarsal heads (*arrows*). The great toe has been amputated because of infection. Note the destruction of the fifth meta-tarsal head (*curved arrow*) and adjacent ulcer (*double arrow*) from current osteo-myelitis. **C:** Anterior views of the knees in a patient without specific trauma. There is a depressed fracture of the right tibial plateau (*arrow*). The left proximal tibial has a metaphyseal fracture with some sclerosis, which indicates there has been some healing and likely some persistent motion. The patient's mild pain was disproportionate to the appearance of the fractures.

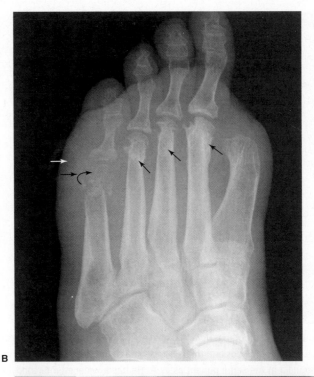

B

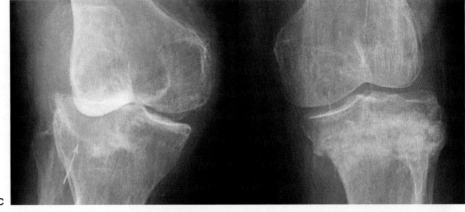

C

FIGURE 6.106. Left shoulder AP radiograph with the humerus in external rotation. Calcific tendinitis. There is dystrophic calcification (*arrow*) in the region of the supraspinatus tendon.

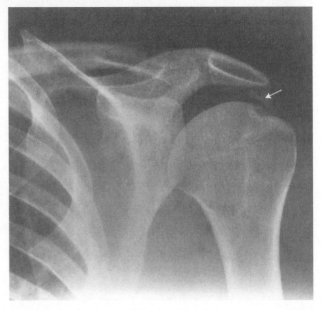

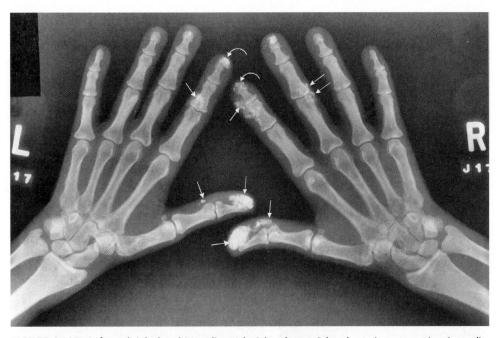

FIGURE 6.107. Left- and right-hand PA radiograph. Scleroderma. Scleroderma is a connective tissue disease that may involve the musculoskeletal system. There are soft tissue calcifications (*straight arrows*) and the soft tissues at the tip of the fingers are atrophic (*curved arrows*). The joints are normal.

arthritis. Bone spurs, which typically occur at tendon or ligament attachments, may cause pain and be clinically difficult to differentiate from arthritis. Also, bursitis may cause periarticular pain and can sometimes be demonstrated radiographically if the bursal distension can be identified, such as the olecranon bursa at the elbow. Scleroderma is a connective tissue disorder that potentially involves the musculoskeletal system. Multiple soft tissue calcifications are commonly seen in these patients (Fig. 6.107). Other radiographic changes in scleroderma include atrophy of the fingertips and loss of bone at the tips of the distal phalanges. If joint changes are present, they may simulate rheumatoid arthritis.

TUMORS

Benign

There are a number of benign bone lesions and it is important to recognize them as such (Table 6.17). A bone island, or enostosis, is the most common bone lesion. It is essentially cortical bone that is found in the medullary cavity and appears as a small sclerotic focus. It blends with the surrounding trabeculae and has no aggressive features (see Figs. 6.14 and 6.107D). Fibrous cortical defects or nonossifying fibroma may appear similar to an enostosis in adults but are closely related to the cortex. These are fibroosseous lesions that are lucent and may expand the cortex in children and adolescents. They are typically small and found incidentally but are occasionally large and may focally weaken the cortex where fractures may occur. They heal or involute as the child matures with a resultant sclerotic area

that may appear as an area of cortical thickening (Fig. 6.108). An osteochondroma or osteocartilaginous exostosis is a common benign bone lesion, which can occur in nearly all bones. They are bony projections of the cortical surface of a bone with a cartilage cap and are most commonly found in the metaphysis of long bones, especially around the knee and shoulder. These lesions can result in bone deformities and/or cause pressure on surrounding structures. The cartilaginous cap of osteochondromas undergoes malignant transformation to chondrosarcoma in less than 1% of the cases. Multiple osteochondromas are seen in familial multiple exostoses a hereditary autosomal-dominant disorder (Fig. 6.109). Growth abnormalities and malignant transformation (5% to 15%) are more common in multiple osteochondromas than in a single osteochondroma. Growth of an osteochondroma in a skeletally mature individual and pain are factors that may make one suspicious of malignant transformation.

A simple benign bone cyst (Fig. 6.110) is commonly found in the metaphysis or metadiaphysis of the proximal humerus and femur, but it can occur in almost any bone. Usually this lesion occurs in patients before the age of 25 years and a common complication is a pathologic fracture. A lucent lesion in an older adult should not be considered a simple bone cyst. However, lucent lesions adjacent to joints with arthritis are likely degenerative cysts or, if large, termed geodes. Another benign bone lesion is the enchondroma (Fig. 6.111A,B). It is a slow-growing cartilaginous tumor usually found in the hand phalanges and in the distal metacarpals. Small calcifications may be present within the lesions, and, occasionally, they may be difficult to

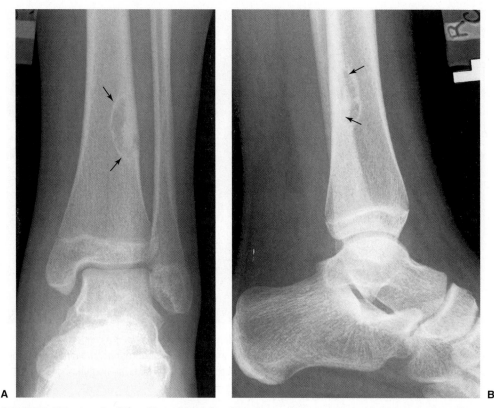

A   **B**

FIGURE 6.108. Anterior **(A)** and lateral **(B)** left ankle radiographs in a 12-year-old girl. Nonossifying fibroma. The bony lesion has a sclerotic margin (*arrows*), is slightly lobulated, and arises from the cortex. This benign fibro-osseous lesion will eventually become sclerotic and appear as a focal area of cortical thickening when she is an adult.

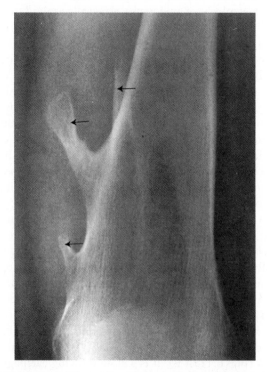

FIGURE 6.109. Left femur AP radiograph. Multiple osteochondromas or familial multiple exostoses. The osteochondromas (*arrows*) point away from the knee joint, simulating a coat hook.

differentiate from bone infarcts. Bone infarcts (Fig. 6.111C) are most frequent in long bones and they may or may not be symptomatic. Bone infarcts (osteonecrosis, AVN) usually have a well-defined and sclerotic border, whereas enchondromas are more likely to have central calcification. Some etiologies of bone infarcts include trauma, steroid use, sickle-cell anemia, renal transplant, therapeutic radiation, and pancreatitis.

Table 6.17
Some Benign Bone Lesions
Bone island
Nonossifying fibroma/fibrous cortical defect
Osteochondroma
Osteoma
Osteoid osteoma
Enchondroma
Bone cyst
Fibrous dysplasia
Chondroblastoma
Osteoblastoma
Hemangioma

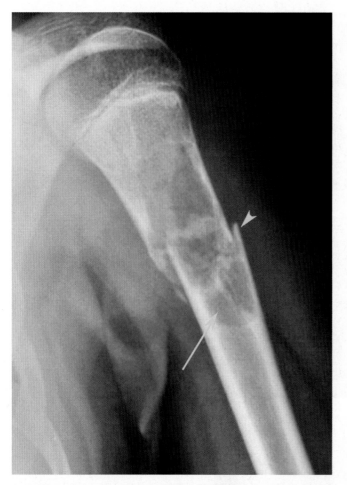

FIGURE 6.110. Left shoulder AP radiograph. Benign cyst (*arrow*) with pathologic fracture in a 10-year-old child. There is mild lateral offset of the distal fracture fragment. Note the thinning of the bone cortex (*arrowhead*) caused by the expanding, benign cyst.

Fibrous dysplasia is a benign fibrous–osseous lesion that arises centrally in the bone, and it can affect one bone (monostotic) or multiple bones (polyostotic). The exact etiology is unknown and these lesions may or may not be symptomatic. The radiographic features include expansive bone lesions, bone cortex thinning, radiolucent lesions of variable density, and pathologic fractures. The differential diagnosis includes Paget disease, hyperparathyroidism, and simple bone cyst.

Osteoid osteoma (Fig. 6.112) is a benign bone lesion of unknown etiology and the typical symptom is night pain relieved by aspirin. It can occur in almost any bone but is most often found in the femoral neck and the tibia. Approximately 75% to 80% of these lesions are intracortical and have multiple radiographic appearances, but the classic appearance is sclerosis surrounding a small radiolucent center or nidus. In some instances, there may be calcifications within this lucent zone mimicking a sequestrum of osteomyelitis. The differential diagnosis would

Table 6.18
Radionuclide Bone Scan to Differentiate Bone Lesions

Positive Bone Scans
Osteoid osteoma
Primary bone tumors
Metastases
Paget disease

Negative (or Nearly Negative) Bone Scans
Multiple myeloma
Bone island
Enchondroma

also include stress fracture, bone island, infection, and metastatic disease.

Osteoid osteoma has intense activity on a radionuclide bone scan (Fig. 6.112B), whereas bone islands have none or very little activity (Table 6.18). CT is usually diagnostic, demonstrating the classic nidus (Fig. 6.112C). MRI may also show the nidus but may be confusing because of the large amount of bone edema surrounding it (Fig. 6.112D).

A chondroblastoma (Fig. 6.113) is an uncommon benign bone lesion found in the epiphysis, usually before skeletal maturity. These radiolucent lesions generally have sclerotic borders and sometimes contain scattered calcifications. The differential diagnosis should include infection, osteoid osteoma, eosinophilic granuloma, and metastatic disease.

Giant cell tumors occur in young adults following skeletal maturity (Fig. 6.114). These lesions are eccentrically located in the end of long bones such as the tibia, femur, radius, and humerus. They usually have sharp nonsclerotic borders without periosteal reaction and usually abut the articular surface. Approximately 15% will recur following simple curettage and packing of the defect. Based on their radiographic appearance, it is difficult to determine whether they are benign or malignant. However, they are rarely malignant and only documentation of distant metastases are considered a reliable radiographic documentation to differentiate malignancy.

Malignant

Metastatic lesions (Fig. 6.115A–C) are the most common malignant bone tumors and represent spread from a wide variety of primary neoplasms. Bone metastases may be single, multiple, osteolytic (radiolucent or black), osteoblastic (white), or mixed. The majority of metastases are osteolytic radiolucent, but osteoblastic metastases frequently result from cancers of the prostate and breast (Table 6.19). A bone island (Fig. 6.115D) should not be confused with an osteoblastic metastatic lesion. Bone islands are benign,

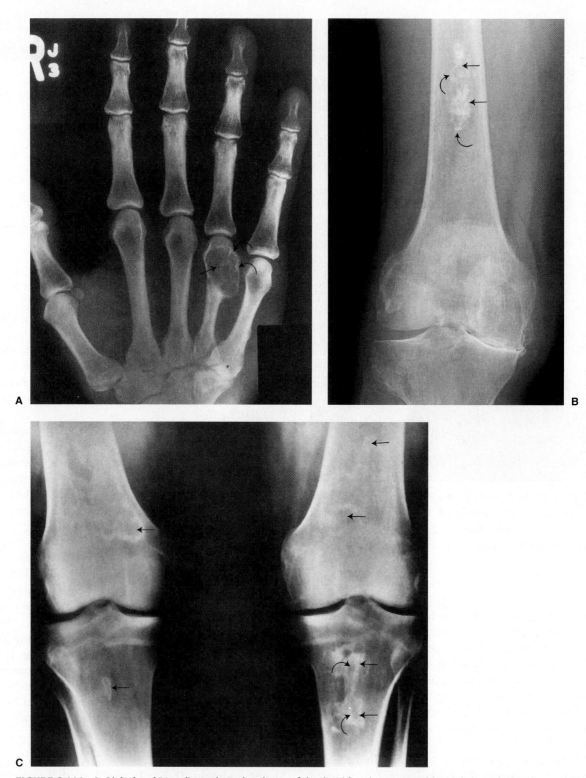

FIGURE 6.111. A: Right-hand PA radiograph. Enchondroma of the distal fourth metacarpal (*straight arrow*). This slow-growing tumor typically causes thinning and scalloping (*curved arrows*) of the inner bone cortex. **B:** Right knee radiograph. Enchondroma. In a large bone, scalloping of the cortex is less common. The calcification of cartilage often appears as small balls (*straight arrows*) or as arcs (*curved arrows*) and rings and occurs in the central part of the lesion. Note osteoarthritis predominantly in the medial compartment of the knee. **C:** Right and left knees AP radiograph. Multiple bone infarcts. The multiple infarcts are manifested by thin zones of sclerosis surrounding lucencies (*straight arrows*) and marrow calcifications (*curved arrows*). The more peripheral calcification pattern helps distinguish infarcts from enchondromas. The etiology in this patient is unknown.

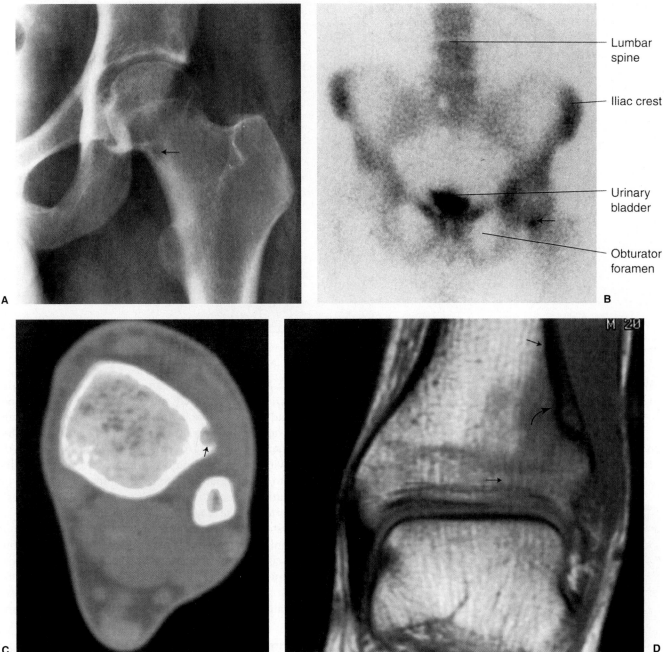

FIGURE 6.112. A: Left hip AP radiograph. Osteoid osteoma in a 20-year-old patient. The patient experienced left hip night pain that was typically relieved by aspirin. The lucent zone (*arrow*) in the inferior aspect of the left femur subcapital region is the osteoid osteoma. **B:** Anterior pelvis radionuclide scan on the same patient. The single area of increased radionuclide uptake (*arrow*) in the left femoral neck corresponds to the radiolucent abnormality visualized in **A.** The bone scan is otherwise normal. Typically, the activity would be much greater, but is less in this patient since the lesion is within the joint. **C:** Axial CT distal tibia. Osteoid osteoma. The cortical lucent nidus (*arrow*) is nicely demonstrated by CT. Rarely, there is a central dot of calcification in the lucency. **D:** Coronal T1 MR in the same patient does not show the nidus as well as CT (*curved arrow*), but the large amount of edema (*gray*) is easy to see (*straight arrows*).

FIGURE 6.113. Right shoulder AP radiograph. Benign chondroblastoma (*straight arrow*) of the proximal humerus epiphysis in a 14-year-old patient. The typical sclerotic border is present (*curved arrows*).

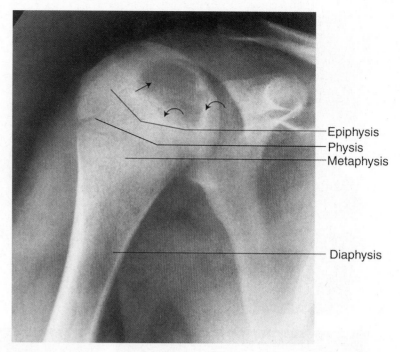

Epiphysis
Physis
Metaphysis

Diaphysis

asymptomatic, and distributed widely and usually sparingly in the skeletal system. Bone islands are essentially cortical bone located in the medullary space.

Multiple myeloma originates in the bone marrow and is the most common primary malignant bone tumor (Table 6.20). The patient usually complains of pain in

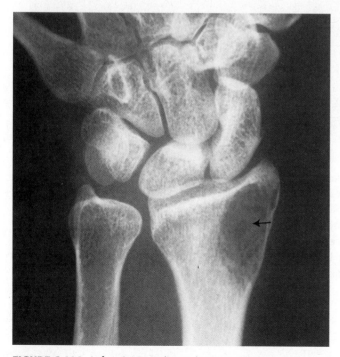

FIGURE 6.114. Left wrist PA radiograph. Giant cell tumor (*arrow*) of the distal radius. This is the classic appearance and common location of this tumor.

the involved area. Although any bone can be involved, the most commonly affected sites include the skull, spine, ribs, and pelvis. Unlike Ewing sarcoma, this disease occurs in the age group over 40 years. The typical radiographic appearance (Fig. 6.116) consists of multiple osteolytic areas with a "punched-out" appearance. At times it is difficult to differentiate multiple myeloma from osteolytic metastatic disease. *Urine and serum protein electrophoresis is important in the diagnosis of multiple myeloma.*

Osteosarcoma is a primary malignant bone tumor that commonly occurs during the second decade of life but has a second peak in later age. It can occur in many locations but is usually found in the metaphysis of a long bone. It has a wide variety of radiographic appearances but classically produces an abundance of new, irregular bone

Table 6.19
Radiographic Appearance of Bone Metastases

Osteoblastic or Sclerotic
Prostate
Breast
Carcinoid
Neuroblastoma

Mixed (Lytic and Blastic)
Breast
Cervix
Bladder

Osteolytic
Nearly all neoplasms

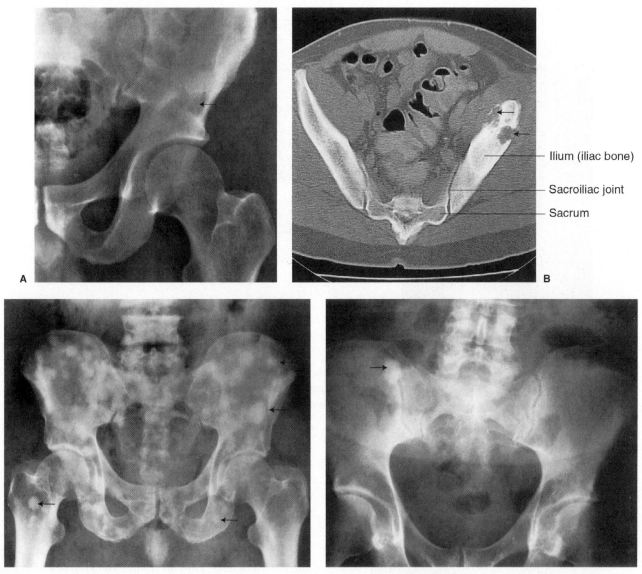

FIGURE 6.115. A: Left hip AP radiograph. Metastatic carcinoma of the lung. The radiolucent area in the left iliac bone (*arrow*) represents a suspected osteolytic metastasis. **B:** Pelvis axial CT image in the same patient. Two osteolytic metastases (*arrows*) in the left iliac bone. The CT image confirmed the presence and extent of two bone lesions. **C:** Pelvis AP radiograph. Osteoblastic metastases from carcinoma of the prostate. The *arrows* indicate multiple bilateral osteoblastic *(white)* metastatic lesions (*arrows*). **D:** Pelvis AP radiograph. Bone island (*straight arrow*). Bone islands are usually ovoid or oblong with a spiculated contour that blends into the bone trabecula. They are benign and generally asymptomatic.

Table 6.20
Some Malignant Bone Lesions

Primary
Multiple myeloma
Osteosarcoma
Ewing sarcoma
Chondrosarcoma

Secondary
Metastases

(Fig. 6.117). In some primary bone tumors, a Codman triangle may be identified and the triangle represents periosteal new bone formation reacting to the growing tumor. Osteosarcomas may have a Codman triangle as well as a sunburst or ray appearance that is secondary to bone formation in the tumor. On occasion, it can be difficult to differentiate osteosarcomas from metastatic disease and other primary bone tumors, especially Ewing sarcoma.

Ewing sarcoma usually occurs in children and young adults (Fig. 6.118). The classic appearance is a permeative or moth-eaten pattern, but it may have a variety of other

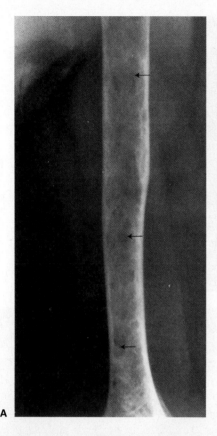

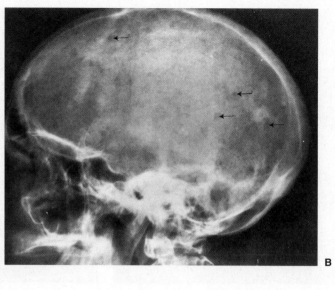

FIGURE 6.116. Left humerus AP radiograph **(A)** and lateral skull radiograph **(B)**. Multiple myeloma. The lucent or black areas indicated by the *arrows* represent the classic appearance of multiple myeloma in bone.

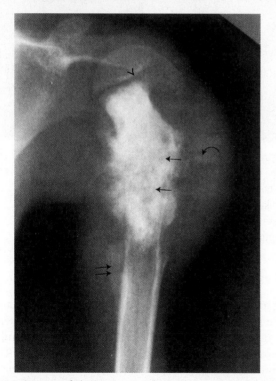

FIGURE 6.117. Left humerus AP radiograph in a 6-year-old. Large osteosarcoma of the humerus metaphysis and diaphysis. The tumor (*single straight arrows*) has not crossed the physis (*arrowhead*). Codman triangle (*double straight arrows*) represents periosteal new bone formation reacting to the tumor growth, and the sunburst or ray appearance (*curved arrow*) represents tumor bone.

associated bone changes such as sclerosis. Occasionally, Ewing sarcoma has a layered periosteal reaction secondary to the tumor's presence that looks like onionskin. Other lesions in children with periosteal reaction include osteomyelitis, fracture, eosinophilic granuloma, neuroblastoma, and osteosarcoma. The soft tissue extension of Ewing's sarcoma usually will not contain bone or cartilage calcification, whereas the soft tissue extensions of osteosarcomas tend to produce bone.

METABOLIC DISEASES

Some metabolic diseases have the potential to affect bones. A few examples are listed in Table 6.21.

Table 6.21
Some Metabolic Diseases That May Affect Bones
Paget disease
Hypothyroidism
Hyperparathyroidism
Rickets
Diabetes mellitus
Scurvy

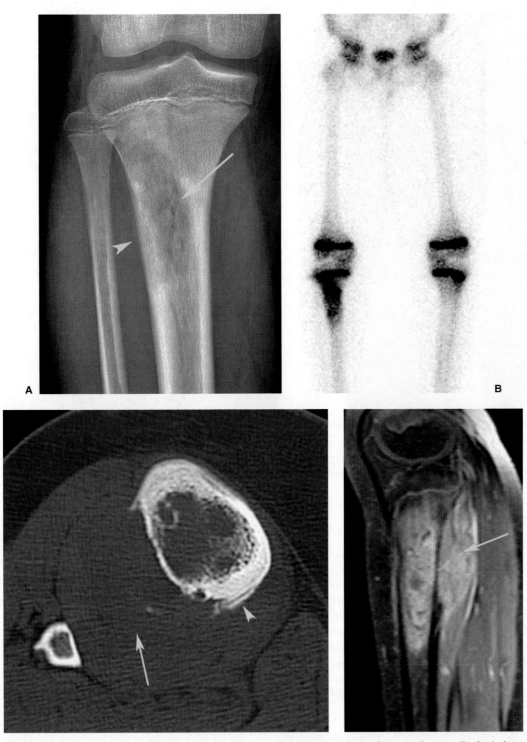

FIGURE 6.118. Ewing sarcoma. **A:** AP view of the right tibia demonstrates a lucent lesion in the metadiaphysis (*arrow*). There is subtle periosteal reaction laterally (*arrowhead*). Note the open physes. **B:** Anterior images from a radionuclide bone scan show normal increased activity of the growing physes and bladder (*black*), but abnormal increased activity in the right proximal tibia. **C:** Axial CT image through the lesion reveals that the normal marrow fat has been replaced by soft tissue density and some cortical thinning and destruction. There is periosteal reaction (*arrowhead*) and a large soft tissue mass (*arrow*). **D:** Sagittal fat-suppressed T1-weighted MR image was obtained after the injection of MR contrast. The tumor enhances both in the bone and soft tissue components (*arrow*).

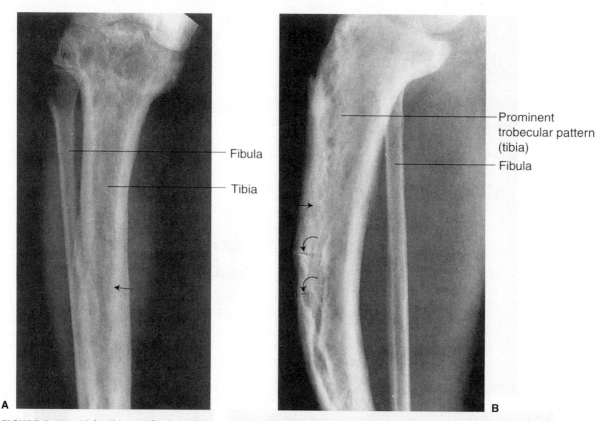

Fibula

Tibia

Prominent trobecular pattern (tibia)

Fibula

A

B

FIGURE 6.119. Right tibia and fibula AP **(A)** and lateral **(B)** radiographs. Paget disease. The tibia cortices are sclerotic in appearance (*straight arrows*) because of widening and thickening of the cortices and a prominent trabecular pattern. The tibia is bowed anterolaterally. The fibula is spared. The typical transverse pathologic fractures are best visualized on the lateral radiograph (*curved arrows*) and they are the most common complication of this disease. There is osteoporosis.

Paget Disease

Paget disease is a fairly common, chronic, and progressive bone disease of unknown etiology that occurs in adults usually over the age of 40 years. This disease can involve any bone (Fig. 6.119). The radiographic features of Paget disease are listed in Table 6.22. On radiographs, the bone cortices are thick and sclerotic in appearance and the trabecular pattern is thickened and prominent. Early in the disease, rarefaction, bone expansion, and bone destruction may occur. Bone deformities such as bowing of long bones and protrusio acetabuli may be the result of softening of the involved bones. The two most significant complications are pathologic fractures and sarcomatous degeneration. The differential diagnosis should include osteoblastic metastatic disease, fibrous dysplasia, lymphoma, and osteosclerosis.

Osteoporosis and Osteomalacia

Osteoporosis (e.g., Figs. 6.20, 6.94–6.99) is secondary to a reduced amount of bone matrix (osteoid) with normal mineralization, whereas osteomalacia is a normal bone matrix (osteoid) with a reduced amount of mineralization. Osteoporosis has become a major public health problem. Osteoporosis is estimated to affect 10 million Americans, 70% to 80% of these women, and 2 million related fractures per year costing an estimated $19 billion per year in 2005. Of those fractures, nearly 300,000 are hip fractures and roughly 550,000 are vertebral fractures. Osteoporosis affects all races and ethnicities, but it is thought to affect 20% of non-Hispanic Caucasians and Asian women over the age of 50 years. There is a long list of osteoporosis etiologies and a partial list of etiologies is shown in Table 6.23. Radiographs are insensitive for evaluation of osteoporosis. Dual x-ray absorptiometry is currently the standard screening method (Fig. 6.120) and is used to determine

---

Table 6.22

Radiographic Features of Paget Disease

Thick and sclerotic bone cortices with enlarged bone
Thick and prominent trabecular pattern
Long bone bowing
Acetabular protrusio
Pathologic fractures
Focal lucent area in the skull (osteoporosis circumscripta)

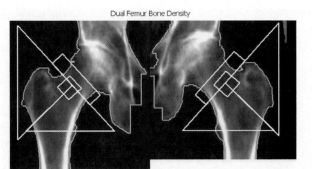

Dual Femur Bone Density

Image not for diagnosis

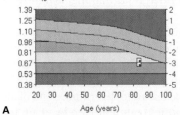

Reference: Total

BMD (g/cm²)   YA T-Score

A   Age (years)

Region	BMD (g/cm²) [1,6]	Young-Adult (%) [2,7]	T-Score	Age-Matched (%) [3]	Z-Score
Neck					
Left	0.685	64	-3.0	79	-1.4
Right	0.667	62	-3.1	77	-1.5
Mean	0.676	63	-3.0	78	-1.4
Difference	0.018	2	0.1	2	0.1
Total					
Left	0.705	64	-2.7	77	-1.5
Right	0.654	59	-3.1	71	-1.9
Mean	0.679	62	-2.9	74	-1.7
Difference	0.052	5	0.4	6	0.4

FIGURE 6.120. A: Dual x-ray absorptiometry evaluation of bone mineral density in the hips in an 83-year-old man. A *T*-score value of −2.5 or less indicates osteoporosis. This gentleman's is −3.0 on the left and −3.1 on the right. **B:** Coronal T1-weighted MR image of the hips obtained after a minor fall on the same gentleman demonstrates an incomplete intertrochanteric hip fracture (*arrow*). **C:** Dual x-ray absorptiometry evaluation of the left hip in an 86-year-old woman. A *T*-score value between −1.5 and −2.5 (this woman's is −2.1 for the femoral neck) indicates osteopenia.

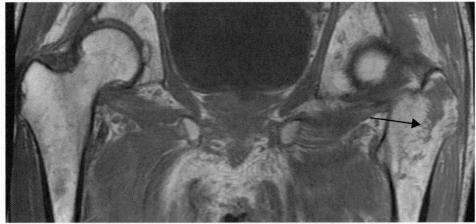

B

Patient:			Patient ID:		
Birth Date:	9/18/	86.0 years	Physician:		
Height / Weight:	58.0 in.	101.0 lbs.	Measured:	9/16/	11:46:29 AM (6.70)
Sex / Ethnic:	Female	White	Analyzed:	9/16/	11:49:12 AM (6.70)

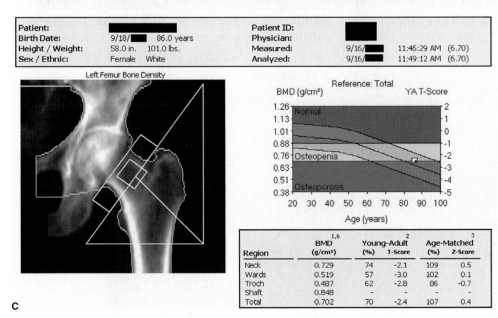

Left Femur Bone Density

Reference: Total

BMD (g/cm²)   YA T-Score

Age (years)

Region	BMD (g/cm²) [1,6]	Young-Adult (%) [2]	T-Score	Age-Matched (%) [3]	Z-Score
Neck	0.729	74	-2.1	109	0.5
Wards	0.519	57	-3.0	102	0.1
Troch	0.487	62	-2.8	86	-0.7
Shaft	0.848	-	-	-	-
Total	0.702	70	-2.4	107	0.4

C

Table 6.23
Some Causes of Osteoporosis
Age-related (senile)
Estrogen deficiency or postmenopausal
Steroid or heparin therapy
Cushing disease
Hyperparathyroidism
Diabetes mellitus
Anemia
Malnutrition
Osteogenesis imperfecta

normal versus osteopenia versus osteoporosis using the *T*-score, which compared the patient's values to a normal young adult.

Rickets

Rickets is a good example of osteomalacia and osteopenia in children. It is found in the growing portions of infant bones and is caused by poor calcification of the osteoid matrix that may result from vitamin D deficiency, renal disease, or intestinal malabsorption diseases. The radiographic findings include widened and irregular physes, cupping of the metaphyses, bowing of the legs, and osteopenia (Fig. 6.121). Rickets only occurs in growing bone and when this disease occurs in adults, it does not affect the growth plates and is termed osteomalacia.

INFECTION

Osteomyelitis (Fig. 6.122) can occur in all age groups and the classic clinical presentation is bone or joint pain and fever. There are multiple etiologies including trauma and hematogenous spread of infection (see Fig. 6.115). In adults, particularly diabetics, the bone destruction is usually adjacent to a soft tissue ulcer and known infection (see Fig. 6.97B). However, barring an adjacent ulcer, the radiographic appearance of osteomyelitis can be similar to a bone tumor with bone and joint destruction, periosteal reaction, and a soft tissue component. Unlike tumors, infections may occasionally have gas in the soft tissues secondary to gas-forming organisms. Osteomyelitis can also be confusing when found in the center of bone, such as at a site of prior fracture when one is tempted to think changes are related to the prior fracture fragments. It is important to remember that when a fracture heals, the bone density should return to normal; persistent sclerosis is suggestive of chronic osteomyelitis. MRI is a very useful tool for the demonstration of bone and soft tissue involvement by infection. However, it can be a confusing picture in a diabetic foot, which may also have abnormalities such as fractures and neuropathic changes (Fig 6.123 and Fig. 6.97B). MRI may be useful to determine a site of amputation, but when antibiotic treatment is to be given for the soft tissue component, serial radiographs are usually sufficient for the diagnosis of osteomyelitis. Osteomyelitis in children is more likely from hematologic seeding and is most often found in the metaphyseal regions of bones where it is thought that the normal loop in the bone's feeding blood vessels creates a slow flow of blood and increased chance for bacteria to deposit.

APPROACH TO COMMON CLINICAL PROBLEMS

When evaluating the musculoskeletal system, a thorough physical examination should dictate the next appropriate steps in imaging. Radiographs are typically the initial screening tool but should be used appropriately. For example, if a patient presents with pain after falling on an outstretched arm, one would not order radiographs of the

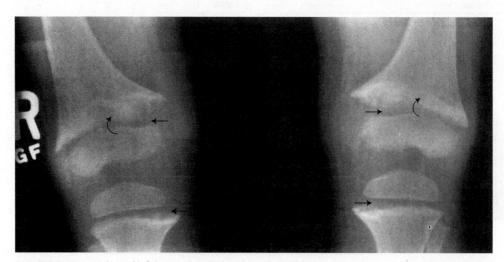

FIGURE 6.121. Right and left knees AP radiographs. Rickets. The physes are widened (*straight arrows*) and the metaphases are cupped (*curved arrows*).

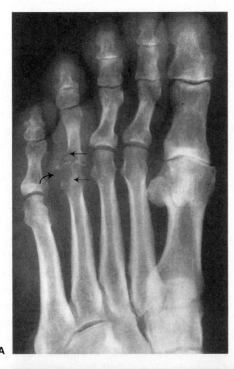

A

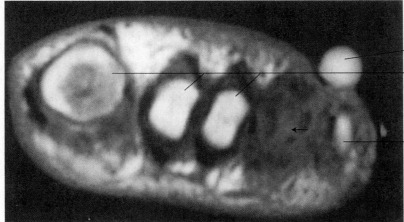

B

FIGURE 6.122. **A:** Left foot AP radiograph. Osteomyelitis in a patient with diabetes mellitus. There are destructive changes (*straight arrows*) involving the base of the proximal phalanx of the fourth toe as well as the fourth metatarsal head. Also, there are destructive changes in the fourth metatarsophalangeal joint manifested by narrowing of the joint space. The infection has characteristically caused destructive joint changes as well as bone destruction on both sides of the joint. Loose bone fragments have resulted from the osteomyelitis (*curved arrow*). **B:** Left foot axial T1 MR image in the same patient. When compared to the other metatarsal heads, the fourth metatarsal head is not visible because the infection (*arrow*) has destroyed and replaced the bone marrow.

Skin marker

1st, 2nd, 3rd metatarsal heads

5th metatarsal head

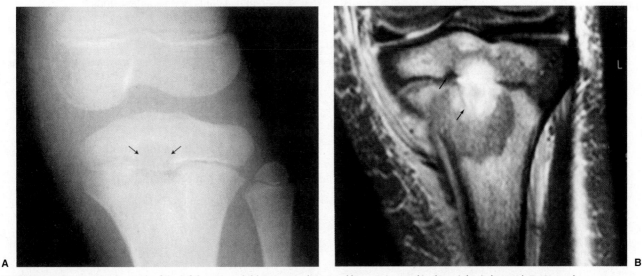

A
B

FIGURE 6.123. **A:** AP radiograph of the left knee in a child. Osteomyelitis. Focal lucency is noted in the epiphysis (*arrows*). **B:** Coronal fat-suppressed T2 MR in the same patient shows the abscess crosses the physis and involves the metaphysis as well (*arrows*).

humerus and forearm in an attempt to screen for injuries to the shoulder, humerus, elbow, forearm, and wrist. A bone is best imaged when the x-ray beam is centered at that bone or joint. Elbow joint effusions are typically not seen on films of the humerus and forearm. Similarly, radial head fractures or scaphoid fractures may be seen only on specialized dedicated views. If our hypothetical patient has focal tenderness over the radial head or has pain with pronation and supination, a dedicated elbow radiographic series is the appropriate choice. If a shoulder dislocation is suspected, a shoulder series to include an axillary or transcapular Y-view is the appropriate study of choice.

When the radiographs are normal, the clinical setting and degree of suspicion of injury will dictate how to proceed. Often, immobilization with repeat radiographs in 1 week is sufficient to evaluate for an occult fracture. This is not appropriate, however, for a potential hip fracture in an elderly person as immobilization could have devastating effects as would weight bearing as this could turn a nondisplaced into a displaced fracture. An emergent MRI has been shown to be the imaging procedure of choice in this circumstance.

Key Points

- It is important to recognize sesamoid bones and ossicles as normal variants. Sesamoids are bones within a tendon or volar plate. Ossicles are extra or supernumerary bones next to the skeleton and usually named after the neighboring bone.
- MRI is useful for injuries to the shoulder rotator cuff, knee ligaments and menisci, ankle ligaments, and Achilles tendon. CT imaging is good for bone detail, fracture diagnosis, locating fracture fragments, and evaluating matrix formation in bone tumors.
- The Salter–Harris classification describes fractures around the physis, which is considered the weakest point in a growing bone.

- Because fractures and other abnormalities may not be visualized on all radiographic views, always insist on at least two views of an injured or diseased area that are 90 degrees to each other.
- Fractures may not be visible on the first radiographs but may become visible after time (7 days) because of bone resorption at the ends of the fracture fragments.
- Osteoarthritis is the most common form of arthritis and often results from asymmetric cartilage wear.
- The radiographic features of osteoarthritis include irregular joint narrowing, sclerosis, absence of osteoporosis, and osteophyte formation.
- The radiographic features of rheumatoid arthritis include periarticular soft tissue thickening, symmetric joint narrowing, marginal erosions, periarticular osteoporosis, and joint deformity.
- Metastatic cancer is the most common malignant bone tumor. The majority of metastatic lesions are osteolytic or radiolucent. Osteoblastic metastatic lesions most commonly are secondary to prostate and breast neoplasms.
- Multiple myeloma is the most common primary malignant bone tumor, and it originates in the bone marrow.
- Ewing sarcoma usually occurs in children and young adults. They may have a permeative type of lesion and an onionskin-like periosteal reaction.
- Osteomyelitis and septic joints typically present with localized pain and fever. The radiographic features include bone and joint destruction, periosteal reaction, and occasionally, a soft tissue component.

FURTHER READINGS

Chew FS, Kline MJ, Bui-Mansfield LT. *Core Curriculum: Musculoskeletal Imaging,* Philadelphia, PA: Lippincott Williams & Wilkins, 2003.

El-Khoury GY. *Essentials of Musculoskeletal Imaging.* New York, NY: Churchill Livingstone, 2003.

Pope T, Bloem HL, Beltram J, et al. *Imaging of the Musculoskeletal System,* Philadelphia, PA: Saunders, 2008.

QUESTIONS

1. The second digit of the hand, when starting on the radial side is properly called
   a. ring finger
   b. index finger
   c. long finger
   d. second finger

2. Bones form by
   a. endochondral bone formation
   b. intramembranous bone formation
   c. periossification bone formation
   d. a and b
   e. a and c

3. A small bone just lateral to the lateral epicondyle of the humerus in an 8-year-old is likely
   a. an apophysis
   b. an epiphysis
   c. a fracture
   d. a normal variant

4. In a child, a fracture line extending through the physis into the epiphysis is a Salter–Harris
   a. I
   b. II
   c. III
   d. IV
   e. V

5. Which finding is most common with a shoulder dislocation?
   a. Anterior location
   b. Greater tuberosity fracture
   c. Posterior location
   d. Glenoid fracture

6. The most appropriate imaging modality to better evaluate a calcaneal fracture is
   a. ultrasound
   b. CT
   c. MR
   d. bone scan

7. An elderly patient with a fall and hip pain has a fracture on radiograph. The next course of action is to
   a. get an MR imaging study
   b. obtain a CT scan to evaluate the fracture
   c. call an orthopedic surgeon
   d. order a bone scan

8. The best study to look at all the internal structures of the knee would be
   a. radiograph
   b. ultrasound
   c. computed tomography
   d. magnetic resonance imaging

9. Periarticular osteoporosis, marginal erosions and morning stiffness best describes
   a. osteoarthritis
   b. gout
   c. rheumatoid arthritis
   d. septic arthritis

10. Which of the following is a malignant bone tumor?
    a. Osteoid osteoma
    b. Multiple myeloma
    c. Enostosis
    d. Osteochondroma

Brain

Wilbur L. Smith • T. Shawn Sato

■ ■ ■ ■ ■ **Chapter Outline**

Brain Imaging	**Tumor**
Trauma	**Congenital Anomalies**
Vascular Disease	**Key Points**

BRAIN IMAGING

Neuroradiology was a relatively unsophisticated branch of imaging prior to 1970. Plain radiographs of the skull were insensitive for predicting neurologic disorders, and obtaining more useful diagnostic imaging information about the brain and spinal cord was cumbersome, painful, and yielded images that were difficult to interpret without advanced knowledge of neuroanatomy. The early brain imaging techniques were at best minimally invasive and many involved such gruesome activities as injecting air into the spinal canal (pneumoencephalography) and rolling the patient about in a specially devised torture chair. Few patients willingly returned for another one of those examinations! The highest level of comfort that the poor patient who needed brain imaging could anticipate was a direct puncture carotid arteriogram or a spinal tap.

The invention and widespread use of the technique of computerized axial tomography (CAT), or computed tomography (CT), allowed relatively painless access to the processes inside the skull and allowed the field of neuroradiology to become a premier subspecialty within radiology. The early CT scanners were slow, lacking in detail, and hard to manage (Fig. 7.1), but they were such a marvelous advance that they were embraced as a revolution in medical imaging. Indeed, Sir Godfrey Hounsfield, the pioneer of CT imaging, won many international awards and was knighted for his work. While magnetic resonance imaging (MRI) advances have supplanted CT in many applications, CT still is the technique of choice for the many of the diagnostic studies of the brain and spine and is still the most common neuroimaging study performed

in the United States. The CT scanners of today are capable of obtaining nearly simultaneous multiple slices documenting cerebral perfusion and with new image processing techniques can produce reconstructed anatomical images in any plane desired. CT scans are routinely performed either with or without intravenous contrast enhancement, and the enhancement produced coupled with the speed of the new scanners makes real-time vascular mapping of the brain a practical clinical tool (Fig. 7.2). Certain clinical indications are generally predictive of the need for iodinated CT contrast, although there are many variations. Table 7.1 gives the usual indications for contrast use; however, if in doubt, radiologists are always available for consultation on individual cases.

In CT scanning, images of the brain are usually acquired in axial (horizontal) planes and then viewed at different digital levels so that one can see the bones of the face and skull as well as the tissues of the brain itself. Two image acquisitions are not required to get these data, but rather, two different methods of viewing the same digital data. The sections that result from the CT scans depict the anatomy at predetermined intervals depending on the parameters of reconstruction of the slices (thickness), speed of table movement (pitch), and timing of acquisition of the data. Generally, the thicker the slices and/or the faster the table speed the fewer the sections needed to get through the brain, but as the slices are thickened, anatomy is depicted in less detail. In the standard brain CT scan, there are several key landmarks to observe for proper orientation. Figure 7.3 illustrates some of the highlights for which you should look in orienting yourself to the anatomy depicted by the slices.

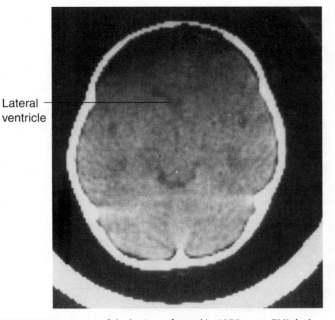

Lateral ventricle

FIGURE 7.1. A scan of the brain performed in 1976 on an EMI device. This single section took about 1 minute to acquire. The coarse pixels make anything but the larger brain structures such as the ventricles difficult to appreciate. This was, however, a huge improvement over the pneumoencephalogram.

Let us begin with the caudal sections and work cephalad. The fourth ventricle, a cerebrospinal fluid (CSF) space located dorsal to the brain stem and in the midline of the posterior fossa, is a good marker for identifying the level of the pons, cerebellar vermis, and the base of the anterior cranial fossa (Fig. 7.3A). On the same section lying ventral to the brain stem are the suprasellar cistern and the dorsum sellae. Note that the figures depict the anatomy of the posterior fossa less sharply than some of the more

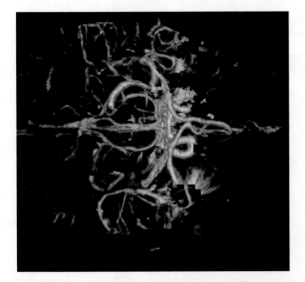

FIGURE 7.2. CT arteriogram of the brain obtained after intravenous contrast shows detail of the intracerebral vessels of the circle of Willis.

Table 7.1	
Some Common Indications for CAT Scanning and Use of Intravenous Contrast Enhancement	
Indications for CAT Scan	**Intravenous Contrast**
Trauma	No
Infection	Yes
Congenital anomalies	No
Tumor	Yes
Metabolic disorder	No
Multiple sclerosis	Yes
Hydrocephalus	No

cephalad sections of brain. CT scans in the posterior fossa are often degraded owing to the absorption of x-rays by the large amount of dense surrounding bone; therefore, detail of the cerebellar hemispheres may be obscured. This technique limitation is mitigated to some degree by faster and better scanners, but bone artifact is a limitation of CT scanning.

Proceeding to sections cephalad from the fourth ventricle, one encounters the ambient cistern and cephalad portion of the suprasellar cistern (Fig. 7.3B). The former is an important landmark for the point where the cerebral peduncles (an extension of the brain stem) pass through the tentorium cerebri. Ventral to this landmark and slightly cephalad are located the third ventricle and the anterior horns of the lateral ventricles. At the lateral margins of the anterior horns of the ventricles are the basal ganglia, identifiable as masses of gray matter bordering the lateral and third ventricles (Fig. 7.3C). The caudate nuclei protrude into the anterior horns of the lateral ventricles.

Further cephalad the scans depict the brain cortex and the orderly interfaces between the gray and white matter (Fig. 7.3D). Note that each section of gray matter has an accompanying area of white matter arranged in a predictable pattern. Symmetry is everything in looking at CT scans of the brain. Provided that the patient is properly positioned, structures should match up from side to side.

Despite its immense success, CT has limitations that inhibit its value. For example, CT is inherently limited in its ability to display high degrees of tissue contrast. If two tissues absorb roughly the same number of photons, even though the tissues may be chemically very different, CT cannot discriminate between them. Bone or other high-density items such as aneurysm clips degrade the CT image. Although the time needed to obtain a section by CT has declined substantially in recent years, there are still physical limitations to CT scanning, and motion artifacts abound in uncooperative or combative patients.

The newer major technique in the imaging of the brain and spinal cord is MRI. This technique also had humble beginnings; the first scanners were used to quantify fat in livestock coming to market. MR images are wonderfully

FIGURE 7.3. A: CT scan of a normal adult at the level of the fourth ventricle. The brain stem structure ventral to the fourth ventricle is the pons. Further anterior lies the five-pointed star representing the suprasellar cistern. Lying within the suprasellar cistern are the vessels of the circle of Willis and the dorsum sellae or back of the sella turcica. **B:** A cut cephalad to **(A)** demonstrates the ambient cisterns as curved black cerebrospinal fluid densities just posterior to the cerebral peduncles. If you use your imagination, the cistern is the mouth, the anterior horns of the lateral ventricles the eyes, and the third ventricle the nose of a smiling man! This is an important landmark as it is the point where the cerebral peduncles pass through the tentorium. **C:** Proceeding cephalad we leave the posterior fossa and image the lateral ventricles, third ventricles, aqueduct of Sylvius, and the cerebral hemispheres.

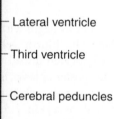

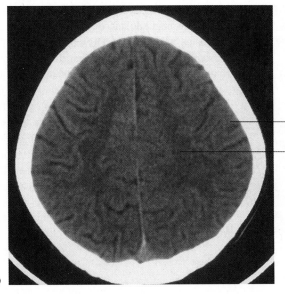

FIGURE 7.3. (*Continued*) **D:** A scan near the vertex of the head depicts the white matter (black on CT) and its relationship to the gray matter. Note that each area of gray matter has an associated column of white matter.

— Gray matter

— White matter

D

detailed and yield unique anatomical and functional data. Generally, the MRI studies require more time and are more expensive to carry out than CT scans. MRI has much better tissue contrast than CT, although special resolution is less. New imaging sequences, improved imaging speed, and enhanced capabilities of MRI to show metabolic, vascular, and functional changes in tissues make it likely that MRI will ultimately be the imaging modality of choice for many neurologic conditions.

MRI imaging depends on alterations in the physical behavior of protons (hydrogen is the most abundant natural proton in our water-filled tissues) when first magnetized, then exposed to a pulse of radio frequency energy. The major variables are, therefore, the strength of the magnetic field, the ability to apply energy to disrupt magnetic equilibrium (gradient coils) the way the radio frequency waves are applied (pulse sequences). Table 7.2 is a very simplified overview of the current major pulse sequences and the color of lesions and the CSF on the currently used human MRI scans. There are many exceptions to the data in Table 7.2, and new sequences are rapidly being developed; therefore, this table should be used only as a rough (90% accurate)

guideline to get you in the ballpark when looking at MRI images. Despite the great potential of MRI and its progression from a research device in the early 1980s to a staple of most imaging departments in the United States, at present CT scans still provide the bulk of diagnostic brain images. Table 7.3 compares the strengths and limitations of CT and MRI. A series of images showing both sequences and typical anatomic structures are demonstrated (Fig. 7.4).

TRAUMA

Perhaps the most common indication for brain imaging is trauma. Human heads are extremely vulnerable to injury; consequently, the trauma CT scanner rarely lacks sufficient business. In assessing a CT performed for trauma, one has a finite number of search parameters for major findings that represent conditions likely to demand immediate intervention. MRI is excellent for subacute trauma detection, but the speed and availability of CT makes it the usual primary imaging device for trauma patients.

The presence of blood in the head but outside the vascular system is often a key to the correct diagnosis.

Table 7.2

MRI Pulse Sequences

Sequence	Cerebrospinal Fluid Color	Lesion Color
T1-weighted	Black	Variable
T2-weighted	White	White
Inversion recovery	Black	White
Diffusion	Black	White
Gradient (susceptibility)	Black	Black

Table 7.3

A Comparison of Indications and Factors Affecting the Choice of CT or MRI

Factor	CT	MRI
Cost	++	+++
Availability	+++	++
Tissue differentiation	+	+++
Multiplanar sequences	+++	+++
Speed of examination	+++	++
Bone reconstruction	+++	+

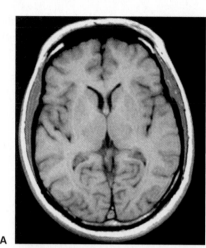

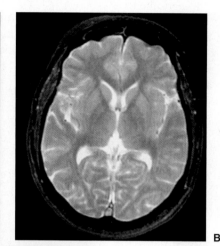

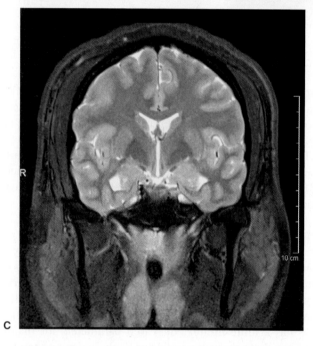

FIGURE 7.4. A: Axial T1-weighted (left) and T2-weighted MRI images at the level of the foramen of Monro. On T1-weighted images, the cerebrospinal fluid in the ventricles is black and on T2-weighted images it is white. Notice the superb anatomical detail, much better than CT. **B:** Coronal T2-weighted image at the level of the foramen of Monro in the same patients. The anatomical definition rivals that of a brain section in the neuroanatomy laboratory. **C:** Sagittal midline T1-weighted image of the same patient. The midline structures, face and foramen magnum, are seen in fine detail. Note how well you see the cerebellum and brain stem without the beam hardening artifacts of CT.

Fortunately, when blood is loose in the head, it usually appears as a conspicuous white blob on the CT scan. Therefore, the first rule of looking at trauma CT scans is to look for the white collections inside the skull (Fig. 7.5). Your diagnosis often can be even more specific because the white (or blood) had an absorption number greater than 50 HU (Hounsfield units) and tends to align in certain predictable ways according to its anatomic location. As an overview, the locations of intracranial bleeding whether by CT or MRI are first separated into intra-axial, meaning within the brain tissues themselves, or extra-axial. The extra-axial hemorrhages occur in spaces with characteristic shapes that can assist in localizing the hemorrhage. Fluid in the epidural space, between skull and dura, usually presents as a crescentic mass, convex to the brain (Fig. 7.6). The subdural space between dura and arachnoid membranes, however, is usually concave to the brain surface, paralleling the surface of the skull; therefore,

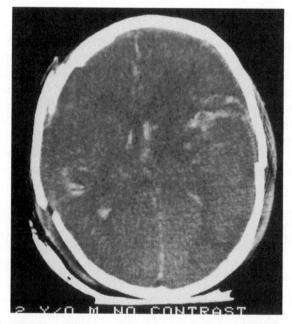

FIGURE 7.5. A child injured in a severe auto accident shows multiple white areas in the brain as well as disruption of the skull. The white areas are intraparenchymal hemorrhage. Also note the disruption of the normal brain architecture (compare to Fig. 7.3D, which shows a section at roughly the same level), reflecting the severe cerebral edema.

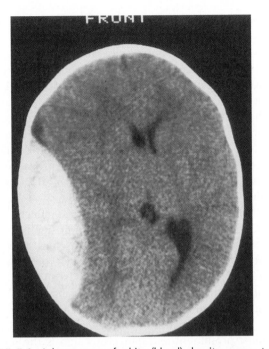

FIGURE 7.6. A large mass of white (blood) density convex toward the brain is characteristic of an epidural hemorrhage. Most of these occur because of traumatic tear of an artery and are surgical emergencies. The brain is shifted by the hematoma as evidenced by the shift of midline.

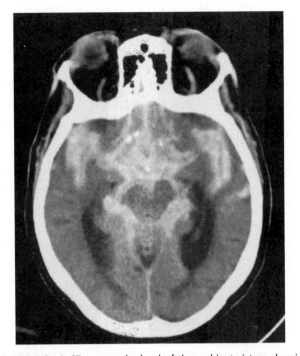

FIGURE 7.8. A CT scan at the level of the ambient cistern showing the cistern as white (blood) instead of black (cerebrospinal fluid; compare to Fig. 7.3B). Note that the white density also surrounds the brain stem. When blood mimics cerebrospinal fluid distribution, it is usually extra-axial and in the subarachnoid space flowing around and over the brain tissues.

subdural hematomas are differentiated from epidural bleeding by their shape (Fig. 7.7). Subarachnoid blood diffuses over the surface of the gyri and fills the CSF cisterns around the brain (Fig. 7.8). Intra-axial bleeding is often confined to the area of the ruptured vessel and is entirely enclosed within the substance of the brain. Intraventricular hemorrhage lies within the ventricles, often pooling in the dependent portion of the ventricle to form a blood–CSF level. By first finding the "white" blood, then looking at its

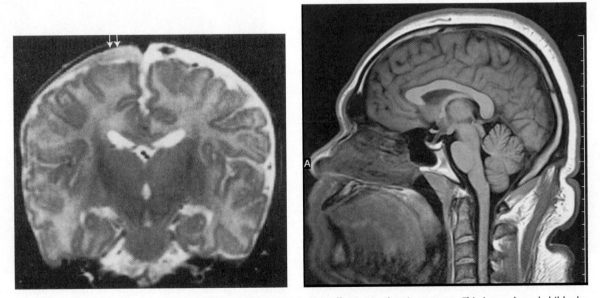

FIGURE 7.7. MRI of the brain, shown to illustrate that MRI is also effective in showing trauma. This is an abused child who has a subdural space hematoma (*arrows*). Note that the surface is concave, reflecting the contour of the cerebral cortex, but not extending among the gyri. This configuration is typical for a subdural hematoma. Also note that the signal densities are different on MRI. Imaging of bleeding is more complex on MRI than by CAT.

Table 7.4

Characteristics of Intracranial Blood by Imaging

		MRI	
Time of Bleed	CT	T1-weighted	T2-weighted
Immediate	White	Black	Black
Acute	White	White	Black
Subacute	Gray–white	White	White

shape and anatomic location, one can be pretty precise about the diagnosis and the location of the blood. As the hematoma ages, the blood assumes different image characteristics. Table 7.4 provides a description of the differing appearances of blood in the head with age of the bleed.

After looking for bleeding in trauma patients, the next step is to look for mass effect, a clue that there is pressure impinging on an area of the brain. For most injuries, the best way to find significant mass effects is to look for asymmetry with displacement of the midline or paramedian structures, the most prominent of which are the falx cerebri, lateral ventricles, and interhemispheric fissure (Figs. 7.6 and 7.9). A midline shift away from a lesion, for example, an epidural blood collection, is usually an emergent situation, particularly in the context of trauma. However, a word of caution is advisable: Midline shift does not always signal a need to take out your pocketknife to perform emergent, kitchen table-type neurosurgery. Diffuse edema of one hemisphere of the brain (Fig. 7.9) or even atrophy of the contralateral hemisphere can cause apparent (or real) shift. The important concept is midline shift. When the brain structures are shifted away from the side of the evident abnormality, such as a hematoma, increase your level of suspicion and urgency in evaluating your patient.

After searching for blood and mass effects on the brain CT scan or MRI, the next important step is to assess the densities of the brain tissues themselves. Earlier we described how the gray and white matter components of the brain should be visible on the CT scan (Fig. 7.3D). The lateral ventricles and CSF spaces are black and should be easily distinguished as separate from the tissues of the brain. Variations on this theme are generally bad news. The most prominent and dangerous sign is the obliteration of the distinction between the gray and white matter, which indicates profound edema in the area. If this is a universal pattern, there is a special name for the profound edema that occurs, obliterating all brain landmarks—the "bad black brain" (Fig. 7.10). This finding usually portends a poor outcome, representing diffuse breakdown of

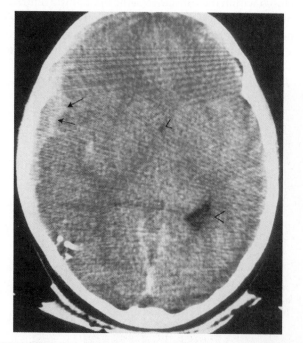

FIGURE 7.9. Intra-axial or intraparenchymal hemorrhage of the brain in a trauma patient. The white densities (blood) do not conform to any definable space and are actually within and between the tissues of the brain. A subdural hematoma (*arrows*) is also present in this patient. Note that the lateral ventricle and its temporal horn (*arrowheads*) are displaced by the mass effect.

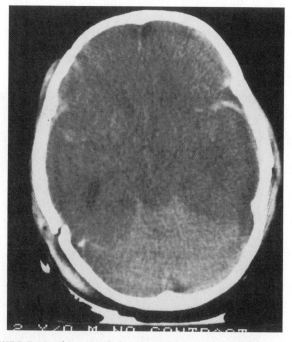

FIGURE 7.10. This severely brain-injured child has neither recognizable ventricles nor gray/white matter differentiation (compare with Fig. 7.3D). In fact, the whole neocortex, except for the areas of hemorrhage, is a uniform shade of black. This severe brain edema portends a poor prognosis.

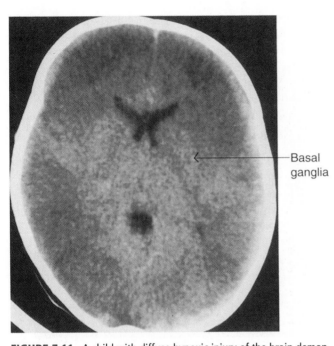

FIGURE 7.11. A child with diffuse hypoxic injury of the brain demonstrates the reversal sign. Note that the basal ganglia are gray and the neocortex black, particularly in the frontal and parietal regions.

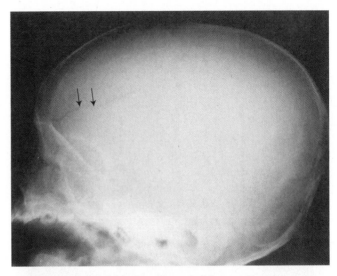

FIGURE 7.12. This child with a linear skull fracture (*arrows*) was completely asymptomatic (except for a palpable bump on his skull) because the brain underlying the skull was not affected. The presence of the skull fracture documents trauma but is of little importance in patient management.

tissue integrity with ensuing cerebral edema. The cause of this catastrophic chain of events is almost always a limitation of the oxygen supply to the brain tissues, owing to either a compromise of the blood supply or a loss of oxygen to the brain cells. In the latter instance, as the brain swells, cerebral blood supply is compromised by loss of the arterial perfusion gradient, and ultimately there is no circulation to the brain. Owing to different tissue densities and less vulnerable perfusion, the basal ganglia and brain stem are often particularly conspicuous against the uniform density of the bad black brain, and their conspicuity results in the so-called reversal sign (Fig. 7.11).

Please note the intentional lack of a detailed discussion of skull fractures in this section on trauma. That is because, in general, skull fractures are not very important in the immediate outcome of a patient. It is the effect of the trauma on the brain that does your patient harm, not the crack in the bone (Fig. 7.12). A significant important exception is the depressed skull fracture, a situation in which the bone is driven directly back into the meningeal coverings and the brain itself. CT imaging and bone windows are of great importance in documenting the depth and extent of this type of injury as well as documenting any intracranial air leaks owing to tears of the dura or meninges (Fig. 7.13). In this type of trauma, surgery is usually needed and the identification of the fracture, depth of the fragment(s), surface brain injury, and pneumocephalus (air inside the skull) are the key observations.

MRI is not to be omitted in any discussion of trauma, but its role, although dramatically increasing, is often secondary. Because of the limitations of patient access

(ventilator limitations, difficulty in patient observation, etc.) and the longer examination times, MRI is often not the first imaging modality used for acute trauma. After the acute, life-threatening emergencies have been handled, MRI is extremely sensitive for assessing the extent of parenchymal injury to the brain (particularly cytotoxic

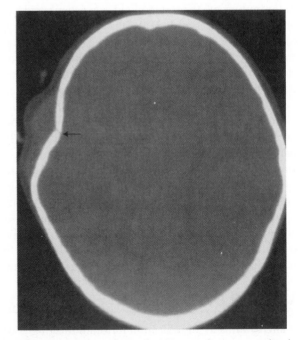

FIGURE 7.13. Bone windows of a CT scan demonstrate the depth of injury in a depressed skull fracture (*arrow*) after this teenager was struck with a hammer.

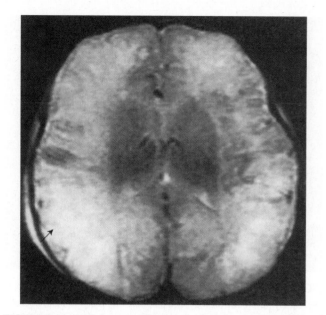

FIGURE 7.14. MRI shows a diffusely increased signal (*white indicated by arrow*) in the posterior parietal lobes of a blunt head trauma victim. This is owing to a cortical contusion that was subtle on the CT scan. Although the finding explained the patient's symptoms and documented the severity of injury, the lesion did not require urgent intervention.

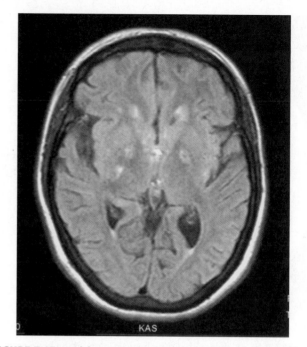

FIGURE 7.15. Widely scattered unidentified bright objects (UBOs) on MRI in the basal ganglia of this octogenarian are not of significance. These UBOs are common near the basal ganglia but can be seen anywhere and are assumed to represent small artery disease with lacunar infarctions.

edema on diffusion-weighted imaging) and for defining more precisely the compartment of localized extra-axial fluid. In each of these instances, the prognosis and etiology of the injury is better defined after MRI. MRI spectroscopy, a study of brain metabolism, holds great promise for predicting the outcome of some injuries. The utility of MRI for finding subarachnoid blood is excellent using susceptibility sequences and MRI is unparalleled in defining precisely which gyrus was smashed in a previous auto accident (Fig. 7.14). The instances in which MRI is critical in deciding the urgent management of a trauma patient are still few, but it is an invaluable secondary tool in selected patients.

In summary, a CT scan of an acute trauma patient should be evaluated for the following findings: (a) White densities defining bleeding, including the shape and distribution of the blood collection(s); (b) mass effect, particularly with shift of the midline structures; and (c) loss of normal contrast characteristics (or asymmetry) of the normal tissue and CSF interfaces. These rules will not get you every answer on every trauma patient, but they will help you in almost 95% of the cases you see. For the other 5%, you may have to do a radiology or neurosurgery residency!

VASCULAR DISEASE

Just after trauma as an indication for brain imaging is vascular disease, and the most prevalent form is stroke. A stroke results from occlusion of the vascular supply (usually arterial but occasionally venous as well) to a focal area

of the brain causing tissue ischemia. Many "strokes" are small and not even detected clinically. Most people in their fifth or sixth decade have small areas of abnormal signal called unidentified bright objects (UBOs) on MRI of the brain (Fig. 7.15), and there are some who ascribe the origin of UBOs to silent strokes. We have a lot of brain tissue that we do not fully use; the loss of these small areas is not necessarily perceived as a clinical problem.

Only when either a large or a particularly critical area of brain becomes ischemic do emergent symptoms appear and neuroimaging comes into play. CT scans are often the first examination; however, their use is problematic as there is a definite incidence of false-negative CT scans in the first 24 hours after a stroke. The size, severity, and presence of hemorrhage clearly affect the CT picture of stroke and so some strokes appear almost immediately; however, the sensitivity of CT scan for the diagnosis is considerably higher after the first 24 hours, unfortunately outside the window for "clot buster" or other stroke prevention treatments (Fig. 7.16). That said since hemorrhage in a stroke is a contraindication for "clot busters" and CT is sensitive for hemorrhage, a CT without contrast is usually the first study for a suspected stroke patient.

The most reliable finding in stroke on CT scan is the loss of the normal architecture of brain substance. The area of the stroke is depicted as a dark (edematous) blotch obliterating the normal tissue density. Occasional strokes will have associated bleeding, particularly in patients with

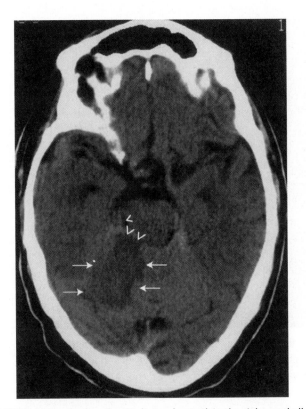

FIGURE 7.16. The low-density lesion (*arrows*) in the right cerebellar hemisphere represents an acute stroke owing to arterial occlusion. Note that there is swelling of tissues involved in the stroke as evidenced by effacement of the ambient cistern on the right (*arrowheads*). The lesion does not contain blood because there is no white signal on CT.

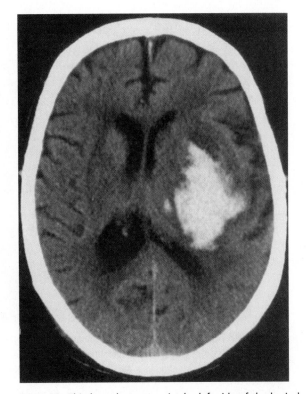

FIGURE 7.17. This huge hematoma in the left side of the brain has an irregular margin and edema surrounding the white area of fresh hemorrhage. This is a 53-year-old hypertensive executive who suffered a fatal acute hemorrhagic stroke.

hypertension, and the blood will show up on CT as a white density within the darker area of infarct (Fig. 7.17). A stroke may also change in nature as the tissue is destroyed and revascularization takes place. Bleeding may ensue such that initially nonhemorrhagic strokes can develop high signal characteristic of internal bleeding. This change often portends a poor prognosis. Newer CT perfusion techniques enabled by faster scanners and better computers may well supersede the current CT for stroke protocols.

There is a developing body of knowledge suggesting that early treatment of stroke may restore circulation and limit brain tissue damage. This has led to a change in imaging to emphasize early diagnosis. MRI, particularly with diffusion imaging sequences and diffusion mapping, is more sensitive to the early changes and has assumed a larger role in the imaging of acute stroke. Diffusion imaging is a series of specific inversion recovery sequences that show Brownian motion of the water molecules (cytotoxic edema) released from the damaged brain tissue, which roughly correlates with areas of cell death. This finding is very sensitive and appears within minutes of tissue injury in experimental studies, making it the most useful tool for diagnosing acute stroke (Fig. 7.18). Advances in MRI

sequencing are rapid, so it is likely that these sequences will be further refined possibly even to anticipate cell death, but for now diffusion is the most accurate and early sequence for stroke. Eight hours or more after a stroke, the MRI of the damaged tissues reliably shows white on standard MRI sequences (T2W and FLAIR) owing to the large amount of free water leaked by the ischemic cells (Fig. 7.19). Unfortunately, by this time it is too late to use many of the thrombolytic techniques to limit stroke; therefore, diffusion is critical early in stroke. The use of MRI contrast (gadolinium) has improved detection even further, and MRI may soon be the standard for stroke imaging (Fig. 7.20).

So far we have discussed acute strokes. Chronic strokes result in atrophy of the brain tissue (Fig. 7.21) manifested by either focal or diffuse shrinkage of the brain owing to cell death. Of special note is diffuse multi-infarct dementia, a condition that is difficult to differentiate from Alzheimer disease. Here the strokes are small and confined to the areas near the ventricles and so the ventricles enlarge at the expense of the dead tissue (Fig. 7.22). The patient's CT scan looks like the ventricles are dilated, with the gyri and sulci appearing unusually prominent, a condition sometimes referred to as *hydrocephalus*

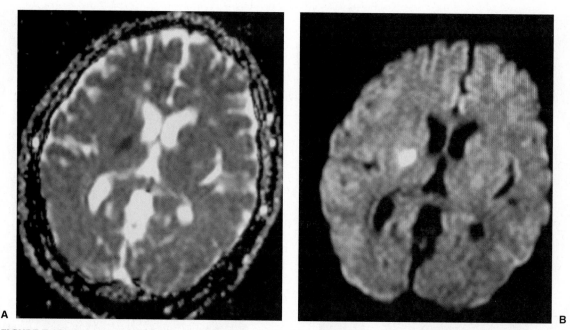

FIGURE 7.18. **A:** An acute stroke in the anterior portion of the right thalamus in this 50-year-old hypertensive executive was detected promptly by diffusion-weighted MRI. The acute diffusion coefficient image shows a low-density (black) lesion in the thalamus on the T2 sequence. **B:** The same lesion is white on the conventional inversion recovery sequence.

ex vacuo. These cases are truly a conundrum because Alzheimer disease, normal pressure hydrocephalus of the elderly, and diffuse brain atrophy from any cause all look the same. Functional brain MRI imaging with spectroscopy, blood perfusion analysis, and/or metabolic measurement is of future consideration for this diagnosis. There is no easy imaging answer, and at present there is no specific treatment with good efficacy for any of these conditions. However, this is a rapidly developing area of medicine and exciting imaging developments are to be anticipated.

TUMOR

The third common application of brain imaging is tumor evaluation. In adults, metastases (Fig. 7.23) constitute the most common tumors, with primary benign or malignant tumors being somewhat less common. The converse is true in children owing to the lower frequency of primary malignancies that metastasize to brain. The location of the tumors also differs with age. A greater proportion of adult tumors are in the cerebral cortex, whereas in children the proportion of tumors originating below the tentorium is much greater (Fig. 7.24).

CT scanning for tumor follows the same general principles as for trauma, with the major exception that most tumor scans are performed after the administration of intravenous contrast. The theory, which works most of the time, is that the abnormal tumor circulation allows contrast to penetrate the blood–brain barrier and enhance the tumor. Because contrast enhancement is white on a CT scan, the tumor becomes conspicuous. However, tumors can bleed, and the white of the contrast may obscure the white of the bleeding. Because the appearance of blood is an important issue in tumor patients, we often have to study them both with and without intravenous enhancement.

FIGURE 7.19. A diffusion-weighted image of a 2-hour-old left parietal stroke. Note that the acute stroke is black on the diffusion image **(B)** and white on the composite ADC "map" **(A).** The patient did not have "clot busters" for other clinical reasons, so a conventional T2-weighted **(C)** image at 12 hours shows the left parietal stroke as a bright signal.

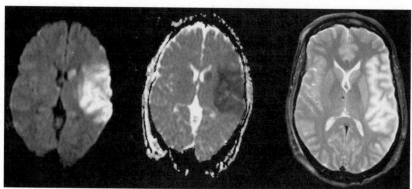

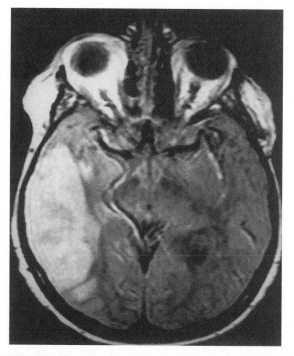

FIGURE 7.20. The white area in the right temporal lobe on this patient is a newly symptomatic stroke as depicted by gadolinium-enhanced MRI.

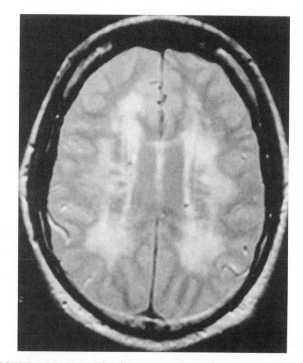

FIGURE 7.22. T2-weighted scan at the level of the lateral ventricles demonstrates multiple high-signal periventricular infarcts owing to lack of perfusion of the deep layers of the brain. These patients present with dementia and movement disorders that may mimic a number of degenerative neurologic conditions.

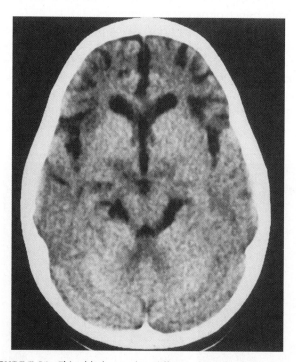

FIGURE 7.21. This elderly man has diffusely dilated ventricles as well as deep sulci over the brain surface because of atrophy presumably associated with multiple prior infarcts.

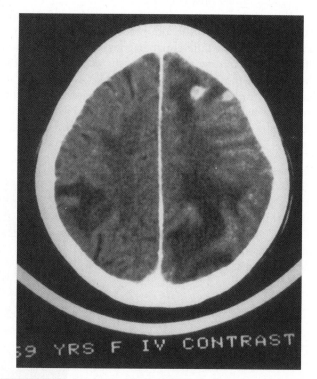

FIGURE 7.23. A contrast-enhanced CT scan of a 59-year-old woman with known lung cancer shows multiple high- and mixed-density lesions. These were metastases from the lung tumor.

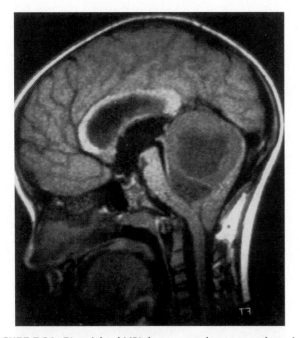

FIGURE 7.24. T1-weighted MRI documents a huge tumor that arises from the cerebellar vermis and pushes the brain stem forward. This is typical behavior of a medulloblastoma.

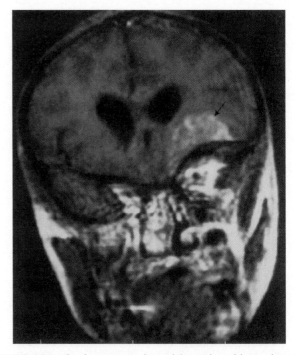

FIGURE 7.26. This large tumor (*arrow*) has a broad base along the roof of the orbit and displaces the frontal lobe of the brain superiorly. This growth is typical of an extra-axial tumor, in this case, a meningioma.

In defining tumor and normal anatomy, MRI equals or surpasses CT in efficacy and few neurosurgeons would tackle a brain tumor without the aid of a with and without contrast (gadolinium) MRI (Fig. 7.25).

Just as with trauma, it is important to differentiate intra-axial masses (within the brain tissues) from extra-axial masses, as the differential diagnosis and approach are different. Determining tumor tissue site of origin is critical but one of the most difficult diagnostic tasks. In general, an extra-axial tumor will display its widest base at the brain surface and will smoothly indent the brain from without (Fig. 7.26). Extra-axial tumors tend to be related to the meninges

or the bones of the skull. Occasionally, a parenchymal brain tumor originates at the brain surface and differentiation is impossible. Conversely, extra-axial tumors sometimes grow from slips of tissues insinuated into the brain, giving the appearance of parenchymal masses.

Tumors that are entirely enveloped within the brain tissues are usually of glial cell origin, with astrocytoma being the most common primary tumor (Fig. 7.27) and metastasis being the most common overall. When the distinction of intra-axial from extra-axial is difficult and critical, using another modality with multiplanar imaging capability,

FIGURE 7.25. A: A T2-weighted image of a brain tumor, a glioma in the right occipital lobe. The central tumor (white) is surrounded by a rim of edema infiltrating the white matter. **B:** After intravenous contrast (gadolinium) a collar of enhancement better defines the boundaries of the tumor for the surgeon.

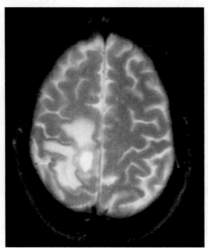

A

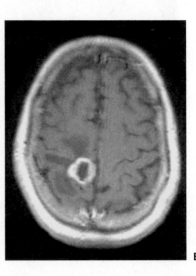

B

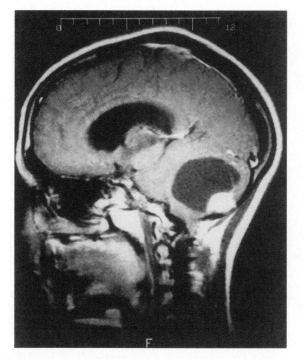

FIGURE 7.27. On gadolinium-enhanced MRI, this cerebellar tumor contains a very bright nidus of tissue within a cystic mass. This is characteristic of a pilocytic astrocytoma.

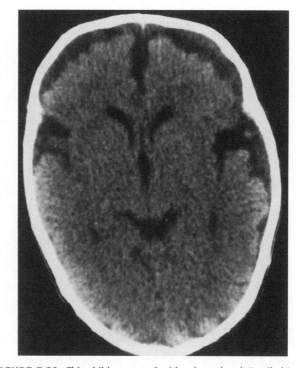

FIGURE 7.28. This child presented with a large head. Family history documented macrocranium in several other family members including the father. The head CT scan shows the ventricles to be slightly enlarged and the subarachnoid spaces to be prominent. This constellation of findings is diagnostic for benign familial macrocranium.

such as MRI, is invaluable. MRI also offers different tissue contrast parameters, and contrast-enhanced MRI adds yet another dimension.

Once the tumor is diagnosed and localized to the proper anatomic location, the next job is to look at the mass effect caused by the tumor and to assess the likelihood of damage to critical centers of the brain requiring emergent action. Here, the principles applied in trauma are useful. Does the tumor cause displacement of the normal structures, such that they are sufficiently compressed to cause compromise of the blood supply or direct pressure damage to the cells of the normal brain tissue? If so, you have to move quickly. Once again, shift away from the tumor and alteration of the normal differentiation of the brain tissues are key to the proper determination.

CONGENITAL ANOMALIES

Although CT is often used for the diagnosis of congenital anomalies of the brain, MRI, with its superior tissue contrast, is invaluable in this area. Congenital anomalies usually present in childhood, either with abnormal physical findings or with seizures. Physical abnormalities most often associated with congenital brain abnormalities include macrocephaly (big head), abnormal appearance of the face (particularly with midline abnormalities such as cleft palate), and meningocele. Each of these findings should tip you off to pursue a specific type of abnormality.

In the case of macrocranium (a big head), the likely differential diagnosis is hydrocephalus or dilatation of the ventricles because of abnormal CSF circulation. Remember, however, that if we use the 95th percentile to define abnormal, 5% of normal kids will have a head that large, so you need to suspect but correlate with other signs before jumping to imaging. If the infant is small enough so the sutures are open ultrasound is a good screening test; however usually a CT will be needed. The lateral ventricles stand out so well owing to their CSF content that CT is well adapted to the initial diagnosis and monitoring of treatment for hydrocephalus (Fig. 7.28). The most critical factor is determining the cause of the hydrocephalus so that you can predict whether or not surgical shunting will be of value for the patient. In most instances the method is straightforward: One looks for the most caudal dilated ventricle and assumes that the obstruction is between that site and the most cephalad normal ventricle. For example, if the lateral and third ventricles are dilated but the fourth ventricle is normal, the obstruction is likely at the outflow area of the third ventricle or the aqueduct of Sylvius (Fig. 7.29).

Often obstructive hydrocephalus can become static owing to equilibration of the CSF dynamics of production and absorption. In this case, it may not be necessary to place a shunt to drain the CSF. Once the dilated ventricles are detected, the need to shunt can be determined by

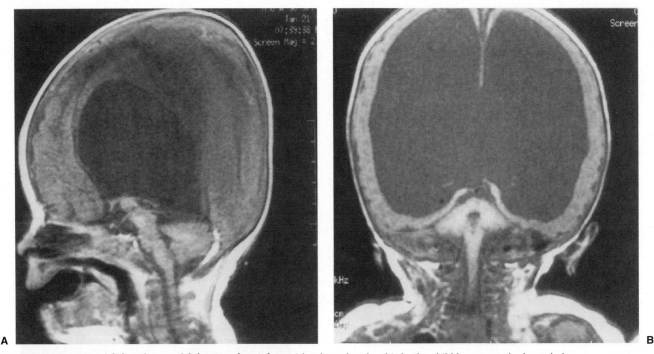

A   B

FIGURE 7.29. Sagittal **(A)** and coronal **(B)** MRIs of an infant with a huge head at birth. The child has severe hydrocephalus involving the lateral and third ventricles but a normal fourth ventricle. This is suggestive of an aqueductal obstruction.

following the ventricular size over time. This should, of course, be coupled with close observation of the patient's clinical status. Do not ever let the imaging hold you back if your patient is deteriorating. CT scans provide sufficient detail for monitoring progression of hydrocephalus. MRI is often of value in the initial evaluation of hydrocephalus, but follow-up monitoring is the domain of CT. Hydrocephalus can occur on other than a congenital basis, but the rules outlined here for evaluation hold for most instances.

MRI is the best method for initial evaluation of most babies with complex defects of the face and brain because the clinical picture is stable and MRI yields better tissue differentiation and multiplanar imaging capability. Holoprosencephaly, or failure of division of the embryonic forebrain, is always associated with facial anomalies and is a good prototype for illustrating the value of MRI. This complex series of anomalies ranges all the way from a totally malformed brain, a condition not compatible with life, to agenesis of the septum pellucidum and optic abnormalities (septo-optic dysplasia), conditions compatible with long life (Fig. 7.30). Whereas CT scans are sufficient for the gross defects of holoprosencephaly, MRI can show sufficient detail to define the absence of the septum pellucidum as well as showing the midline defects of the optic tracts. If you have one test to do in these children, MRI is the best.

Meningocele is a common condition caused by failure of closure of the embryonic neural tube. This condition is almost invariably associated with a complex series of

abnormalities called the Arnold–Chiari II malformation. The reason all of these brain anomalies are associated with what commonly is a spinal abnormality is complex, but the findings are reproducible and best demonstrated by

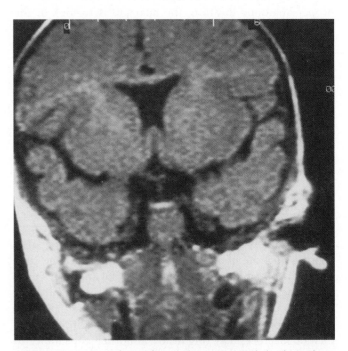

FIGURE 7.30. MRI of an infant with septo-optical dysplasia documents the minimal abnormality of incomplete septation of the lateral ventricles by showing a deficiency of the septum pellucidum.

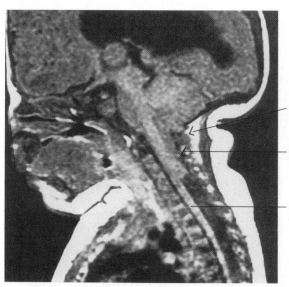

FIGURE 7.31. MRI from a baby with lumbar myelomeningocele. The posterior fossa is small and the cerebellar tonsil protrudes far below the foramen magnum. This is a constant component of the Arnold–Chiari malformation.

— Foramen magnum

— Cerebellar tonsils

— Spinal cord

MRI (Fig. 7.31). The tethering of the spinal cord that occurs with meningocele is associated with protrusion of the cerebellar tonsils below the foramen magnum. As with our other examples, the complex anatomy in developmental brain anomalies is best shown by MRI.

The finding of seizures in a child suggests a congenital defect, either structural or owing to a metabolic problem. In either case, MRI is more likely to yield the correct answers. Structural abnormalities include errors of neuronal migration in which the brain tissues are arrested in their normal growth, leaving focal islands of tissue in abnormal locations throughout the brain (Fig. 7.32).

Other structural abnormalities result from abnormal arrests of neuronal tissues during the proliferating phase of brain development thereby disrupting the normal brain tissue. A good prototype condition here is tuberous sclerosis (Fig. 7.33), although any other phakomatosis can give similar problems. Metabolic abnormalities causing seizures usually cause demyelination, thereby affecting the white matter either diffusely or as focal lesions (Fig. 7.34). MRI is clearly superior to CT here, although the findings are not specific for one disease process; focal infection or demyelinating disorders such as multiple sclerosis can look the same as metabolic defects.

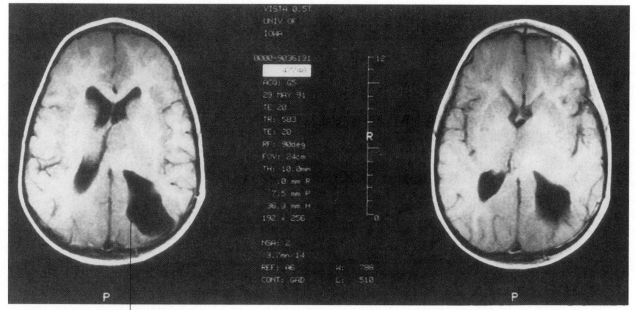

Schizencephalic cleft

FIGURE 7.32. A child with seizures. MRI shows a cleft from the posterior portion of the left lateral ventricle all the way to the brain surface. This condition, caused by a failure of proper migration of neurons as the brain is formed, is called *schizencephaly*.

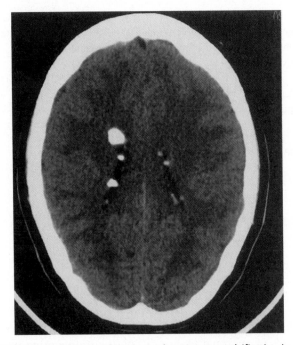

FIGURE 7.33. CT scan of the brain demonstrates calcification in the roof of each lateral ventricle. These calcifications are within the hamartomas or tubers. MRI would also demonstrate the hamartomas as well as showing the lesions that are not calcified.

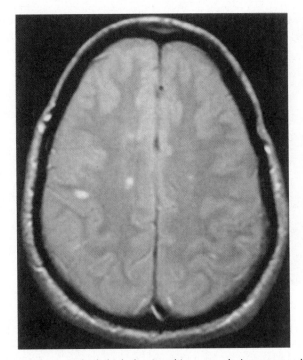

FIGURE 7.34. Multiple high-density white matter lesions are consistent with a myelodegenerative phenomenon, in this case, multiple sclerosis. These findings are not specific and must be combined with the clinical and laboratory results to be diagnostic.

There are many other potential uses for imaging in neurologic disease. However, if you retain the general principles elucidated here, you can make most of the diagnoses needed for patient care, whether or not you completely master all of the nuances of the differential diagnosis.

Key Points

- CAT, or CT, is the most commonly performed neuroimaging study in the United States. CT scans can depict the brain in horizontal planes that can be viewed at different levels.
- When assessing a CT scan for potential trauma, begin by looking for blood in the head outside the vascular system. Blood appears on CT initially as a white blob.
- Mass effect is a clue that pressure is impinging on an area of the brain. The best way to find significant mass effect is to look for asymmetry with displacement of the midline structures.
- Obliteration of the distinction between gray and white matter in the brain represents profound edema. If the edema is universal, you are witnessing a "bad black

brain," which portends a poor outcome and is almost always caused by a limitation of oxygen in the brain.
- On CT, acute strokes often initially appear as a dark edematous blotch obliterating the normal tissue density. On many MRI sequences with inversion recovery or T2 weighting, the damaged tissues are white because of water leaked by the ischemic cells. Diffusion MRI is the most sensitive imaging test for acute stroke.
- Tumors that are entirely enveloped in the brain tissues are usually of glial cell origin, with astrocytoma being the most common primary tumor.
- Complex anatomy in developmental brain anomalies is best shown with MRI.
- Physical abnormalities most often associated with congenital brain abnormalities include macrocephaly (big head), abnormal appearance of the face (particularly with midline abnormalities such as cleft palate), and meningocele.

FURTHER READING

Osborn A. *Diagnostic Neuroradiology*. St. Louis, MO: Mosby, 1994.

▰▰▰▰▰▰▰ QUESTIONS

1. True or false: Considering brain CT
   a. Brain CT uses ionizing radiation techniques
   b. Separate exposures are needed for with and without CT of the brain
   c. Current CT techniques only allow horizontal sectioning of the brain unless the head is repositioned
   d. CT of the brain for trauma is usually performed without intravenous contrast

2. True or false: Regarding brain tumors
   a. The most common malignant brain tumor in adult patients is a metastasis
   b. The theory for contrast enhancement of brain tumors is caused by hypervascularity
   c. Brain tumors in children are usually primary and in the cortex of the brain
   d. MRI has superior tissue contrast to CT and therefore usually gives a more precise location of a tumor

3. True or false: Regarding appropriate brain imaging
   a. Hydrocephalus monitoring, congenital anomaly evaluation, and trauma brain CT usually does not require contrast administration
   b. Most babies with macro-cranium (head circumference above 95th percentile) need evaluation for hydrocephalus
   c. The principal role of MRI in hydrocephalus is usually in specific initial diagnosis and subsequent monitoring is usually done by MRI
   d. MRI is highly useful for demonstrating bone defects and fractures of the calvarium

4. True or false: In suspected vascular disease
   a. MRI is more sensitive than CT for detection of stroke within the first 24 hours after the onset of symptoms
   b. The principal reason for immediate CT after stroke symptoms is to exclude brain hemorrhage
   c. Flair (fluid attenuated inversion recovery) images are the most sensitive diagnostic imaging tool for acute stroke
   d. CT perfusion can only be accurately done on multislice CT devices

Head and Neck

Yutaka Sato

In this chapter, a short overview of head and neck imaging is presented. With the recent advancement and widening availability of sectional imagings, such as CT and MRI, the part played by the plain radiographs has decreased significantly.

As an initial screening of sinusitis or facial trauma, radiographs may be used when more sophisticated sectional imagings are not readily available. For facial bone and paranasal sinus evaluation, routine radiographic views include Waters (Fig. 8.1), Caldwell (Fig. 8.2), and lateral (Fig. 8.3) views. Lack of aeration in the sinus antra is suggestive of sinusitis, and a definitive diagnosis can be made when an air–fluid level is present. CT is the primary modality for the evaluation of sinus infection and facial trauma (Fig. 8.4) because bone detail is best evaluated by CT. Because of multiple horizontally placed buttresses of the facial skeleton, multiplanar reconstructed images in coronal and sagittal planes generated from axial data are essential for the detailed evaluation of facial fractures (Fig. 8.5).

Ultrasound (US), which does not use radiation, is often sufficient to make diagnosis of nonsurgical mass lesions.

When surgery is contemplated, MRI or CT becomes necessary. MR imaging is the modality of choice for the evaluation of neoplastic lesions of the head and neck, because of its superior soft-tissue characterization and multiplanar capability. MR imaging is essential to evaluate skull-base involvement by head and neck tumors.

SINUSITIS

Clinical presentation of pain, swelling over the paranasal sinuses, and leukocytosis are sufficient for the diagnosis of sinusitis and, in the majority of cases, imaging is not necessary. When intraorbital or intracranial extension of the inflammatory process is suspected and surgical intervention is contemplated, imaging becomes necessary. CT is the modality of choice. Acute fluid collection in the sinus cavity is diagnostic, and associated findings include mucosal thickening (Fig. 8.6) and erosive or destructive changes of the sinus wall. Extension of the inflammatory process into the orbits (Fig. 8.7) or cranial cavity may be seen and helps to determine the therapeutic approach.

For evaluation of children, the developmental sequence of the paranasal sinus should be taken into consideration. Generally, the ethmoid and maxillary sinuses are present at birth, but may not be aerated. The sphenoid and frontal sinuses start to be seen at about 3 and 6 years of age, respectively.

TRAUMA

For the evaluation of facial fractures, CT is also the modality of choice. Nasal fractures are the most common, followed by zygomatic fractures. Zygomatic fractures commonly involve: The lateral orbital wall at the frontozygomatic suture, maxillozygomatic suture, and the zygomatic arch, and is named a "trimalar" or "tripod" fracture

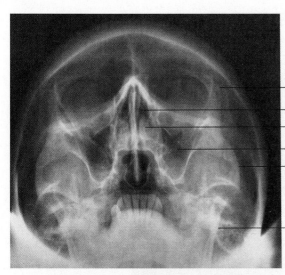

FIGURE 8.1. Normal Waters view of the face, showing the good delineation of the maxilla. The maxillary sinuses are optimally displayed, and the anterior portions of the orbit and the nasal cavity are clearly outlined.

- Frontal zygomatic process
- Nasal cavity
- Nasal turbinate
- Maxillary sinus
- Zygomatic arch
- Mandible

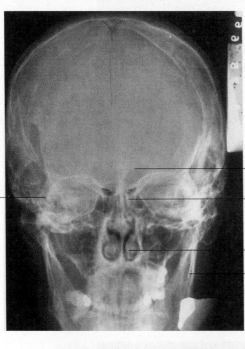

FIGURE 8.2. A Caldwell, or posteroanterior, view of the face. Note how well the orbits and frontal bone are seen. The maxilla is superimposed on the skull base to some degree. The structures of the internal auditory canals are visible through the orbits.

Orbit

- Frontal sinus
- Ethmoid sinuses
- Nasal turbinates
- Ramus of mandible

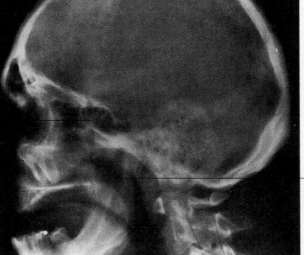

FIGURE 8.3. Lateral view of the skull shows the posteriorly located sphenoid sinus and the nasopharyngeal airway. This view complements the others, adding the third dimension to the structures of the head and the neck.

Frontal sinus

Sphenoid sinus

Anterior wall maxillary sinus

Hard palate

- Nasopharynx

FIGURE 8.4. Normal axial CT images: Inferior plane **(A)**, middle plane **(B)**, and superior plane **(C)**.

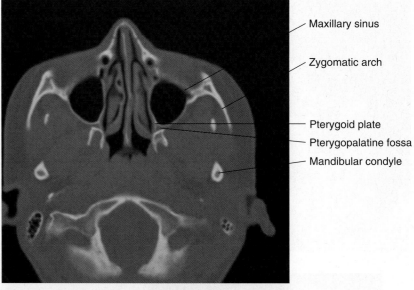

— Maxillary sinus

— Zygomatic arch

— Pterygoid plate
— Pterygopalatine fossa
— Mandibular condyle

A

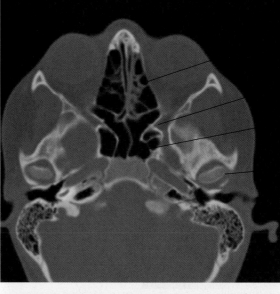

— Ethmoid sinus

— Inferior orbital fissure

— Sphenoid sinus

— Temporomandibular joint

B

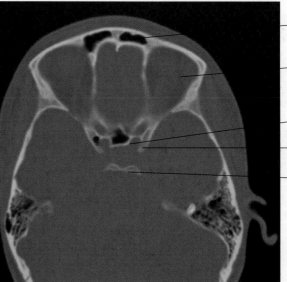

— Frontal sinus

— Orbit

— Optic foramen

— Anterior clinoid process
— Dorsum sella

C

FIGURE 8.5. Reconstructed coronal CT images: Anterior plane **(A)**, middle plane **(B)**, and posterior plane **(C)**.

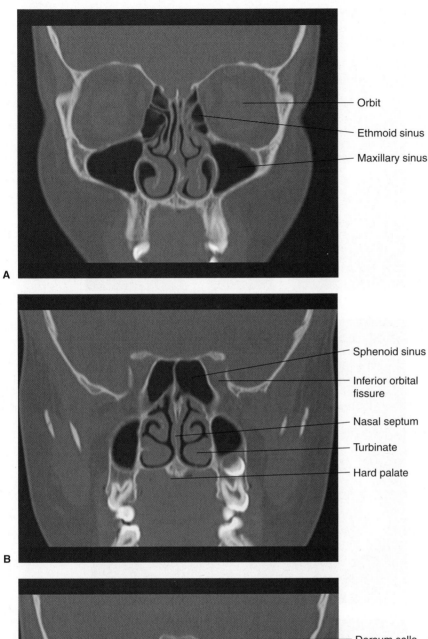

A

— Orbit

— Ethmoid sinus

— Maxillary sinus

B

— Sphenoid sinus

— Inferior orbital fissure

— Nasal septum

— Turbinate

— Hard palate

C

— Dorsum sella

— Sphenoid sinus

— Foramen ovale

FIGURE 8.6. Chronic maxillary sinusitis. The right maxillary sinus is opacified by thickened mucosa, and mucosal thickening extends into the right nasal cavity. Also, notice sclerotic thickening of the sinus wall, suggestive of the chronic nature of the sinusitis.

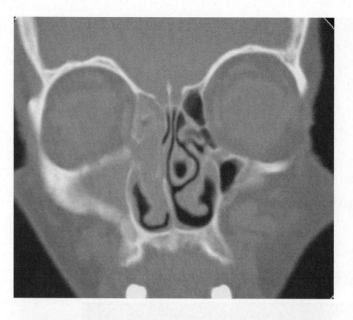

FIGURE 8.7. Orbital cellulitis, **(A/B)** axial/coronal CT. Inflammation of the ethmoid sinus extends into the orbit through the thin wall, lamina papyracea, forming a subperiosteal abscess.

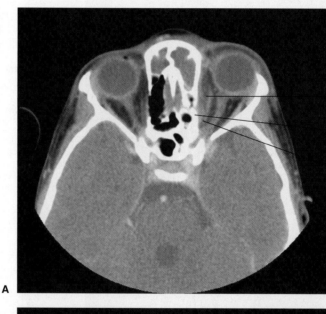

Subperiosteal abscess

Lamina papyracea

Medial rectus muscle

A

Ethmoid sinus

Lamina papyracea

Medial rectus muscle

Maxillary sinus

B

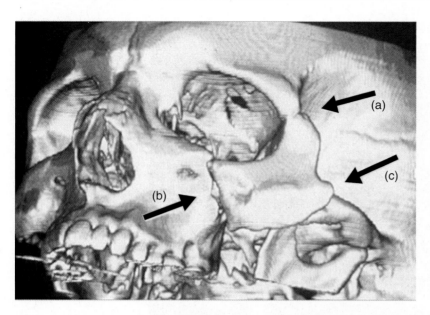

FIGURE 8.8. Tripod fracture. Three-dimensional reformatted CT. Note the fractures involved: (a) The lateral orbital wall, (b) the maxillozygomatic suture, and (c) the zygomatic arch.

(Fig. 8.8). If the facial fracture extends posteriorly and violates the pterygoid plate, the fractured facial bones are detached from the cranium. Depending upon the level of the fracture line traversing the central midface, these fractures are classified as Le Fort I, II, or III fractures (Figs. 8.9 and 8.10).

CT is essential to evaluate the entrapped soft tissue and nerves by the fracture fragments, which may require urgent decompression.

Orbital blowout fracture occurs when an object larger than the orbit, such as a fist or a baseball, hits the eye. The impact is transmitted to the orbital contents and raises the

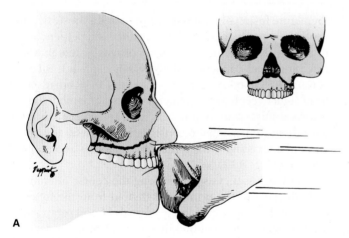

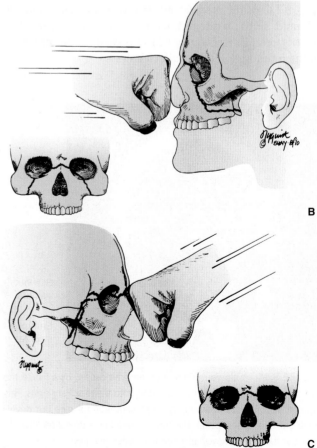

FIGURE 8.9. A: Le Fort I fracture. **B:** Le Fort II fracture. **C:** Le Fort III fracture. (From Langland OE, Langlais RP, McDavid WD, et al. eds. *Panoramic Radiology.* 2nd ed. Philadelphia, PA: Lea & Febiger, 1989, with permission.)

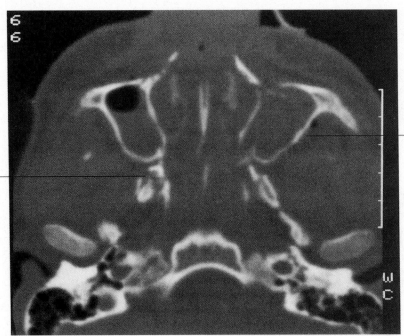

FIGURE 8.10. CT scan of an auto accident victim who struck the windshield. There are multiple fractures including disruption of the deeper structures of the face (pterygoid plates illustrated). This is a complex fracture pattern of the Le Fort type and can be defined well only with CT.

intraorbital pressure enough to shatter the weakest wall of the orbit, either the inferior wall into the maxillary sinus (Fig. 8.11) or the medial wall (lamina papyracea) into the ethmoid sinus, without fracturing the orbital rim. The inferior rectus muscle may be trapped and cause paralysis of the inferior gaze of the affected eye.

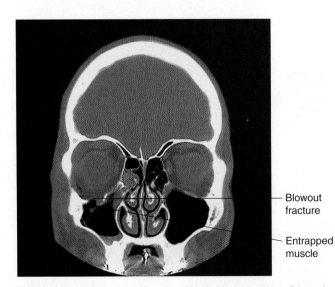

FIGURE 8.11. A blowout fracture of the orbit caused by a fist to the eye. Note the soft tissue mass protruding into the maxillary sinus. This woman had no gaze abnormality on presentation for care but developed one shortly thereafter. The fracture required surgical reconstruction, but the patient now has a normally functioning eye.

CONGENITAL ANOMALIES

Premature fusion of a cranial suture (craniosynostosis) prevents the growth of cranium in the direction perpendicular to the involved suture. Sagittal synostosis results in a narrow long head (dolichocephaly, scaphocephaly). Bilateral coronal or lambdoid synostosis results in a broad short head (brachycephaly). Unilateral coronal or lambdoid synostosis results in an asymmetric head (plagiocephaly). CT with three-dimensional reconstruction is useful for evaluation of coexisting intracranial abnormalities and surgical planning (Fig. 8.12).

Thyroglossal cysts occur along the course of embryologic dissents of the primordial thyroid from the foramen cecum of the tongue base to the normal cervical paratracheal location and is most commonly seen as an anterior paramedian cystic mass closely related to the strap muscle (Fig. 8.13).

Branchial cleft cysts are prototypical congenital lateral neck masses seen at the bifurcation of the carotid artery anterior to the sternocleidomastoid (SCM) muscle (Fig. 8.14).

Venolymphatic malformations (aka cystic hygroma) are developmental vascular malformations most commonly seen as a multilocular cystic mass often associated with hemorrhagic fluid–fluid levels in the posterolateral neck centered around the posterior triangle (Fig. 8.15).

Fibromatosis colli is a benign fibrous proliferation of the SCM muscle and the most common cause of neonatal torticollis. US is diagnostic, demonstrating spindle-shaped enlargement of the lower one-third of the SCM muscle (Fig. 8.16). It is treated conservatively with physiotherapy.

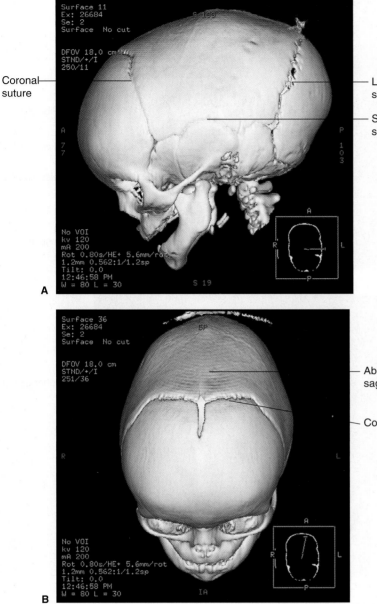

A

B

FIGURE 8.12. Sagittal synostosis, **(A,B)** lateral/anterior view of the three-dimensional reconstructed CT images. The sagittal suture is fused and the head is dolichocephalic.

Coronal suture

Lambdoid suture

Squamosal suture

Absent sagittal suture

Coronal suture

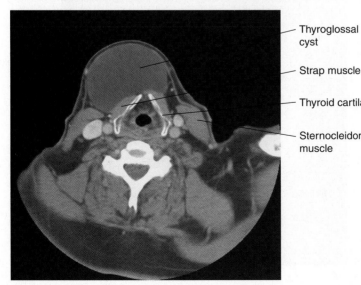

Thyroglossal cyst

Strap muscle

Thyroid cartilage

Sternocleidomastoid muscle

FIGURE 8.13. Thyroglossal cyst. CT of the infrahyoid neck shows a paramedian cystic mass anterior to the strap muscle.

FIGURE 8.14. Branchial cleft cyst. CT at the hyoid level shows a lateral neck cystic mass anteromedial to the sternocleidomastoid muscle, lateral to the carotid artery and internal jugular vein.

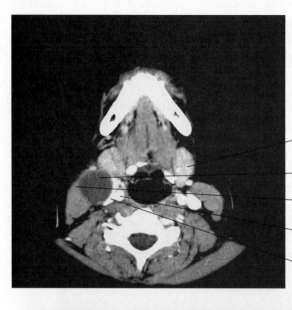
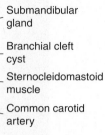

Submandibular gland

Branchial cleft cyst

Sternocleidomastoid muscle

Common carotid artery

Internal jugular vein

FIGURE 8.15. Venolymphatic malformation. MR images (**A/B,** coronal/axial T2-weighted images) show multicystic mass lesion in the base of the neck posteromedial to the sternocleidomastoid muscle extending into the axilla. Note also multiple fluid–fluid levels (*arrows*) caused by intracystic hemorrhage.

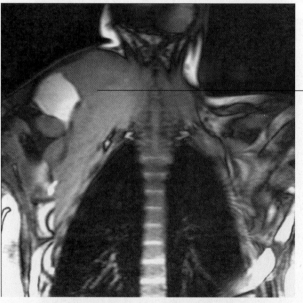

Lymphangioma

A

Sternocleidomastoid muscle

B

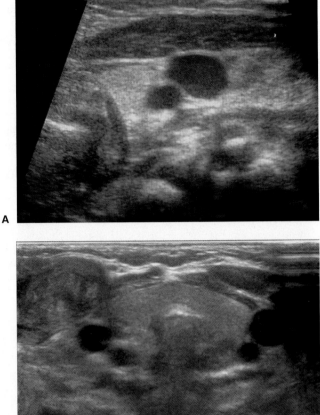

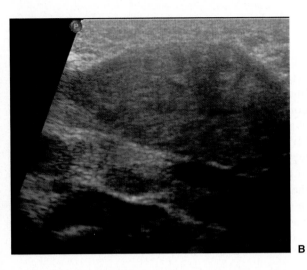

FIGURE 8.16. Fibromatosis colli of the right SCM muscle. **A:** US longitudinal along the normal left sternocleidomastoid muscle. **B:** Along the right SCM muscle. **C:** Transverse. US images along the sternocleidomastoid muscle show a spindle-shaped enlargement of the lower one-third of the right SCM muscle.

TUMORS

MRI is the modality of choice to evaluate the neoplastic lesions of the head and neck. The histologic diagnosis of head and neck neoplasms are usually made by fine-needle biopsy and imagings are primarily used to evaluate the extent of the disease, to delineate the relationship of the tumor to the adjacent anatomic structures, and to evaluate metastasis to the regional lymph nodes. All of this information is essential to determine the optimal mode of therapy. MRI

is essential, particularly for the evaluation of skull-base involvement by head and neck tumors (Fig. 8.12).

In adults, squamous cell carcinoma is the most common malignant head and neck mass. Among the pediatric age group, benign masses are more common than malignant ones. Benign masses include congenital cystic lesions such as thyroglossal cysts and branchial cleft cysts. Benign neoplasms seen in this age group include teratoma and juvenile angiofibroma. Rhabdomyosarcoma is the most common pediatric head and neck malignancy (Fig. 8.17).

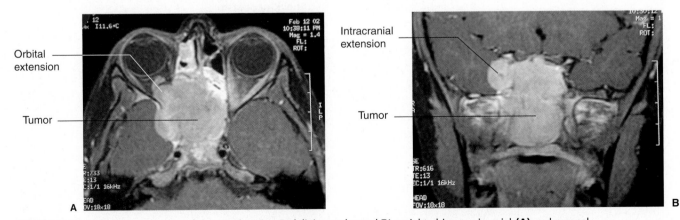

FIGURE 8.17. Rhabdomyosarcoma of the nasal cavity. Gadolinium-enhanced T1 weighted images in axial **(A)** and coronal plane **(B)** show avidly enhancing nasal cavity mass extending into the right orbit and into the cavernous sinus.

Key Points

- CT is the imaging modality of choice in the evaluation of sinusitis and facial bone fractures.
- Imaging features of sinusitis include acute fluid collection of the sinus cavity, mucosal thickening, and erosion of the bony wall of the sinus.
- "Tripod" fractures involve the lateral orbital wall, maxillozygomatic suture, and zygomatic arch.
- In Le Fort fractures, the facial bones are detached from the cranium by the fracture of the pterygoid plates.
- In orbital blowout fractures, the inferior rectus muscle may be trapped by the fracture fragments of the orbital floor, requiring surgical release.

- MR is the imaging modality of choice in evaluating head and neck tumors. A skull-base extension of the tumor requires MR imaging.
- In adults, malignant mass lesions are common. In children, benign masses are more common.

FURTHER READINGS

Harnsberger HR, Glastonbury CM, Michel MA, et al. *Diagnostic Imaging: Head and Neck.* 2nd ed. Salt Lake City: Amirsys, 2010.

Som PM, Curtin HD, eds. *Head and Neck Imaging.* 5th ed. St. Louis, MO: Mosby, 2011.

QUESTIONS

1. What is the most appropriate imaging modality to examine facial fractures?
   a. Radiographs
   b. Ultrasound
   c. CT
   d. MRI

2. What is the correct sequence of sinus development?
   a. Maxillary/ethmoid–frontal–sphenoid
   b. Maxillary/ethmoid–sphenoid–frontal
   c. Frontal–sphenoid–maxillary/ethmoid
   d. Sphenoid–maxillary/ethmoid–frontal

3. Which is the component not affected by tripod fracture of the facial bone?
   a. Zygomatic arch
   b. Frontozygomatic suture
   c. Lamina papyracea
   d. Maxillozygomatic suture

4. Which cranial suture synostosis is responsible for dolichocephaly?
   a. Bilateral coronal sutures
   b. Bilateral lambdoid sutures
   c. Sagittal suture
   d. Metopic suture

5. Differential diagnosis of a cystic neck mass in the neck on US examination include following entities except
   a. venolymphatic malformation
   b. branchial cleft anomalies
   c. thyroglossal duct anomalies
   d. fibromatosis colli

6. Choose all the correct statements from below.
   a. Majority of pediatric neck masses are benign
   b. Thyroglossal cyst is paramedian in location
   c. Branchial cleft cyst is lateral neck in location
   d. Rhabdomyosarcoma is the most common pediatric neck neoplasm

Spine and Pelvis

Carol A. Boles

The axial skeleton consists of the skull (which is covered separately), the spine, and the pelvis. It is the main structural support for the body and, as a result, is subjected to many stresses. The spine consists of cervical, thoracic, lumbar, and sacral divisions composed of bones, joints, ligaments, muscular attachments, and nerves. The pelvis articulates with the sacrum on each side, supports many soft tissue structures, articulates with the femurs, and is the proximal attachment for many muscles involved in locomotion.

Back pain is a problem for the majority of patients at some time in their lives. Most people recover from their back pain with little or no medical care. Occupational-related back injuries are not uncommon and other common etiologies of back pain are listed in Table 9.1. When patients do seek medical care for back pain, radiologic imaging is frequently overutilized. Following a thorough history and physical examination, anteroposterior (AP) and lateral radiographs often are the first radiologic consultation to be requested to evaluate the symptomatic region of the spine. These images may be supplemented

with oblique and coned-down views to better visualize an area, and occasionally lateral flexion and extension views are requested to document spine motion and stability. Yet according to the American College of Radiology Appropriateness Criteria, imaging is usually not appropriate for uncomplicated acute low back pain and/or radiculopathy with a nonsurgical presentation.

Magnetic resonance imaging (MRI) can be a useful, noninvasive diagnostic tool in visualizing the spine, discs, and nerves, and its use is increasing while utilization of the invasive myelogram with CT is decreasing. CT delineates anatomy and pathology, particularly lateral disc herniations, more clearly than does myelography with only radiography. CT can demonstrate disc disease and degenerative facet disease, but has largely been replaced by MRI for this purpose. MRI is very good for imaging soft tissues and the bone marrow, spinal cord, and the intervertebral discs.

CT is, however, quite helpful for localizing the exact position of vertebral fracture fragments following acute trauma, particularly important when the fracture fragments are displaced into the spinal canal. MRI is also used

Table 9.1

Back Pain Etiology

Congenital/Developmental
Meningocele and myelomeningocele
Syringomyelia
Transitional vertebra with pseudarthrosis
Sickle cell anemia
Scheuermann disease

Acquired
Discs Herniation, Annular Tear
Arthritis–degenerative, rheumatoid, ankylosing
    spondylitis
Infection–staphylococcus, tuberculosis
Metabolic–osteoporosis, osteomalacia, Paget disease
Neoplasm–benign and malignant primary bone
    tumors, metastatic
Trauma–fracture, muscle and ligament injury,
    spondylolysis, and spondylolisthesis

Extraspinal
Cardiovascular system–referred myocardial pain,
    aortic aneurysm
Gastrointestinal disease
Genitourinary system–renal and ureteral pain
Muscle strain
Psychosomatic or functional

Table 9.2

Indications for the Use of Imaging Modalities in the Spine and Pelvis

Radiographs (in the setting of trauma)
Cervical spine—lateral
Pelvis–AP

CT
Fractures

MRI
Soft tissues and bone marrow (tumor, infection)
Spinal cord and disc disease
Fractures with suspected cord injury

Myelogram
Disc disease, spinal stenosis

---

when a spine fracture is present and an associated cord injury is suspected (Table 9.2). However, MRI costs at least twice as much as CT imaging. In addition, some patients may not be able to have an MRI because the strong magnetic field may disrupt a pacemaker, displace an aneurysm clip, or the patient may not tolerate the relatively confined space.

NORMAL IMAGES

Despite a decreasing need for radiography of the spine, a thorough understanding is necessary, particularly since post injury follow-up examinations are typically radiographs. Normal versus abnormal as well as detection of subtle changes may have profound effects on patient outcome.

Cervical Spine

As previously emphasized in other anatomic regions, a systematic approach for evaluating the spine is needed. You will eventually develop your own system, but the following one will work until you do (Table 9.3). Start with the lateral radiograph (Fig. 9.1A) as it is the most important cervical spine radiograph. Glance at the entire image to see if something obvious jumps out at you. If it does, put that aside and force yourself to look at the entire study.

It is not uncommon to stop looking once one abnormality is found. This can lead to serious consequences! On the lateral radiograph the normal cervical curve should be mildly convex anteriorly (lordotic). When the patient has pain, straightening of the spine may occur secondary to muscle spasm. A patient in a hard cervical collar also has a straightened curvature. Make note of the normal lines that should be intact on this view (Fig. 9.1B). Now simply count the cervical vertebrae. Things you must see in the setting of trauma include: All seven cervical vertebrae, the entire C7 and T1 intervertebral disc space, and, ideally, the T1 vertebral body. This is especially important as a fracture could be lurking in nonvisualized areas of the spine, and the result could be catastrophic. For example,

---

Table 9.3

Checklist for Spinal Radiograph Observations

Lateral Radiograph
Alignment (three lines in cervical spine)
Must visualize seven cervical vertebrae
Vertebral body heights
Disc space heights
Osseous density
Facet joints/pars interarticularis

AP Radiograph
Alignment
Vertebral body heights
Disc space heights
Bone density
Pedicles (lower cervical, T- and L-spine)
Facet joints

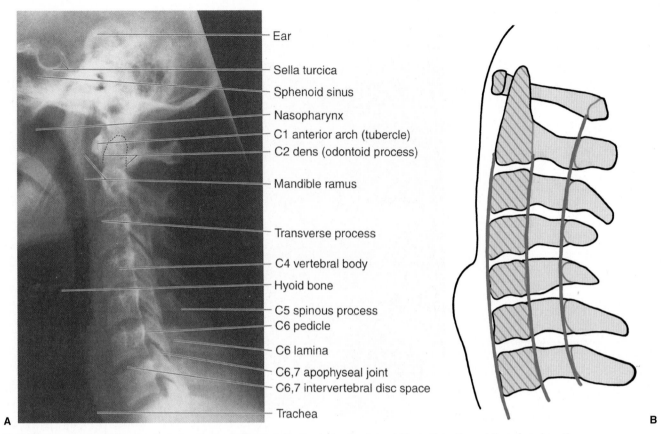

A   **B**

FIGURE 9.1. A: Cervical spine lateral radiograph. Normal. **B:** Cervical spine lateral illustration. Normal lines found on the normal lateral radiograph.

if the C7 vertebra is not included on the lateral cervical spine radiograph, a fracture of C7 might go unrecognized. An unrecognized and displaced fracture has the potential to cause a serious cord injury (see Fig. 9.28). *Always* gauge the vertical heights of the vertebral bodies and the intervertebral disc spaces. The vertical heights of each vertebral body and intervertebral disc space should be approximately equal to those immediately above and below. Note the osseous densities in general. Some common causes for decreased (osteopenia) and increased bone density are shown in Table 9.4. Metastatic bone disease from prostate, breast, and other malignancies can result in an increased bone density or osteosclerotic appearance. The transverse foramina may appear as focal, round lucencies projected over the vertebral body; this is most common at C2.

Next, look at the AP radiograph (Fig. 9.2A) and again check the alignment of the cervical spine. The spine should be straight on this view. Again note the heights of the vertebral bodies and intervertebral disc spaces. When disease or injury is suspected at the C1 and C2 levels, an AP radiograph of the upper cervical spine is obtained by directing the central x-ray beam through the patient's open mouth. This is called the *open mouth view* (Fig. 9.2B), and it allows visualization of the dens, or odontoid process, of

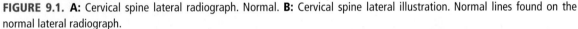

Table 9.4

Some Common Causes for Increased and Decreased Bone Density

Decreased
Osteolytic metastases
Osteomalacia
Osteomyelitis
Osteoporosis
Primary bone tumor, especially multiple myeloma
Rheumatoid arthritis, ankylosing spondylitis

Increased
Bone infarcts
Bone island
Callus formation–fractures
Endplate sclerosis–disc degeneration
Fibrous dysplasia
Lymphoma
Osteoblastic metastases (prostate and breast)
Osteopetrosis
Paget disease
Primary bone tumors (5% of multiple myeloma)

FIGURE 9.2. A: Cervical spine AP radiograph. Normal. **B:** Cervical spine AP open mouth radiograph of the upper cervical spine. Normal.

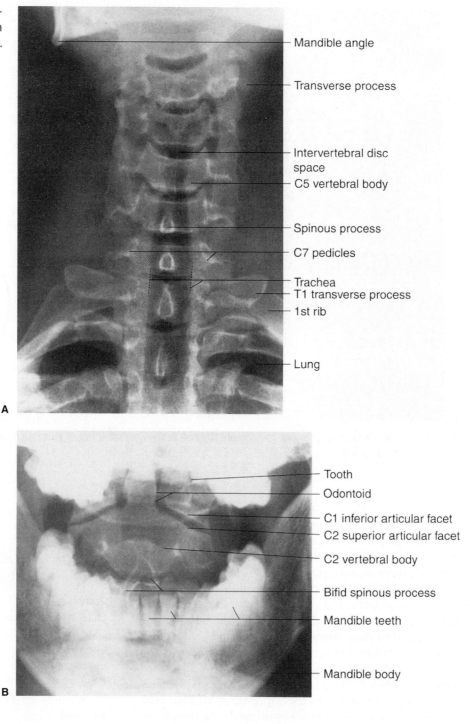

A

- Mandible angle

- Transverse process

- Intervertebral disc space
- C5 vertebral body

- Spinous process

- C7 pedicles

- Trachea
- T1 transverse process
- 1st rib

- Lung

B

- Tooth
- Odontoid

- C1 inferior articular facet
- C2 superior articular facet

- C2 vertebral body

- Bifid spinous process

- Mandible teeth

- Mandible body

the C2 vertebra and the C1 and C2 alignments and joints. An extremely important observation to make is the presence or absence of the vertebral pedicles. Pedicles look like the headlights of the vertebrae in the low cervical, thoracic, and lumbar regions, but are obliquely oriented in the upper and mid cervical spines and best seen on cervical oblique views. They are often involved by metastatic diseases because of their abundant blood supply. *If one or more pedicles are absent, metastatic involvement or some other destructive process must be strongly suspected.* There

are benign causes such as a meningocele or congenital absence of the pedicle, but these need to be proven rather than assumed.

Occasionally, oblique views (Fig. 9.3) are obtained and the same observations are made as on the other views. The intervertebral foramina, through which the spinal nerves pass, are well seen on these views. Any disease process that narrows the foramina could potentially cause pressure on the nerve exiting through that neural foramen, resulting in radiculopathy, or pain along the distribution

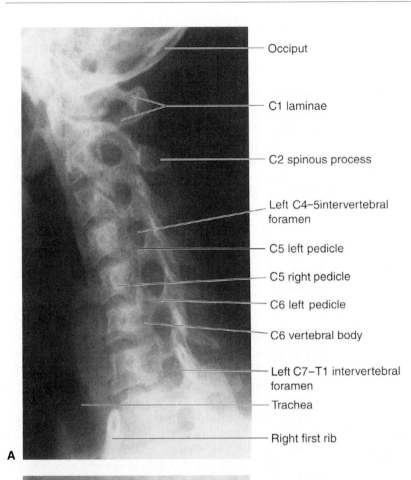

Occiput

C1 laminae

C2 spinous process

Left C4–5intervertebral foramen

C5 left pedicle

C5 right pedicle

C6 left pedicle

C6 vertebral body

Left C7–T1 intervertebral foramen

Trachea

Right first rib

A

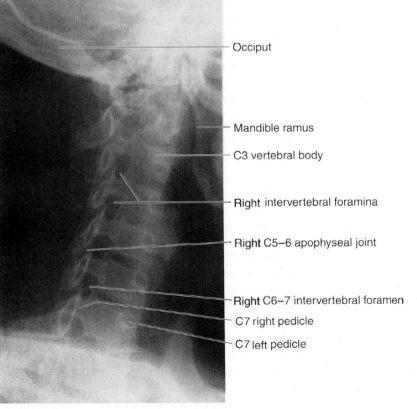

Occiput

Mandible ramus

C3 vertebral body

Right intervertebral foramina

Right C5–6 apophyseal joint

Right C6–7 intervertebral foramen

C7 right pedicle

C7 left pedicle

B

FIGURE 9.3. Cervical spine right **(A)** and left **(B)** oblique radiographs. Normal.

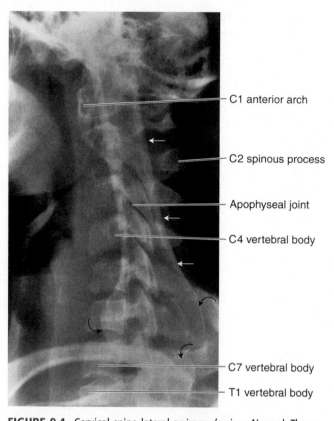

C1 anterior arch

C2 spinous process

Apophyseal joint

C4 vertebral body

C7 vertebral body

T1 vertebral body

FIGURE 9.4. Cervical spine lateral swimmer's view. Normal. The patient is almost always radiographed supine with one arm, usually the left, abducted upward alongside the head whereas the other arm is lowered. This position makes patients appear as if they are swimming the backstroke. The central x-ray beam is directed to the C7–T1 level from the patient's side on which the arm is lowered, usually the right. The *straight arrows* indicate the raised arm humerus projecting over the spine. The *curved arrows* outline the humeral head. Note how well the C7 vertebra is visualized as well as a portion of the T1 vertebra and the apophyseal joints. In this view, it is considered a good technique when you can see the entire C7 vertebra and at least the upper one-third of the T1 vertebral body.

of the involved nerve. Some processes that can impinge on the intervertebral foramina include intervertebral disc disease, arthritis, and primary and secondary neoplasms. In the trauma setting, these oblique views allow for evaluation of the facet joints to look for fractures or dislocations.

Lateral flexion and extension views may be necessary to evaluate stability of the spine and assess for ligamentous injury. They should not routinely be obtained when a fracture is present. The majority of motion occurs in the upper cervical spine. When the lower cervical vertebrae cannot be visualized on the lateral view, a swimmer's view is indicated (Fig. 9.4). CT is typically used to diagnose cervical spine fractures, determine the extent of fractures, and localize fracture fragments. High-level trauma patients are routinely screened with a CT of the entire cervical spine. The CT data can then be reformatted into coronal and sag-

ittal plane images. As already mentioned, MRI is especially useful to evaluate the spinal cord, the intervertebral discs, and assess ligamentous injury (Fig. 9.5).

Thoracic Spine

Radiographic study of the thoracic spine consists of AP and lateral radiographs (Fig. 9.6). When viewing the thoracic spine, it is easiest to begin with the lateral view and follow the same method of evaluation as used for the lateral cervical spine radiograph. The normal dorsal curve should be mildly convex posterior (kyphotic). Again, assess the vertical heights of the dorsal vertebral bodies and intervertebral disc spaces. As always, check the overall densities of the bones. The lamina and spinous processes are not well seen because the ribs project over them (see Fig. 9.6B). It is difficult to number the vertebral bodies without using the anterior view to determine the size of the twelfth rib.

Next, evaluate the AP thoracic spine radiograph; the spinal alignment should be straight. Assess the vertical height of each dorsal vertebral body and each dorsal intervertebral disc space. The paraspinal line along the left side of the vertebra should be narrow and straight. A focal bulge may be your first indication of a fracture. The pedicles look like headlights on the vertebral bodies, and every attempt should be made to visualize all of them. On AP radiographs, the spinous processes project over the mid vertebral bodies at all levels in the spine. Assess the number of rib-bearing vertebra. T12 typically has two short ribs, but transverse processes may instead be present. Similarly, L1 may have rudimentary ribs so it is important to count from the top down. Occasionally, C7 will have short ribs, but these do not have the typical curved appearance of the true first rib and is usually not a cause of mislabeling.

MRI and CT (Fig. 9.7) imaging are useful in the thoracic spine for the same indications as in the cervical spine.

Lumbar Spine

Pain in the lumbar spine region is a major cause of disability, lost work time, and health–dollar expenditure. The etiology of back pain is complicated, varied, and poorly understood. When obtained, lumbar radiographs generally consist of AP and lateral views (Fig. 9.8). As previously noted, look first at the lateral view using the same system as described for the lateral cervical and dorsal spine radiographs. In general, note the lumbar spine alignment, which is normally convex anterior (lordotic). When muscle spasm or disease processes are present, this normal curvature may be lost and the spine appears straight. In addition, observe the overall osseous densities. Next, carefully evaluate the vertical heights of the lumbar vertebral bodies and the intervertebral disc spaces; they should be approximately equal to those immediately above and below, but gradually become taller as you progress distally. As a general rule, the L4–L5 intervertebral disc space

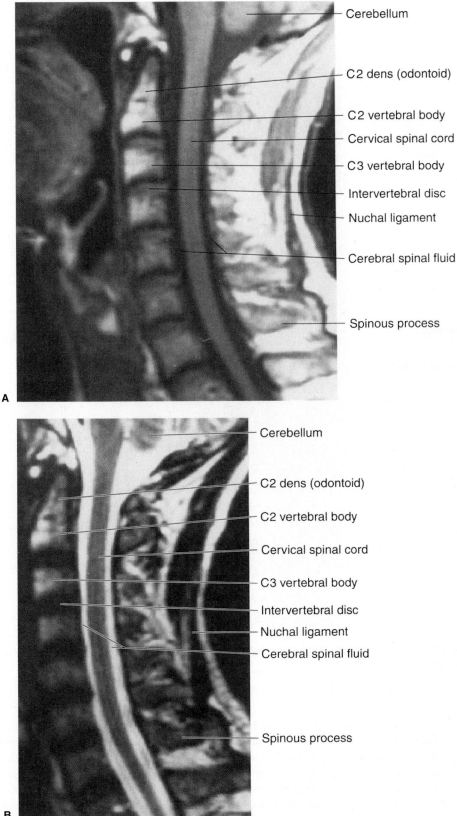

— Cerebellum

— C2 dens (odontoid)

— C2 vertebral body
— Cervical spinal cord
— C3 vertebral body
— Intervertebral disc
— Nuchal ligament

— Cerebral spinal fluid

— Spinous process

A

— Cerebellum

— C2 dens (odontoid)

— C2 vertebral body

— Cervical spinal cord

— C3 vertebral body

— Intervertebral disc
— Nuchal ligament
— Cerebral spinal fluid

— Spinous process

B

FIGURE 9.5. A: Cervical spine midline sagittal T1 MR image. Normal. The cerebral spinal fluid is nearly black on a T1-weighted image and white on a T2-weighted image. The bone marrow fat appears whiter (high-intensity signal) on a T1 image than on the T2 image. **B:** Cervical spine midline sagittal T2 MR image. Normal.

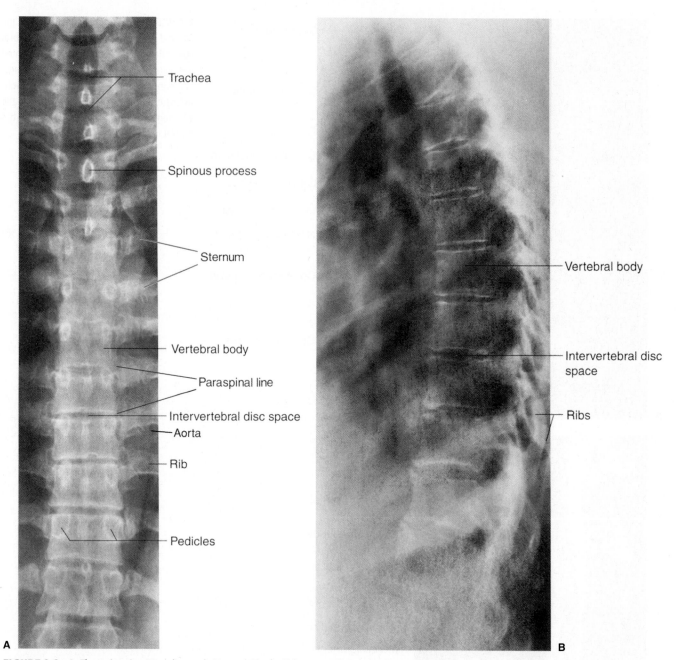

FIGURE 9.6. **A:** Thoracic spine AP radiograph. Normal. The pedicles on each vertebra have an appearance similar to automobile headlights. **B:** Thoracic spine lateral radiograph. Normal.

height is greater than the other lumbar disc spaces. This also means that the L5–S1 disc level is typically narrower than that at L4–L5 and should not be considered abnormal because of decreased height alone. It should be noted that an isolated decreased disc space has no association with clinical symptoms as decreased disc space height is so prevalent. Approximately 15% of the population will have variability in the appearance at the lumbosacral junction. There may be partial or complete lumbarization of S1 or sacralization of L5. Numbering of the lumbar spine can be very difficult and every attempt should be made to number

correctly using chest radiographs if needed to count the number of ribs. It is incorrect to assume that the first non-rib-bearing vertebra on the anterior view is L1 and the vertebra above the sacrum on lateral view is L5. I have seen the same vertebral body numbered differently on the AP and lateral views! Finally, observe the facet joints since facet joint arthritis can be a cause of back pain.

Similar observations are made on the AP radiograph regarding alignment, density, vertical heights of the lumbar vertebral bodies, and the lumbar intervertebral disc spaces. Again, be certain that all of the pedicles are present.

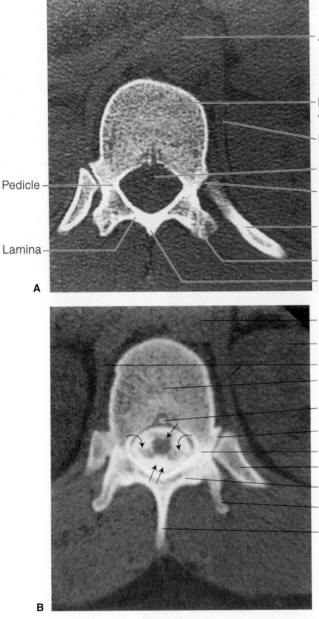

Aorta

Dorsal vertebral body

Diaphragm crus

Spinal canal

Costovertebral articulation

12th rib

Transverse process

Spinous process

Pedicle

Lamina

A

Aorta

Left kidney

Diaphragm crura

Vertebral body

Basivertebral vein

Costovertebral joint

Pedicle

12th rib

Lamina

Mamillary process

Spinous process

B

FIGURE 9.7. A: Thoracic spine axial CT image at the T12 level. Normal. **B:** Thoracic spine axial CT image at the T12 level. Normal. The spinal cord (*single straight arrow*), nerve roots (*curved arrows*), and the contrast-filled subarachnoid space (*double straight arrows*) are well visualized. The contrast media was introduced into the subarachnoid space as part of a myelogram while the CT imaging followed the myelogram. Note how well the osseous structures of the spine are demonstrated.

Depending on the angulation at L5–S1, it may be difficult to see the L5 pedicles. Occasionally, an angled anterior view is obtained to better evaluate L5 (Fig. 9.9). This view also nicely displays the sacroiliac (SI) joints. Always observe the pars interarticularis region of each vertebra for a possible defect, as an interruption of bone continuity in the pars interarticularis is abnormal and called *spondylolysis*. The pars can be seen on lateral view, but is quite difficult on the anterior projection. It is easiest to see on the oblique view also that, oblique radiographs (Fig. 9.10) are sometimes necessary to better assess the pars interarticularis when spondylolysis is suspected. Once again, the observation checklist for spine radiographs is outlined in Table 9.3.

MRI of the lumbar spine is often requested to evaluate the vertebrae, intervertebral disc spaces, and the spinal cord (Fig. 9.11), which usually ends at the level of L1. As elsewhere in the spine, CT imaging may be requested to determine the presence and extent of fractures and the presence of intervertebral disc disease (Fig. 9.12).

In the past, the myelogram was the gold standard for the diagnosis of disease in and around the neural canal. The myelogram is an invasive procedure that is accompanied by discomfort. It is accomplished by injecting contrast material into the intrathecal space via a lumbar or cervical puncture and typical images are shown in Figure 9.13. Fortunately, water-soluble myelographic contrast agents do not require physical removal as oil-based

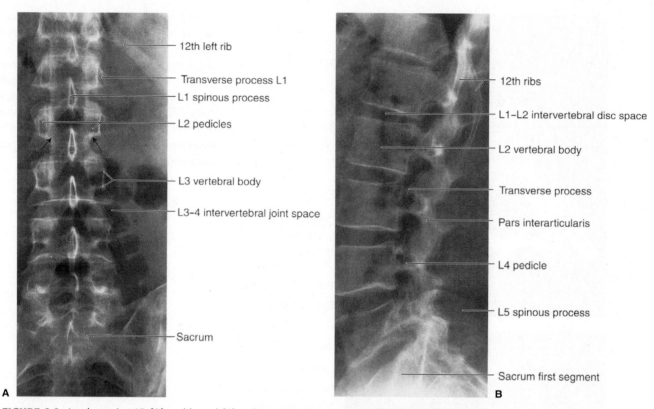

FIGURE 9.8. Lumbar spine AP **(A)** and lateral **(B)** radiographs. Normal. The arrows on the AP radiograph indicate the pars interarticularis region.

FIGURE 9.9. Lumbar spine angled view of lumbosacral junction. Note how the L5–S1 disc is now easily seen when compared to Figure 9.8. The facets are prominent due to arthritis. The *small straight arrows* show the arcuate line of the right S1 anterior sacral foramen.

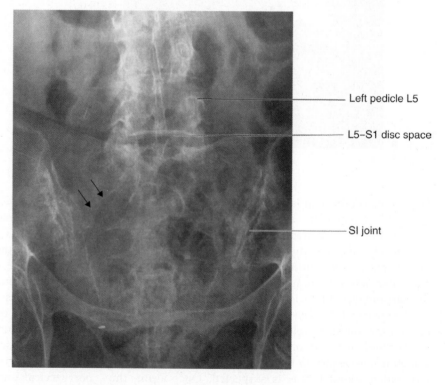

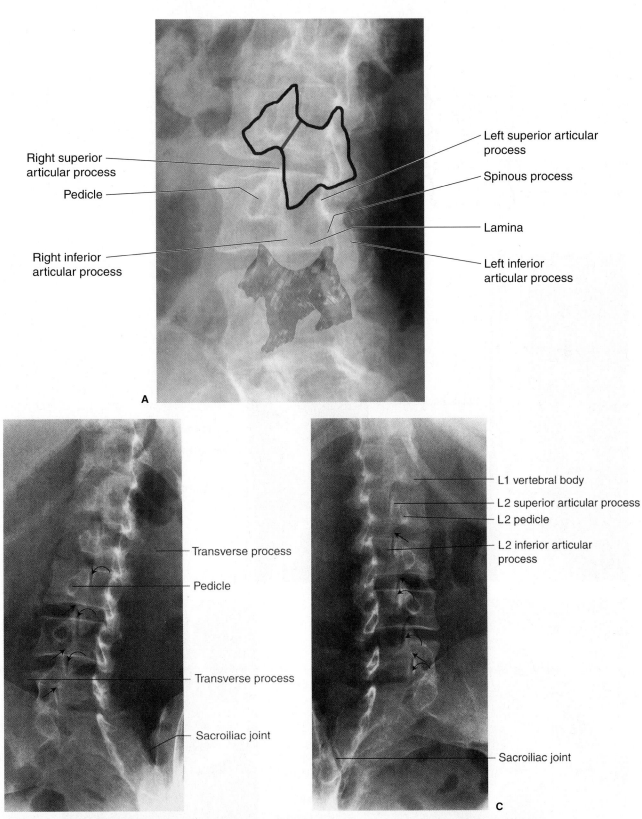

Right superior articular process

Pedicle

Right inferior articular process

Left superior articular process

Spinous process

Lamina

Left inferior articular process

B

Transverse process

Pedicle

Transverse process

Sacroiliac joint

C

L1 vertebral body

L2 superior articular process

L2 pedicle

L2 inferior articular process

Sacroiliac joint

FIGURE 9.10. A: Visible "Scotty dog" and the anatomy that it represents on oblique lumbar spine radiographs. The neck of the Scotty dog represents the pars interarticularis. When the Scotty dog neck is disrupted, the condition is called spondylolysis. **B,C:** Lumbar spine right **(B)** and left **(C)** oblique radiographs. Normal. Note on these oblique views how well you visualize the normal pars interarticularis or the neck of the Scotty dog (*straight arrows*) and the normal apophyseal (facet) joints between the superior and inferior articular processes (*curved arrows*).

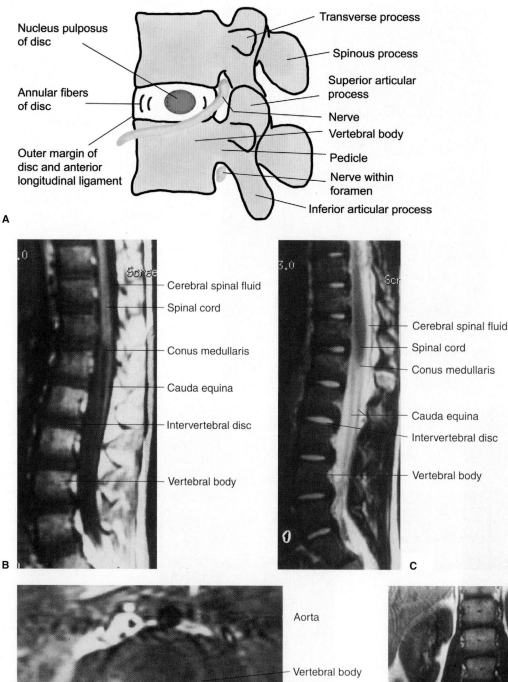

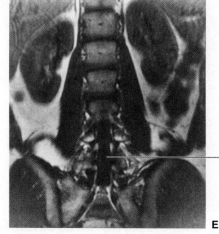

FIGURE 9.11. A: Lumbar spine lateral illustration. Normal. **B,C:** Lumbar spine T1 **(B)** and T2 **(C)** sagittal MR images. Normal. Notice again that the cerebral spinal fluid is black on a T1 image and white on a T2 image. Also, the bone marrow fat is whiter (high-intensity signal) on the T1 image. The intervertebral disc is whiter on the T2 image. **D:** Lumbar spine T1 axial image. Normal. Note that the nerve roots (*curved arrows*) are well visualized. **E:** Lumbar spine T1 coronal MR image. Normal. The coronal plane passes through the upper lumbar vertebral bodies and the lower lumbar neural sac. Illustration by CBoles Art.

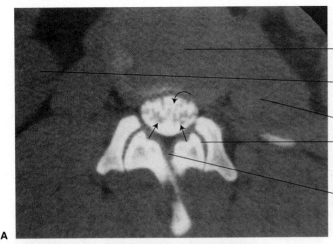

Lumbar
intervertebral
disc

Right kidney

Psoas muscle

Apophyseal
joint

Ligamentum
flavum

A

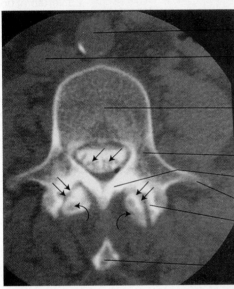

Aorta

Inferior vena cava

Lumbar
vertebral body

Pedicle

Lamina

Transverse process

Inferior articular
process

Spinous process

B

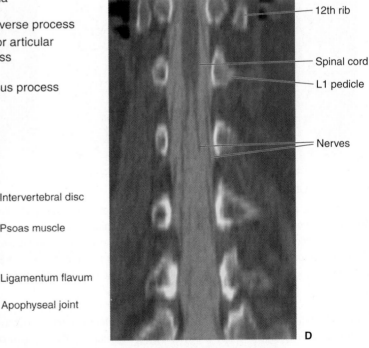

12th rib

Spinal cord

L1 pedicle

Nerves

D

Intervertebral disc

Psoas muscle

Ligamentum flavum

Apophyseal joint

C

FIGURE 9.12. **A:** Lumbar spine axial CT image through the L1–L2 intervertebral disc level. Normal. The *straight arrows* indicate the cauda equina surrounded by contrast media in the subarachnoid space cerebral spinal fluid (*curved arrow*). **B:** Lumbar spine axial CT image through a lumbar vertebra. Normal. The *single straight arrows* indicate multiple nerve roots. Notice how the inferior articular processes of the vertebra articulate with the superior articular processes (*curved arrows*) from the vertebra below to form the apophyseal joints (*double straight arrows*). **C:** Lumbar spine axial CT image through a lumbar intervertebral disc. Normal. The *straight arrow* indicates nerve roots in the posterior aspect of the subarachnoid space whereas the *curved arrows* indicate nerve roots about to exit through the neural foramina. **D:** Lumbar spine coronal reformatted CT. The image was obtained following a myelogram and reformatted through the thecal space from a series of axial images. This has a similar appearance to the conventional myelogram radiographs and shows the conus quite well.

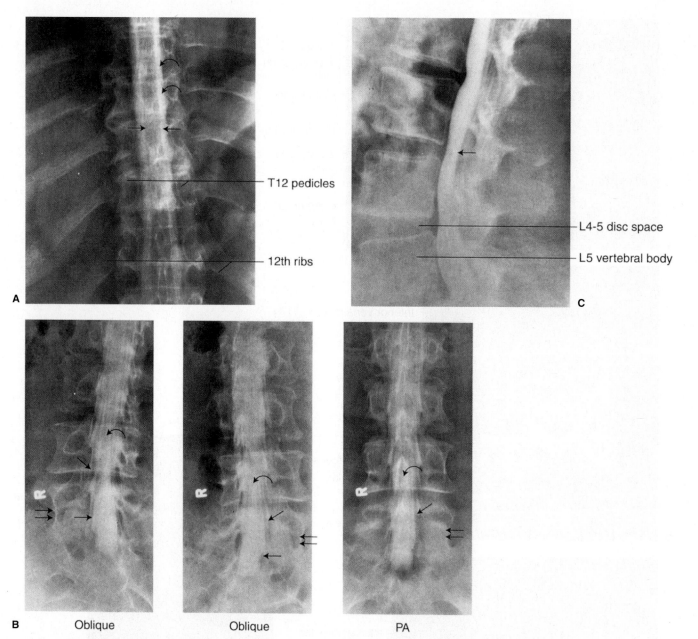

FIGURE 9.13. A: Thoracic spine PA (posteroanterior) myelogram radiograph. Normal. The spinal cord (*between the straight arrows*) is outlined by the injected subarachnoid contrast media (*curved arrows*). **B:** Lumbar spine oblique and PA myelogram radiographs. Normal. The *single straight arrows* indicate the nerve roots surrounded by contrast media exiting the spinal canal. The *curved arrows* indicate nerve roots within the thecal sac. The *double straight arrows* indicate the L5 lumbar vertebra. **C:** Lumbar spine lateral myelogram radiograph. Normal. The thecal sac contains contrast media (*arrow*).

contrast once did. CT routinely follows the injection to better define the disc and nerve pathology. Understandably, CT and MR examinations are generally more acceptable to the patient than the invasive spinal puncture associated with myelography. However, some surgeons still find a myelogram of benefit in certain circumstances, so they are still occasionally performed.

The sacrum should be evaluated with both the spine and the pelvis, playing a role in both. Unfortunately, it may be difficult to evaluate, especially in an older patient with

osteoporosis or constipation. The normal sacrum has an anterior concavity and is tilted posteriorly at the L5–S1 junction. The arcuate lines of the neural foramina should be evaluated closely on the AP view. They should be smoothly curved and symmetric (Fig. 9.14). Asymmetry may be the result of fracture or tumor involvement. The SI joints should be evaluated as they are important in the evaluation of several arthritides and may be widened as a result of trauma. Both CT and MRI can be useful in the evaluation of the sacrum and SI joints.

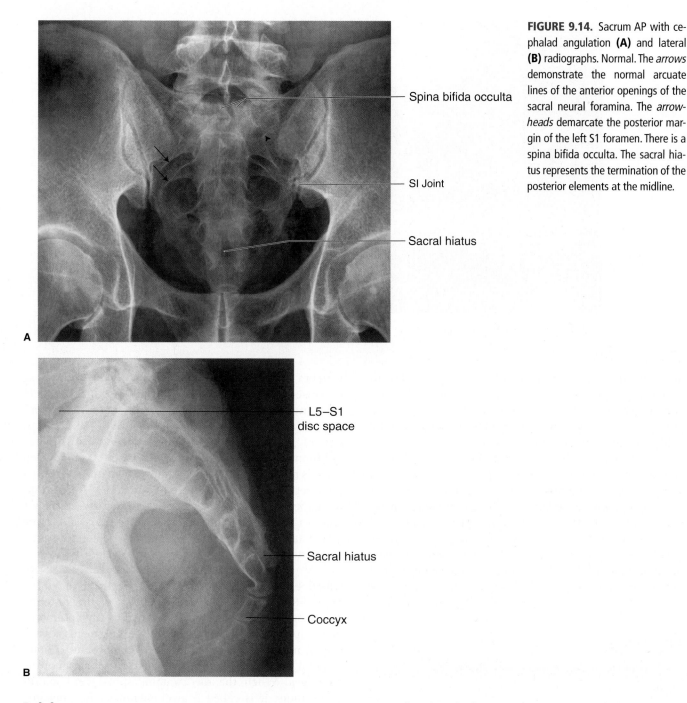

Spina bifida occulta

SI Joint

Sacral hiatus

L5–S1 disc space

Sacral hiatus

Coccyx

A

B

FIGURE 9.14. Sacrum AP with cephalad angulation **(A)** and lateral **(B)** radiographs. Normal. The *arrows* demonstrate the normal arcuate lines of the anterior openings of the sacral neural foramina. The *arrowheads* demarcate the posterior margin of the left S1 foramen. There is a spina bifida occulta. The sacral hiatus represents the termination of the posterior elements at the midline.

Pelvis

An AP pelvis radiograph is the standard view (Fig. 9.15). A lateral view is not obtained but on occasion up- and downtilt AP (outlet and inlet) views are indicated to assess fracture displacement. Oblique (Judet) views are useful in the evaluation of acetabular fractures. A modified outlet view is also useful to assess the SI joints. As elsewhere, you must know the anatomy and have a system for looking at the pelvis radiograph. First look at the sacrum and coccyx followed by the iliac bones bilaterally. Compare the SI joints as they may be narrowed or even absent in diseases like ankylosing spondylitis (see Fig. 9.50C). Then check out the ischial bones bilaterally as well as the pubic rami and the symphysis pubis.

Remember that the hamstring muscles arise from the ischial tuberosity; this explains why someone with a hamstring injury runs off the athletic field clutching his or her buttock. As you know, all of the pelvic bones must be evaluated for fractures, density, anomalies, and metastatic lesions.

ANOMALIES

Anomalies of the spine and pelvis (Table 9.5) vary in severity from mild to severe. *As a general rule, most mild spinal anomalies are asymptomatic.* Small extra bones or supernumerary bones called *accessory ossicles* are usually asymptomatic, and they may be located near many different bones

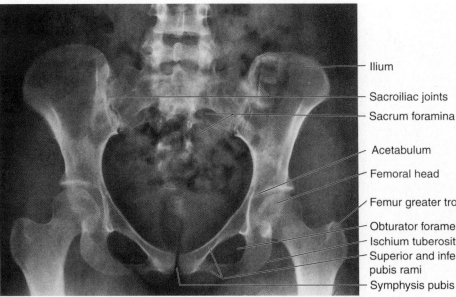

— Ilium

— Sacroiliac joints

— Sacrum foramina

— Acetabulum

— Femoral head

— Femur greater trochanter

— Obturator foramen

— Ischium tuberosity

— Superior and inferior pubis rami

— Symphysis pubis

FIGURE 9.15. Pelvis AP radiograph. Normal.

including the spine. Examples of accessory ossicles are shown in Figure 9.16A,B. Accessory ossicles are simply normal variants and should not be confused with a fracture. The smoothly corticated, usually rounded margins help differentiate them from fractures.

Occasionally, extra ribs arise from the cervical spine, and they are called *cervical ribs* (Fig. 9.16C). Cervical ribs are generally asymptomatic, but have the potential to cause symptoms secondary to extrinsic pressure on the brachial plexus and the vessels of the upper extremities. A common anomaly at the lumbosacral junction is a *transitional vertebra* in which the L5 vertebra begins to have the appearance of the sacrum or the sacrum begins to look like a lumbar vertebra. Partial sacralization of L5 is the term used when fusion exists between a portion of the L5

vertebra and the sacrum. Usually one of the L5 transverse processes is enlarged and fused with the sacrum, but there are many variations. Occasionally, the anatomic L5 is completely sacralized, having the appearance of the first portion of the sacrum. Transitional vertebra may become symptomatic especially after excessive back strain or when there is a *pseudarthrosis* (two bones articulating without a joint between them) as seen in Figure 9.17A. A less common anomaly is an abnormal articulation between the C1 spinous process and the occiput (Fig. 9.17B). A more severe anomaly of the spine is total absence of the posterior vertebral arch as in a meningomyelocele.

An important anomaly is spina bifida (Fig. 9.18), which occurs in approximately 5% of the population. Spina bifida occulta is a midline defect of the vertebral arch (usually posterior), and it is generally asymptomatic. When spina bifida has an associated soft tissue mass associated, it is called a meningocele. Meningoceles contain cerebral spinal fluid and the sac envelope consists of the meninges. When the sac contains spinal cord and/or nerve roots, it is called a myelomeningocele ("myelo-" refers to the cord). A meningocele (Fig. 9.19) is a herniation of neural tissue through a bone defect. The size of these herniations is variable, and the herniation direction most commonly is posterior, but can be anterior or lateral. The symptoms vary from nonexistent to extensive and disabling. Visceral innervation of the bladder and/or rectum may be affected, as well as sensory and motor nerves. Another unfortunate anomaly in this category is complete absence of the sacrum (sacral agenesis), and it is often associated with a variety of other anomalies. Another severe anomaly is exstrophy of the urinary bladder, which is associated with abnormal widening of the symphysis pubis. This widening of the symphysis pubis,

Table 9.5
A Partial List of Spine and Pelvis Anomalies

Mild

Accessory ossicles
Cervical ribs
Hemivertebra
Osteitis condensans ilii
Scoliosis
Spina bifida
Transitional vertebrae

Severe

Absence of the sacrum
Meningocele and myelomeningocele
Scoliosis
Symphysis diastasis

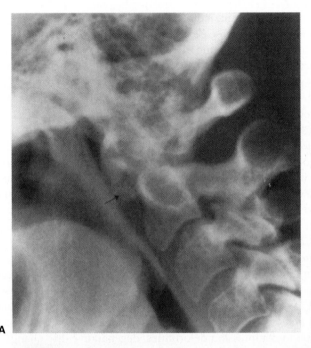

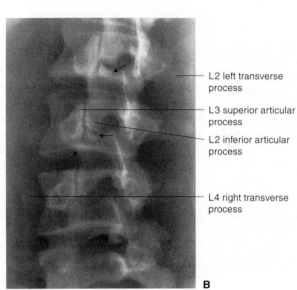

L2 left transverse process

L3 superior articular process

L2 inferior articular process

L4 right transverse process

A   **B**

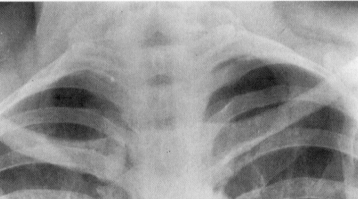

C

FIGURE 9.16. A: Cervical spine lateral radiograph. This accessory ossicle is located inferior to the anterior arch of the atlas or C1. This supernumerary bone or os (*arrow*) is a normal variant. **B:** Lumbar spine right oblique radiograph. Lumbar spine accessory ossicles (*arrows*). This 22-year-old gymnast experienced a sudden onset of back pain. The accessory ossicles are variants of normal and had nothing to do with the patient's back pain. They are usually found around the L2 and L3 levels. **C:** Lower cervical and upper thoracic spine AP radiograph. Bilateral cervical ribs. The small bilateral ribs (*arrows*) arise from the C7 vertebra; hence the name cervical ribs.

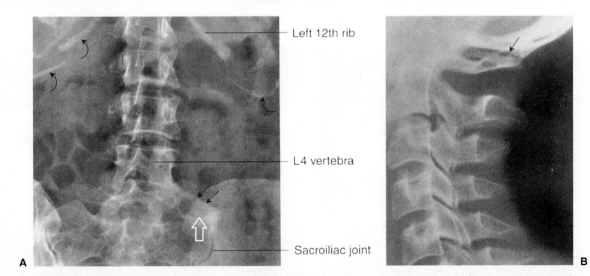

Left 12th rib

L4 vertebra

Sacroiliac joint

A   **B**

FIGURE 9.17. A: Lumbar spine AP radiograph. Partial sacralization of L5. L5 articulates with the left sacrum in an anomalous fashion (*straight arrows*). There is a pseudarthrosis (*white arrow*). Transitional vertebrae describe a situation in which L5 begins to look like a part of the sacrum or the sacrum begins to look like a part of the lumbar spine. The *curved arrows* indicate calcifications within the cartilaginous portion of the ribs. **B:** Cervical spine lateral radiograph. Partial occipitalization of C1. The spinous process of C1 articulates with the occiput (*arrow*). Normally the spinous process of C1 does not articulate with the occiput.

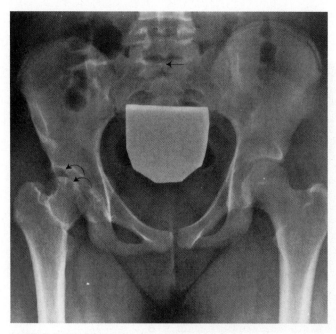

FIGURE 9.18. Pelvis AP radiograph. Spina bifida occulta and developmental dysplasia of the hip. Spina bifida occulta is indicated by the *straight arrow* and represents incomplete fusion of the posterior sacral segments. Right hip developmental dysplasia (*arrows*) is characterized by the steep slant of the acetabulum compared to the left. The femoral head remodels as it grows in the shallow socket. Note the presence of a gonadal shield.

or diastasis, is most often the result of trauma (Fig. 9.20), but can occasionally be associated with a difficult or large baby birth, some bone dysplasias, epispadias, hypospadias, and the prune belly syndrome (loss or absence of abdominal wall muscles).

One of the most clinically important anomalies of the spine is scoliosis. Some of the many etiologies of scoliosis

include idiopathic, disc degeneration and osteoarthritis, neuromuscular diseases, trauma, infections, tumors, radiation therapy, and underlying congenital problems such as hemivertebrae (Fig. 9.21) and pedicle bars. A hemivertebra is a vertebra with formation of only one side secondary to absence of a lateral ossification center. Typically, there is a body, pedicle, lamina, and corresponding rib on only one side (Fig. 9.22). Pedicle bars occur when two or more pedicles on the same side are joined by a bony bridge. While the normal side grows, the absent side of a hemivertebra or side with a pedicle bar cannot grow as much and a curvature develops. Approximately 10% of scoliosis cases are congenital with associated vertebral and rib abnormalities as shown in Figure 9.22, but, by far, most cases are idiopathic (Fig. 9.23). Scoliosis may be associated with abnormalities of the spinal cord, such as a syrinx. When scoliosis is severe or rapidly progressive, it may be treated by fusion of a long segment of the spine (Fig. 9.24). Degenerative lumbar scoliosis (Fig. 9.25) is an increasing problem in the older population. It is likely multifactorial and may be related to altered load due to compression deformities, degenerative disc changes, leg length discrepancies, and lumbosacral anomalies. This deformity may be slow or rapidly progressive and can lead to back pain, radiculopathy, and spinal stenosis. It is occasionally treated by decompression of the stenosis and fusion.

Osteitis condensans ilii (Fig. 9.26) is a well-marginated, triangular-shaped area of increased bone density found predominately in women of childbearing years. It is located in the iliac bone just lateral to the SI joint, but the sacrum and SI joints are not involved. This abnormality may or may not be symptomatic. The differential diagnosis, when not perfectly symmetric, might include osteoblastic metastatic disease, ankylosing spondylitis, and other inflammatory arthritides such as rheumatoid arthritis. It usually can be differentiated from metastatic disease that

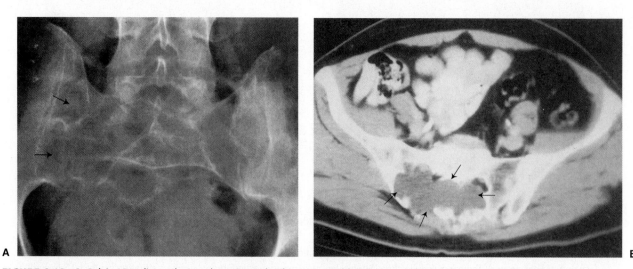

FIGURE 9.19. **A:** Pelvis AP radiograph. Sacral meningocele. This 54-year-old patient consulted a physician because of urinary retention. The lucent areas in the sacrum (*arrows*) indicate the bone defect secondary to the meningocele mass. **B:** Pelvis axial CT image. The full extent of the meningocele mass within the sacrum is indicated by the *arrows*.

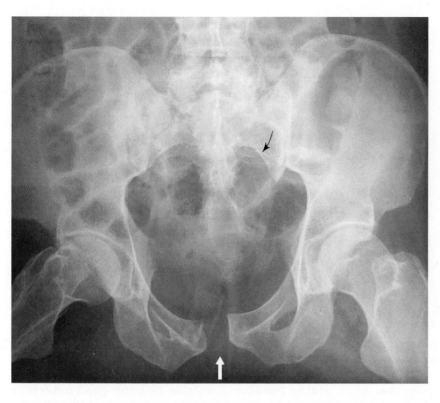

FIGURE 9.20. AP pelvis. Symphysis pubis diastasis. Widening of the normal close relationship of the left and right pubic bones (*white arrow*) is due to trauma in this patient. Note the irregular margin from fracture of the right side of the symphysis. The disrupted arcuate line of the left sacral foramen (*black arrow*) should be searched for since the pelvic "ring" typically breaks in at least two places.

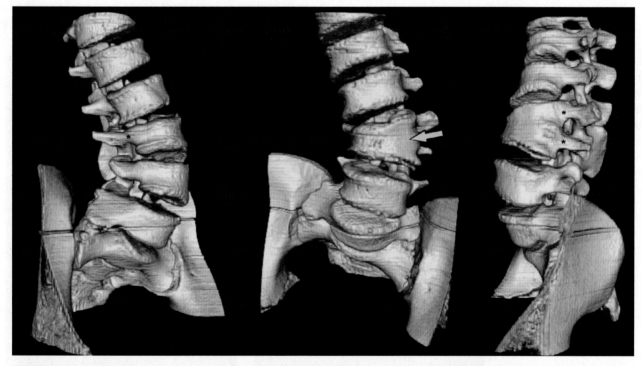

FIGURE 9.21. Lumbar spine 3D reconstruction from axial CT dataset. Midlumbar hemivertebra and fusion anomaly with scoliosis. These images were taken from a video of a rotating spine to best demonstrate the abnormality. Note that the vertebral body is shorter on the left side (patient's right) and has only one pedicle (*asterisk*) while the right side (patient's left) is taller due to fusion of a hemivertebra with the adjacent normal (*arrow*) and has two pedicles (*asterisk*). The cause for the spine curvature is obvious. The line going through L5 and the iliac bones is an artifact due to a small movement of the patient during the CT scan.

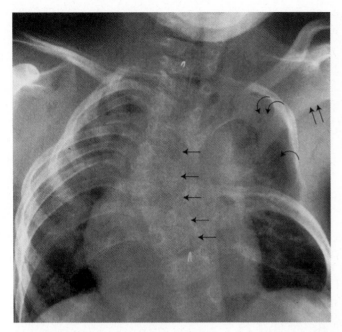

FIGURE 9.22. Thoracic spine AP radiograph. Congenital scoliosis. The thoracic spine is convex to the right, and the thorax is markedly asymmetric. Underlying the scoliosis are multiple hemivertebrae or incompletely formed thoracic vertebrae (*single straight arrows*). There are multiple absent left ribs (*curved arrows*) and several left upper ribs are fused (*double curved arrows*). The left scapula is abnormally elevated (*double straight arrows*).

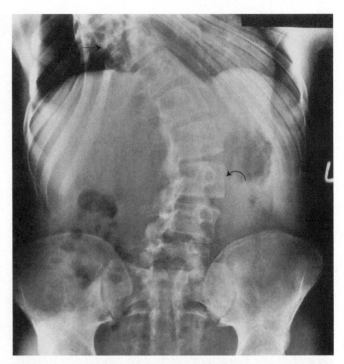

FIGURE 9.23. Thoracolumbar spine AP radiograph. Idiopathic scoliosis of the thoracic and lumbar spine. The lumbar spine is convex to the left (*curved arrow*), and the lumbar vertebrae are markedly rotated. This rotation component causes the lumbar vertebra to appear oblique on the radiograph. The lower thoracic spine is convex to the right (*straight arrow*) resulting in asymmetry of the ribs and thorax. Interestingly, the foramen magnum and sacrum usually form a vertical line when a line connects the two.

FIGURE 9.24. AP **(A)** and lateral **(B)** thoracolumbar radiographs. Posterior spinal fusion for idiopathic scoliosis. Fusion rods, screws, and hooks are used to decrease the curvature. Bone graft is usually placed as well to prevent progression of the curves.

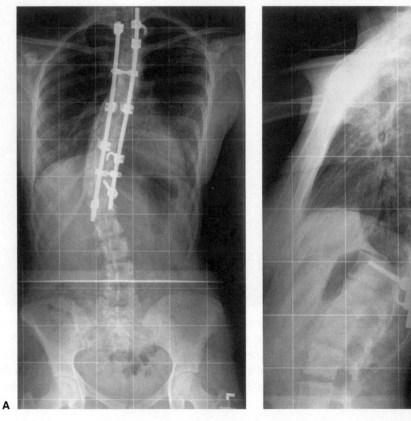

A
B

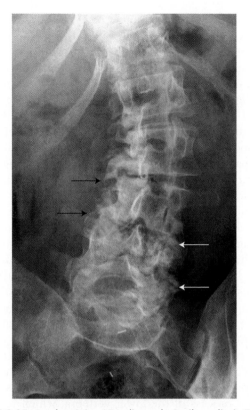

FIGURE 9.25. Lumbar Spine AP radiograph. Senile scoliosis. The lumbar spine is convex to the left. The discs are asymmetrically narrowed and there is prominent osteoarthritis of facets (*arrows*), which is worse on the concave sides.

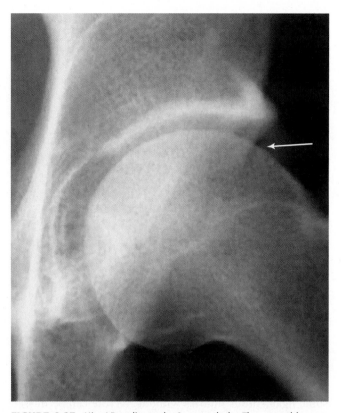

FIGURE 9.27. Hip AP radiograph. Os acetabula. The smoothly marginated, oval density near the superolateral margin of the acetabulum (*arrow*) is a normal variant and should not be confused with a fracture.

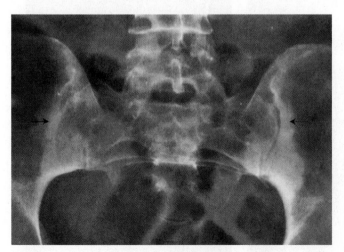

FIGURE 9.26. Pelvis AP radiograph. Osteitis condensans ilii. The sharply marginated, bilateral, increased densities (sclerosis) involve the iliac sides of the SI joints and spare the sacrum. This is a benign condition that is usually found in women in their childbearing years and seldom found in older women. This can be an incidental finding on a radiograph or the patient may present with acute or chronic back pain.

commonly involves multiple widespread sites. The SI joints are usually narrowed or absent in ankylosing spondylitis and often appear irregular in the other inflammatory arthritides such as rheumatoid arthritis.

A sometimes-confusing variant in the pelvis is *os acetabula*. This is an accessory center of ossification at the superolateral margin of the acetabulum (Fig. 9.27). It is typically triangular in shape. The margins are smooth and corticated, which should allow differentiation from a fracture. There has been some association with femoroacetabular impingement, which has been associated with early development of osteoarthritis.

TRAUMA

Fractures

Fractures of the spine and pelvis are common and result from a wide variety of traumas including motor vehicle accidents, sports, falls, and normal activity in those who have osteoporosis or bone loss due to tumor. Fractures of the spine are obviously important as the spinal cord and nerves are vulnerable to injury because of their close proximity to the vertebrae. Roughly 40% of cervical spine fractures have neurologic complications, 10% in the thoracic spine and 4% at the thoracolumbar junction.

Table 9.6
Cervical Spine Injuries
Flexion
Anterior wedge fracture
Facet locking
Ligament disruption
Odontoid process fracture
Teardrop fracture (C5)
Extension
Hangman fracture (C2)
Ligament disruption
Odontoid process fracture
Spinous process fracture
Teardrop fracture (C2)

Cervical Spine Injuries

Most cervical spine fractures occur between C5 and C7, with another peak at C1 and C2. A variety of injuries occur when the cervical spine undergoes acute hyperflexion and hyperextension (Table 9.6). CT is now the preferred method for initial evaluation, its only limitation is that some ligamentous injuries without fracture can be missed due to the supine positioning of the patient during the scan. Findings are the same for radiographs, which will be used for follow-up, and CT and are discussed as one topic. As noted previously, it is important to visualize all the cervical vertebra completely. The junction of C7 and T1 can be an important source of injury between the mobile cervical vertebra and the fixed thoracic vertebral column (Fig. 9.28). Swimmer's views may be obtained on radiographic evaluation while CT of the cervical spine typically includes several upper thoracic vertebrae. The flexion teardrop fracture (Fig. 9.29) is one type of injury that results from acute cervical spine hyperflexion. The teardrop-shaped fracture fragment is the result of compression at the anterior inferior aspect of the vertebral body. This fracture is usually accompanied by disruption of the interspinal ligaments between the spinous processes, thus making the spine very unstable. Other ligaments that may be involved are the supraspinous ligament and the ligamentum flavum. The involved vertebral body may be displaced posteriorly, and this situation is a good indication for CT imaging to determine the extent of the fracture lines and to determine the precise location of the fracture fragments, especially their relationship to the cervical spinal cord. Particularly with neurologic deficit, MRI may be used to evaluate the spinal cord for injury and the soft tissue structures such as the ligamentum flavum and interspinous ligaments.

Facet locking is another hyperflexion injury. Locking will occur when the inferior articular process of the upper vertebra moves forward or anteriorly over the superior articular process of the lower vertebra, which results in an anterior dislocation of the upper vertebra. Once again, the spine is unstable as there usually is posterior and sometimes anterior ligamentous disruption, and cervical spinal cord injury is common. The lateral radiograph is usually sufficient to make the diagnosis (Figs. 9.28 and 9.30A),

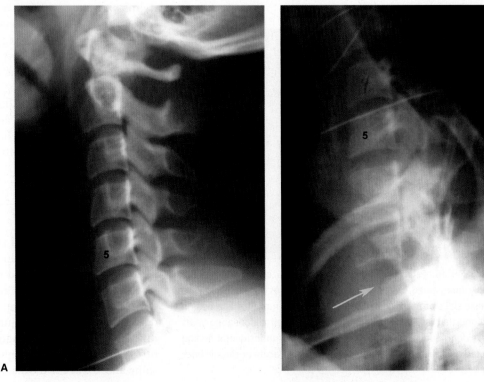

FIGURE 9.28. A: Lateral cervical spine radiograph is normal, but note that the inferior margin of C7 is not visualized. **B:** Swimmer's view in the same patient reveals bilateral jumped facets at the C7–T1 junction (*arrow*).

A

B

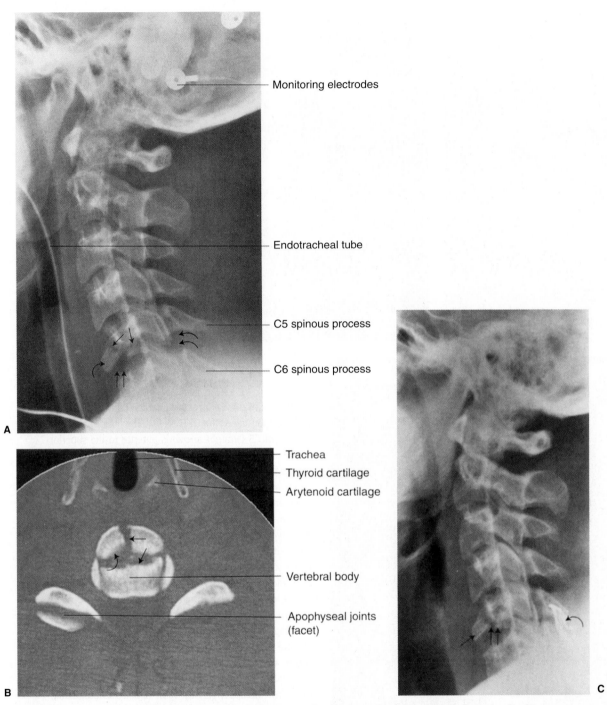

— Monitoring electrodes

— Endotracheal tube

— C5 spinous process

— C6 spinous process

A

— Trachea
— Thyroid cartilage
— Arytenoid cartilage

— Vertebral body

— Apophyseal joints (facet)

B

C

FIGURE 9.29. A: Lateral cervical spine radiograph. C5 flexion teardrop fracture. This 21-year-old man was involved in a motor vehicle accident. There is mild compression anteriorly of the C5 vertebral body secondary to the comminuted fracture (*single straight arrows*), and there is mild separation of the fracture fragments. The major fracture fragment has a teardrop shape (*single curved arrow*) due to avulsion at the site of the anterior longitudinal ligament. The hyperflexion injury has resulted in a mild separation or fanning of the space between the C5 and C6 spinous processes secondary to ligamentous disruption (*double curved arrows*). The disrupted ligaments are the interspinal and supraspinal ligaments and possibly the ligamentum flavum. Also, the hyperflexion injury created minimal widening of the C5–C6 disc space (*double straight arrows*) and mild angulation of the spine at this level with minimal retrolisthesis of C5 on C6. This type of cervical fracture usually is associated with severe cord injury as the vertebral body is often displaced posteriorly into the spinal canal. **B:** Cervical spine axial CT image of the C5 vertebra. The comminuted fracture lines in the vertebral body are separated or distracted (*straight arrows*), and the anterior fracture fragments are displaced anteriorly approximately 3 mm (*curved arrow*). **C:** Lateral cervical spine radiograph. Posterior wire stabilization of the cervical spine between the spinous processes of C5 and C6 vertebrae (*curved arrow*). The major fracture fragment (*single straight arrow*) is in fairly good alignment with mild offset of the fragments (*double straight arrows*), but no attempt is made to reduce this fragment.

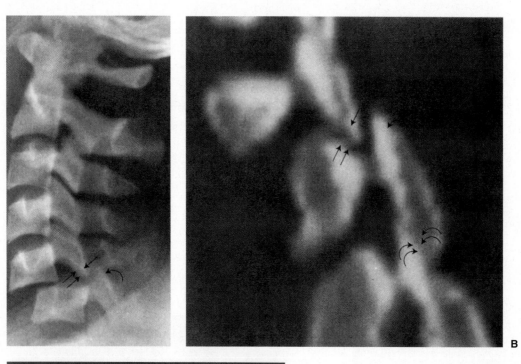

A

B

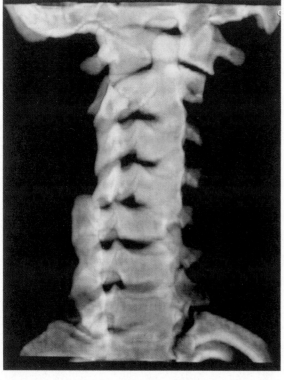

C

FIGURE 9.30. **A:** Cervical spine lateral radiograph. Bilateral facet locking at the C5–C6 level. The inferior articular process of C5 (*straight arrow*) is anterior to the superior articular process of C6 (*curved arrow*). The double *straight arrows* indicate the expected normal position for the superior articular process of the C6 vertebra. There is obvious anterior dislocation of the C5 vertebral body referable to the C6 vertebral body. No fractures are apparent. **B:** Cervical spine sagittal reconstructed CT image on a different patient. Bilateral facet lock. The inferior articular processes of the upper vertebra (*straight arrow*) is in an abnormal relationship with the superior articular process of the lower vertebra (*single curved arrow*). The *double straight arrows* indicate the expected normal location of the displaced superior articular process. A normal apophyseal articulation is visible at the level below (*double curved arrows*). **C:** Reformatted CT image in another patient with unilateral locked facets at C4–C5 on the right. Note how the upper cervical spine appears rotated while the lower cervical spine is straight. The left facets are not shown on this 3D reformat, but had a normal relationship.

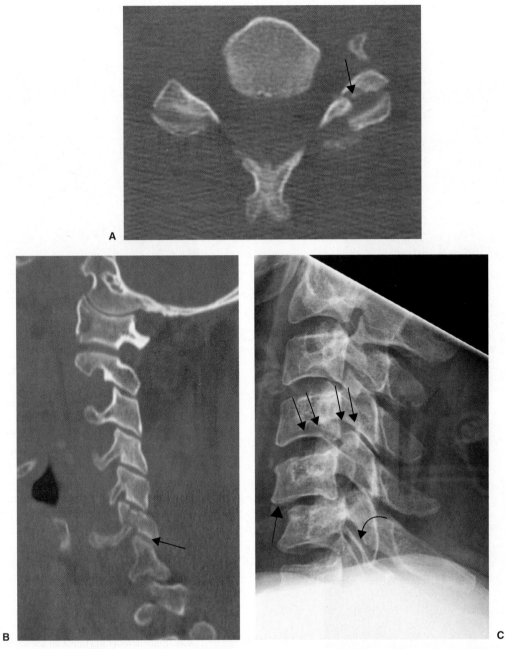

FIGURE 9.31. A: Axial CT image through C6. The left inferior articular process of C5 is broken, but not displaced (*arrow*). **B:** Sagittal reformatted image uses the axial dataset from the CT scan to project a sagittal slice through the facet joints. There is a normal relationship between the fractured C5 inferior articular process and the superior articular process of C6 (*arrow*). **C:** Lateral radiograph of the cervical spine obtained 1 month later demonstrated mild anterolisthesis of C5 on C6 (*single straight arrow*) and rotation of the articular pillar above this level. Note the overlap of bilateral facets below (*curved arrow*) compared to the "bowtie" appearance above with this unilateral facet fracture–dislocation (*double straight arrows*).

but occasionally a reconstructed sagittal CT image (Fig. 9.30B,C) is necessary to confirm the diagnosis. Unilateral locked facet (Fig. 9.30C) has a rotational component and does not have the extensive ligamentous disruption as the bilateral form does. Unilateral facet fracture–dislocation may be a difficult diagnosis since there is less displacement as a result of the fracture of the superior articular process. The rotational component may not be manifested until later and should be looked for on subsequent radiographs (Fig. 9.31).

Occasionally hyperflexion injury results in ligamentous injury without fracture (Fig. 9.32). As with other hyperflexion injuries, this has the potential for spinal instability and cord injury.

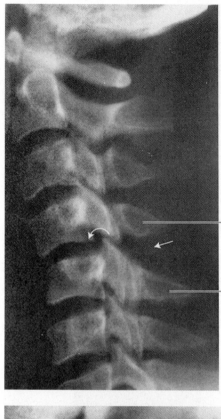

— C4 spinous process

— C5 spinous process

A

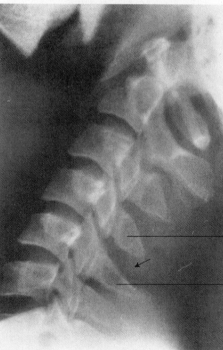

— C4 spinous process

— C5 spinous process

B

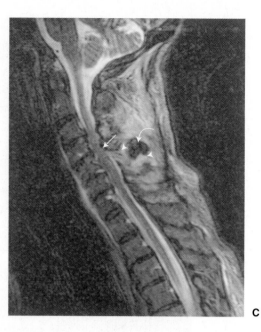

C

FIGURE 9.32. A: Cervical spine cross-table lateral radiograph with the patient supine. Posterior ligament disruption at C4–C5. There is an increase in the height of the interspinous space between the C4–C5 spinous processes (*straight arrow*) secondary to disruption of the C4–C5 interspinal ligament, supraspinal ligament, and possibly the ligamentum flavum. Compare the height of the C4–C5 interspinous space to those above and below. The mild anterior spondylolisthesis of C4 referable to C5 (*curved arrow*) has resulted in mild kyphotic angulation and reverse of the normal cervical curvature at the C4 level. **B:** Cervical spine extension lateral radiograph in the same patient. When the cervical spine is in full extension, the C4–C5 interspinous space (*straight arrow*) is now normal in height and the anterolisthesis of C4 on C5 has been reduced. **C:** Sagittal T2-weighted MRI cervical spine in a different patient. Ligament disruption without fracture. There is widening between the spinous processes at C5–C6 and increased signal (white) (*arrowheads*). Disruption of the ligamentum flavum (*straight arrow*) is also seen. A hematoma (*curved arrow*) can be seen, which would explain persistent widening of spinous processes on radiographs. There is a small amount of high signal within the posterior aspect of the C5–C6 disc which may suggest a disc injury as well.

Dens or odontoid process fractures are relatively common in the older population and they may result from hyperflexion or hyperextension injuries. The fractures are often not displaced initially and may be difficult to detect. The best methods for the diagnosis of odontoid process fracture are AP open mouth and lateral cervical radiographs, and, of course, CT imaging. The odontoid fracture

in Figure 9.33 is probably a hyperextension injury as the odontoid is displaced posteriorly.

Thoracic Spine Fractures

Most fractures of the thoracic spine occur in the lower thoracic region. Fractures of the thoracic spine may result from significant trauma; however, underlying bone diseases can

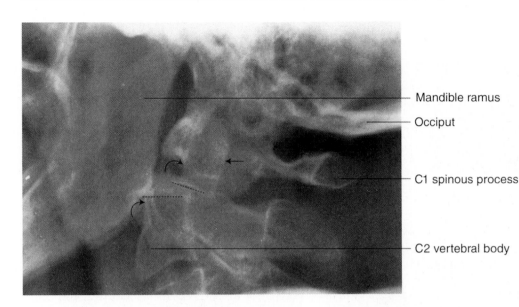

Mandible ramus

Occiput

C1 spinous process

C2 vertebral body

FIGURE 9.33. Cervical spine lateral radiograph. Displaced fracture through the caudad or inferior aspect of the dens or odontoid process of C2. The actual fracture edges are indicated by the dotted lines and the dens (*arrow*) is displaced posteriorly approximately 8 mm. The *curved arrows* indicate the amount of displacement of the dens.

weaken the vertebrae and pathologic fractures may occur with little or no trauma. These fractures are usually wedge-shaped compression fractures, often with no canal compromise and are, by far, the most common thoracic spine fracture. A few of the underlying diseases that may cause pathologic fractures are osteoporosis, primary and secondary bone tumors, Paget disease, osteopetrosis, and osteomalacia (Fig. 9.34). If there are neurologic symptoms, imaging with MR is usually warranted.

Lumbar Spine Fractures

Fractures commonly occur in the lumbar spine and are usually diagnosed by radiography (Fig. 9.35A,B). MRI

may be helpful in assessing the effect of the fracture fragments on the thecal sac (Fig. 9.35C). As in other areas of the spine, CT imaging is helpful to evaluate the extent of the fractures and to precisely locate the fracture fragments within the neural canal and their relationship relative to the thecal sac (Fig. 9.35D,E).

Spondylolysis and Spondylolisthesis

Spondylolysis and spondylolisthesis are difficult and confusing terms for the beginner. To add to the confusion, many will use the term "spondylosis" to describe degenerative changes in the spine. However, an understanding of these conditions and their clinical significance is necessary

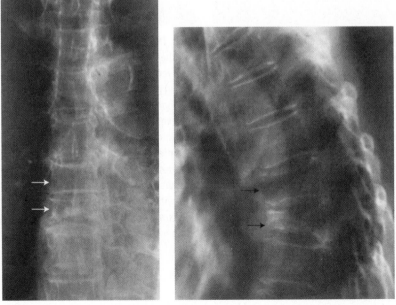

A   B

FIGURE 9.34. Thoracic spine AP **(A)** and lateral **(B)** radiographs. Osteopenia due to senile osteoporosis with secondary pathologic compression fractures of the T7 and T8 vertebral bodies. The compression fractures (*arrows*) are manifest by a decrease in the vertical height of the T7 and T8 vertebral bodies when compared to the other dorsal vertebral bodies. Notice the overall decreased density (osteopenia) of all the osseous structures due to osteoporosis.

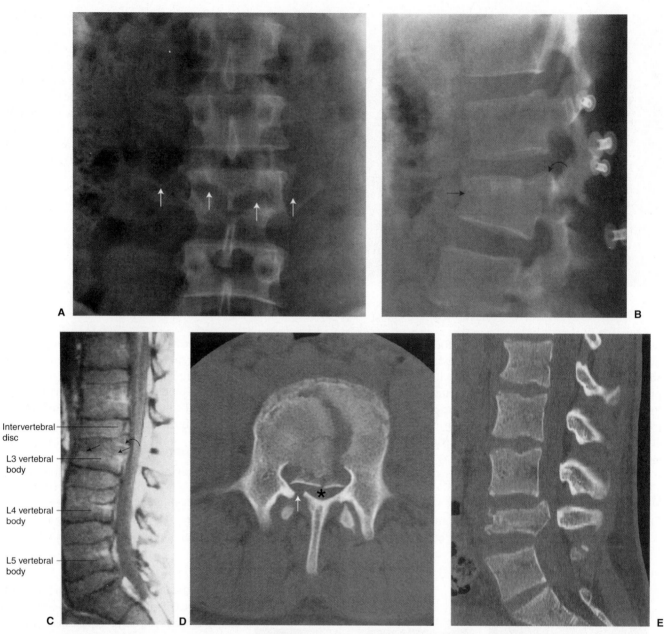

FIGURE 9.35. Lumbar spine AP **(A)** and lateral **(B)** radiographs. Seat belt fracture of the L3 vertebrae. This 30-year-old was wearing a lap seat belt when involved in a motor vehicle accident, and this is a flexion injury caused by the mobile upper body flexing on the lower body that is fixed by the lap seat belt. There is a transverse fracture through the L3 vertebra involving the vertebral body and the transverse processes (*straight arrows* **(A)** *and* **(B)**). A large fracture fragment arising posteriorly from the vertebral body is displaced into the neural canal (*curved arrow* **(B)**). The L3 vertebral body height is less than normal secondary to compression or collapse caused by the fracture. There is mild dorsal angulation of the spine at the level of the L3 fracture. These fractures may be either stable or unstable. The remainder of the lumbar spine is normal. Note the clothing snaps. **C:** Lumbar spine sagittal proton-density MR image. A lap seat belt L3 displaced fracture in another 30-year-old patient. The L3 vertebral body is mildly compressed secondary to a fracture (*straight arrows*), and a posterior fracture fragment resides in the neural canal compressing the neural canal (*curved arrow*). **D:** Lumbar spine axial CT image. L5 vertebra displaced burst-type fracture in a 28-year-old involved in a motor vehicle accident. The mechanism of injury is axial compression with or without flexion and/or rotation. There is severe compromise of the neural canal (*asterisk*) with resultant neurologic injury. The *straight arrow* demonstrates a fracture of the right lamina in this unstable fracture. **E:** Sagittal reformatted CT image on the same patient shows the severity of the canal compromise compared to the other levels.

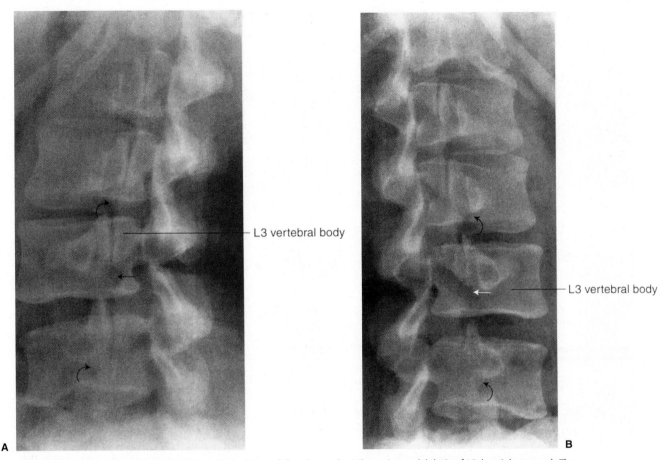

A   B

FIGURE 9.36. A,B: Lumbar spine right **(A)** and left oblique **(B)** radiographs. Bilateral spondylolysis of L3 (*straight arrows*). The pars interarticularis or the Scotty dog neck is disrupted bilaterally in the L3 vertebra. Normal Scotty dog necks or pars interarticulares are present in the L2 and L4 vertebrae bilaterally (*curved arrows*). (*continued*)

as they will commonly be encountered in clinical practice. *Spondylolysis* refers to a defect in the pars interarticularis that lies between the superior and inferior articular processes of a vertebra. In other words, the neck of the Scotty dog is missing or some say that a collar has been placed (see Fig. 9.10A). The defect occurs in about 5% of the population and, in most cases, is thought to be a stress fracture. It is seen on lateral radiographs, but seen particularly well on oblique views (Fig. 9.36). It is seen more often in athletes whose activities require prolonged or forced extension of the lower back. *Spondylolisthesis* is the forward movement of a vertebra relative to the more stable vertebra below. The forward movement may be made possible by a bilateral spondylolysis defect in the vertebra (Figs. 9.36 and 9.37). Actually, with a pars defect, it is the vertebral body, pedicles, and superior articular processes that move forward or ventrally, whereas the laminae, inferior articular processes, and the spinous process remain in their normal positions (see Fig. 9.37). This actually increases the size of the canal at this level. The majority of the spondylolysis with spondylolisthesis cases occur in the lumbar spine, especially at L5–S1 levels, and it is uncommon in the thoracic and cervical spine. Spondylolisthesis may be asymptomatic, and the most frequent symptom is low back pain probably due to muscle spasm and instability. Symptoms, when they occur, are not necessarily related to the severity of the disease.

Spondylolisthesis secondary to spondylolysis must be differentiated from the spondylolisthesis secondary to disc and facet degeneration without spondylolysis. Degenerative spondylolisthesis is best imaged on a lateral radiograph of the lumbar spine (Fig. 9.38) and it most commonly occurs at the L4–L5 level. There are degenerative changes in the disc space and the apophyseal (facet) joints *without a defect in the pars interarticularis*. Because there is no defect in the region of the pars interarticularis, however, there is more likely to be encroachment of bony structures into the neural foramina, which may lead to nerve compression.

Pelvic, Acetabular, and Sacral Fractures

Fractures of the pelvis are common and result from a variety of injuries (Fig. 9.39). Stable pelvic fractures only break the "ring" of the pelvis in one place. These include fractures of unilateral pubic rami, acetabulum, or sacrum. Typically both superior and inferior pubic rami are broken

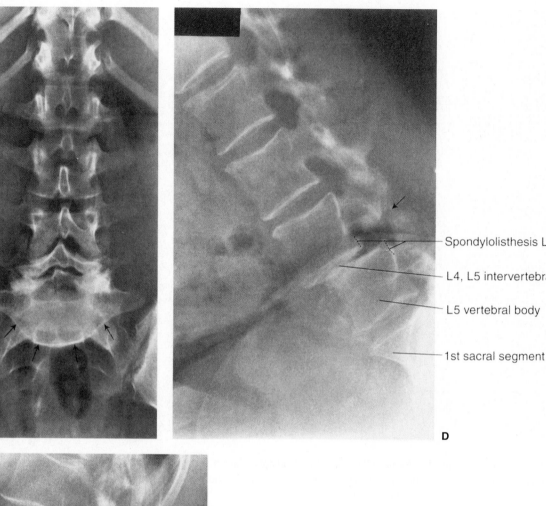

C

Spondylolisthesis L4 on L5

L4, L5 intervertebral space

L5 vertebral body

1st sacral segment

D

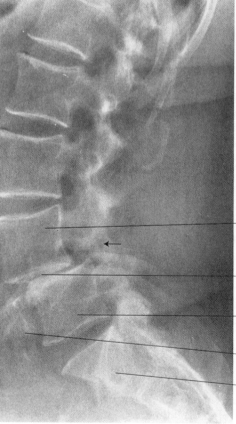

L4 vertebral body

L4, L5 intervertebral space

L5 vertebral body

Artery calcification

1st sacral segment

E

FIGURE 9.36. (*Continued*) **C:** Lumbar spine AP radiograph. The classical appearance of the Napoleon hat sign (*straight arrows*) on an AP radiograph is secondary to severe (grade 4) spondylolisthesis of L5 referable to S1. The Napoleon hat is inverted or upside down. **D,E:** Lumbar spine lateral flexion (**D**) and extension (**E**) radiographs. This is a different patient with L4 spondylolysis and grade 2 anterior spondylolisthesis of the L4 vertebral body referable to the L5 vertebral body. The spondylolysis defect in the pars interarticularis (*straight arrows*) can be visualized on both views but the flexion radiograph opens the defect for easier visibility. The degree of spondylolisthesis is slightly less on the lateral extension radiograph as extension would counteract the forward slip. Notice the marked narrowing of the L4–L5 intervertebral disc space.

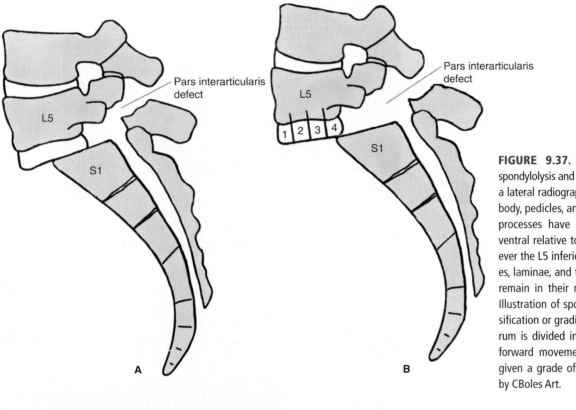

FIGURE 9.37. A: Illustration of spondylolysis and spondylolisthesis on a lateral radiograph. The L5 vertebral body, pedicles, and superior articular processes have moved forward or ventral relative to the sacrum. However the L5 inferior articular processes, laminae, and the spinous process remain in their normal position. **B:** Illustration of spondylolisthesis classification or grading system. The sacrum is divided into fourths and the forward movement of L5 is simply given a grade of 1 to 4. Illustration by CBoles Art.

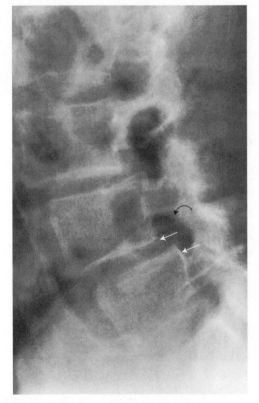

FIGURE 9.38. Lumbar spine lateral radiograph. Degenerative grade 1 spondylolisthesis of L4 on L5 (*straight arrows*). This is a common complication of degenerative spine changes. The pars interarticularis is intact (*curved arrow*). The spondylolisthesis is secondary to the degenerative changes in the intervertebral space and the apophyseal joints that allow L4 to move forward relative to L5.

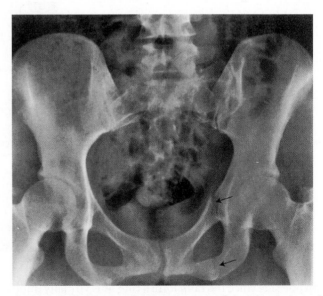

FIGURE 9.39. Pelvis AP radiograph. Fractures of the left superior and inferior pubis rami (*arrows*). Sacral fractures are present but are partly obscured by the overlying intestinal gas. Note how the sacral arcuate lines are poorly seen on the left compared with those on the right.

FIGURE 9.40. Acetabular fractures in three different patients. **A:** Pelvis AP radiograph. Left acetabular fracture (*arrows*). The fracture that involves the iliac wing is considered part of the acetabular fracture. **B:** Axial CT at level of the acetabulum. This 23-year-old was involved in a motor vehicle accident. The right femoral head is dislocated posteriorly, nicely demonstrating the mechanism for a fracture of the posterior wall of the acetabulum. The *arrow* shows the fracture site from which the posterior wall fragment came. **C:** Posterior view of a 3D CT reformatted image in a different patient with a right posterior wall acetabular fracture (*arrow*). These images can sometimes allow better demonstration of the location of fracture fragments.

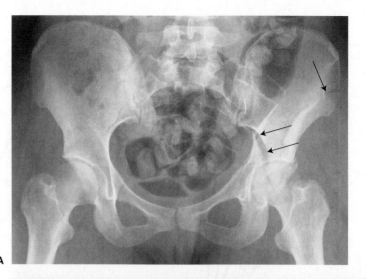

A

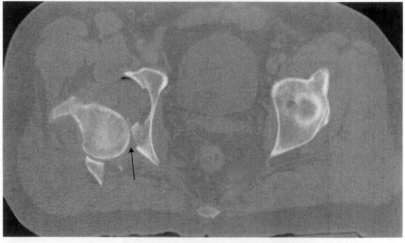

B

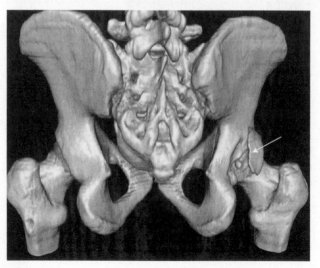

C

on one side since the rami form a ring. It is virtually impossible to break a ring in only one place and most pelvic fractures are unstable, disrupting the pelvic bones, symphysis and/or SI joints. These fractures are better evaluated by CT, which also allows evaluation of many of the soft tissue structures such as the bladder, urethra, and other pelvis soft tissues that may be damaged by fracture fragments. CT reformatted images are often useful to better evaluate the pelvic fractures.

Acetabular fractures result most commonly from motor vehicle accidents as the femoral head is driven into the acetabulum. Depending on the direction of force, the femoral head may dislocate, typically posteriorly, with or without an acetabular fracture. Avascular necrosis (AVN)

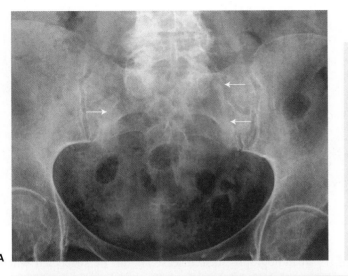

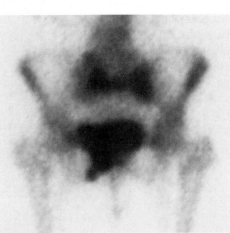

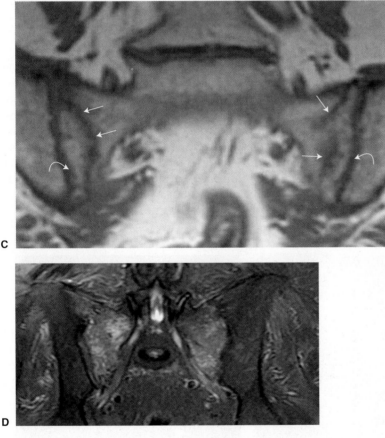

FIGURE 9.41. A: Sacrum AP radiograph. Insufficiency fractures of the sacrum. There is subtle sclerosis in a vertical orientation involving each sacral ala (*arrows*). Compare this to the normal sacrum in Figure 9.14A. **B:** Radionuclide bone scan posterior view of the pelvis in this same patient reveals increased activity (black) due to the healing fractures. The vertical orientation of each side with a horizontal connecting fracture line has been termed the "Honda sign." **C:** Coronal T1-weighted MR pelvis in a different patient. The characteristic sacral insufficiency fracture lines are easily seen (*straight arrows*), but should not be confused with the normal SI joints (*curved arrows*). **D:** Coronal T2-weighted MR image in another patient. Increased signal (white) due to edema and blood is present throughout both sacral ala. A discrete fracture line is not always seen depending on the acuteness of fracture or degree of healing.

is a complication of hip dislocation as the vascular supply to the femoral head is stretched or disrupted during the dislocation. Prompt reduction of the dislocation is imperative to minimize the risk of AVN. Sciatic nerve injury also occurs in up to 20% of cases; the risk greater if there is an associated posterior acetabular wall fracture. Pelvic oblique, or Judet, views and CT, often with two-dimensional (2D) and three-dimensional (3D) reconstructions, are useful in the evaluation of acetabular fractures (Fig. 9.40).

Sacral fractures may occur with major pelvic trauma, but may be an isolated insufficiency-type fracture in the elderly and osteoporotic populations. When the fracture enters the sacral foramina, the arcuate lines are disrupted (see Fig. 9.20). Sacral insufficiency fractures, which occur in weakened, usually osteoporotic bone may occur with little or no trauma. An older patient may present with lower back, buttock, or hip pain. Radiographs frequently will not demonstrate the fracture. Bone scan or MRI may be the next study to evaluate for an occult or developing hip fracture and the sacral fracture discovered (Fig. 9.41). Occasionally, these studies have an atypical appearance, but CT will demonstrate the healing fracture.

FIGURE 9.42. Anterior radiograph of the pelvis. Note the increased space between the apophysis and the remainder of the iliac bone on the right (*single arrow*) compared with that of the left (*double arrow*). There has been an avulsion of the attachment of the abdominal musculature in this young runner following a quick change in direction.

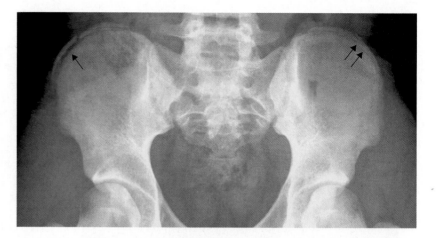

Apophyseal avulsion fractures in the adolescent are due to muscle traction in athletes. Several sports are more closely related to these injuries found in sprinters, long jumpers, cheerleaders, hurdlers, and gymnasts. These are the typical locations and the involved muscles: Anterior inferior iliac spine (rectus femoris attachment), ischial tuberosity (hamstring attachment), and iliac crest (abdominal muscle attachment) (Fig. 9.42). In the more mature athlete, a muscle strain or tear would result from the same type of injury. MRI may be useful to evaluate extent of muscle involvement and degree of retraction, if any.

Herniated Intervertebral Disc Disease

Intervertebral disc herniations may occur at any level in the spine. Although intervertebral discs cannot be visualized on radiographs, disc disease should be suspected whenever there is intervertebral disc space narrowing on radiographs. However, a narrowed disc level identified on radiographs cannot predict whether or not that level is symptomatic. Often the disc spaces are narrowed due to chronic disc degeneration and not an acute herniation. MRI has really become the main imaging tool for diagnosis of disc herniation. CT alone may give some information about morphology of the discs and frequently follows myelography when that is needed. On occasion, a discogram is utilized to try to determine which disc or discs are symptomatic. This is a more invasive test as contrast is placed at multiple levels into the nucleus of the disc. Injection of contrast into an abnormal disc is used to determine if that reproduces the patient's pain (Fig. 9.43).

FIGURE 9.43. Discograms. **A:** Lateral view obtained during a discogram. Needles have been placed into the nucleus of each of three discs. Levels L3–L4 and L4–L5 are normal. L5–S1 disc shows degeneration with multiple annular tears or fissures (*arrow*). **B:** Lateral radiograph following a discogram. Focal posterior herniations are seen at all three levels (*arrowheads*) and diffuse degeneration at L4–L5 with numerous annular tears (*arrow*). The patient's pain was concordant during the injection at L2–L3. The herniation at L3–L4 is likely a protrusion and the other two are extrusions.

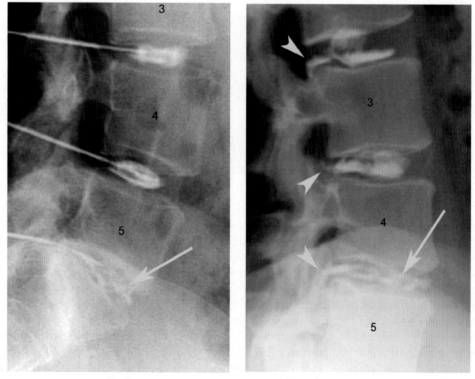

It is not a pleasant study and should be used sparingly in complex, difficult cases.

The normal disc structures are shown in Figure 9.11. Some confusing terms have developed in the classification of herniated intervertebral discs, but the following is the current most accepted approach to this terminology problem. There is some "normal" drying out of discs with aging, which may lead to decreased disc space height. Disc *degeneration* usually refers to this "drying out," narrowing, and/or numerous small tears of the annulus fibrosis in all directions, which allows the nucleus of the disc to spread out. *Annular fissure (tear)* usually refers to a focal tear in the annulus allowing nuclear material to extend toward the outer margin of the disc without extending beyond the margin (Fig. 9.44A). A *bulging disc* means that 50% or more of the circumference of the disc is mildly displaced outward relative to the margin of the vertebral body. Scoliosis often leads to multiple asymmetric bulging discs due to the change in bony alignment. In this instance the appearance is not due to structural problems within the discs. *Herniation* is a general, umbrella term, and it can be divided into three main categories, that is, protruded, extruded, and sequestered discs (Table 9.7; Fig. 9.44B). A *protrusion* implies the depth of disc extension is less than the width of its base at the disc margin. A *broad-based protrusion* involves over 25% of the circumference of the disc while *focal protrusion* involves less than 25% of the disc margin. If the extension of disc material is greater than the width of its base or extends superior or inferior to the endplate, it is termed *extrusion*. If the fragment becomes detached, it is termed a *sequestered fragment*. Herniated lumbar intervertebral disc disease is common especially at the L4–L5 and L5–S1 levels (Fig. 9.44). Therapeutic injections are often performed. These are usually nerve blocks or epidural injections of a steroid and often an anesthetic agent. They have been shown to be useful to allow a patient to tolerate the acute disc pain

long enough for some healing to take place and avoid or delay surgery (Fig. 9.45). MRI with the use of intravenous contrast has proved useful in determining whether or not there has been a recurrent disc herniation (Fig. 9.46). MRI on patients with prior back surgery is most often performed with and without contrast to assist discriminating between disc and scar tissue.

Usually, disc herniations are lateral and/or posterior. However, when the disc herniates anteriorly and into the vertebral body, this results in a vertebral defect with a classical appearance called a limbus vertebra (Fig. 9.47). When the disc herniates into the vertebral endplate, the resulting defect is called a Schmorl node. There are some people who feel that these are congenital or developmental variants. Scheuermann disease is osteochondrosis of the epiphyseal plates in teenagers, who often complain of back pain. The diagnosis of Scheuermann disease usually can be made on lateral spine radiographs. The radiographic features include fragmented and sclerotic epiphyseal plates of the vertebrae, wedge-shaped vertebral bodies with increased AP diameter, and narrowed disc spaces. Limbus vertebrae and Schmorl nodes may both be present.

ARTHRITIDES

Because the spine has multiple joints, it is not surprising that most of the arthritides involve the spine in some fashion (Table 9.8).

Osteoarthritis

Osteoarthritis or degenerative arthritis (Fig. 9.48) is the most common arthritis, and the facet joints of the spine are frequently involved. Patients with osteoarthritis will usually complain of pain and/or limited motion in the involved spine. As in the extremities, the typical radiologic features include irregular joint narrowing, sclerosis, and osteophyte formation. The differential diagnosis of degenerative or osteoarthritis typically includes neuropathic joints and diffuse idiopathic skeletal hyperplasia. Common complications of osteoarthritis are spinal stenosis (Fig. 9.49) and spondylolisthesis.

Spinal stenosis describes a vertebral or neural canal that is too narrow, and the multiple etiologies can be classified as congenital, developmental, and idiopathic. Although myelography dramatically demonstrates this abnormality, MRI enjoys excellent patient acceptance, and determines the causes and precise location (foraminal, lateral recess, or

---

Table 9.7
Intervertebral Disc Herniation Nomenclature
Annular fissure (tear)—focal disruption in the outer fibrous layers of disc
Bulge— > or = 50% width of disc displaced beyond vertebral body margin
Herniation:
Protrusion—depth of extent of disc < width of base at disc margin
Extrusion—depth of extent of disc > width of base at disc margin
Sequestration—detached disc fragment
Limbus vertebra
Schmorl node
Scheuermann disease

Table 9.8
Arthritides
Osteoarthritis
Inflammatory arthritis (rheumatoid arthritis and ankylosing spondylitis, psoriasis, Reiter Syndrome)
Neuropathic joint (Charcot joint)
Infectious arthritis

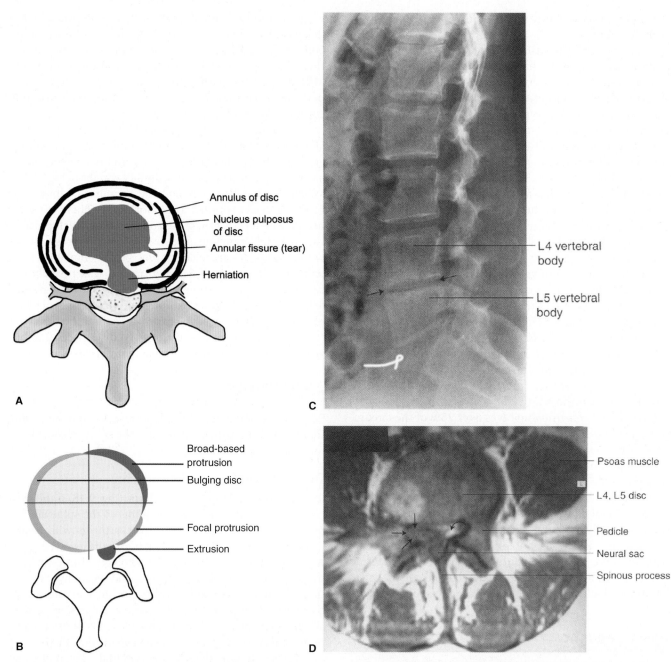

FIGURE 9.44. A: Lumbar intervertebral disc illustration. A disc herniation is a tear extending from the nucleus pulposis through all the layers of the annulus fibrosis. There may be compression of the thecal sac and possibly nerve roots. Smaller annular fissures may or may not cause pain. **B:** Lumbar intervertebral disc illustration. The disc has been divided into quadrants (*blue lines*) to visually aid the terminology of disc herniation based on percentage of disc involved. **C:** Lumbar spine lateral radiographs. Herniated L4–L5 intervertebral disc. The patient is a 30-year-old woman with bilateral leg weakness greater on the right than the left. There is significant narrowing of the L4–L5 intervertebral disc space (*arrows*) suggesting disc disease at this level. Again, the disc is not visible on the radiograph. The disc space narrowing is more apparent when you compare the L4–L5 disc space to the other lumbar disc spaces. Normally the L4–L5 disc space height is greater than the other lumbar spine disc spaces. **D:** Lumbar spine axial T1 MR image in the same patient. Large extruded L4–L5 intervertebral disc. The disc is extruded posterolaterally to the right (*straight arrows*), and it is creating extrinsic pressure on the neural sac and obliterating the epidural fat on the right side. Normal epidural fat is present on the left (*curved arrow*). Illustration by CBoles Art.

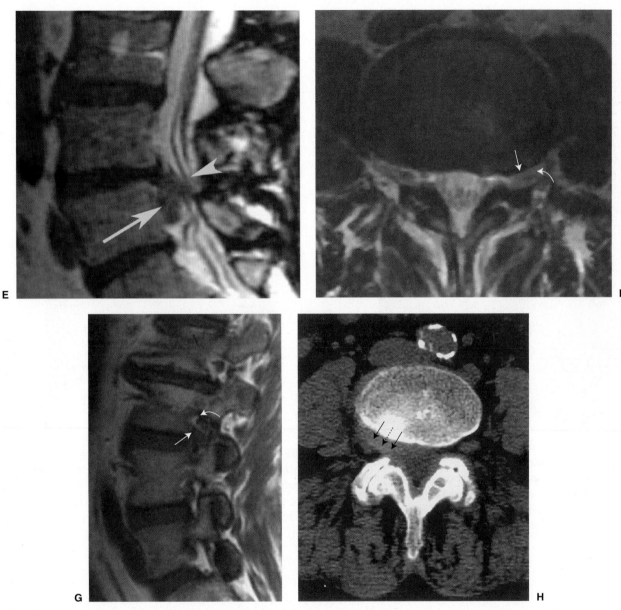

FIGURE 9.44. (*Continued*) **E:** Lumbar spine sagittal T2-weighted MR image in a different patient. Caudally extruded L4–L5 intervertebral disc and a protruding L5–S1 intervertebral disc. Notice that the extruded L4–L5 disc (*arrow*) has migrated inferiorly to the level of the L5–S1 disc space posteriorly and is causing spinal stenosis and displacing nerve roots (*arrowhead*). A bulging disc at L5–S1 does not touch the thecal sac at this level. Note a small vertebral hemangioma in L3 (*rounded bright signal*). **F:** Axial T2 MR image at L3–L4 in a 43-year-old man. Foraminal disc protrusion. The disc protrusion (*straight arrow*) narrows the left foramen and displaces the L3 nerve (*curved arrow*). **G:** Sagittal PD (proton density) MR on the same patient. This view shows the disc extension into the neural foramen (*straight arrow*) and relationship to the nerve (*curved arrow*). There are degenerative disc changes at L2–L3 as well with some foraminal narrowing seen at that level. **H:** Lumbar spine axial CT image. Protruded L4–L5 intervertebral disc. The *arrows* mark the protruded disc with narrowing of the right foramen by the disc and facet arthritis.

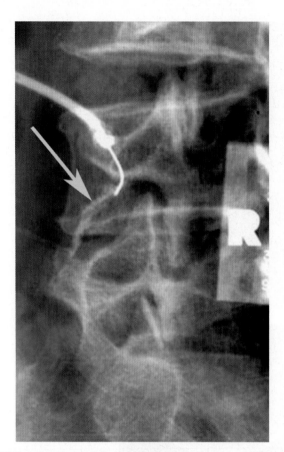

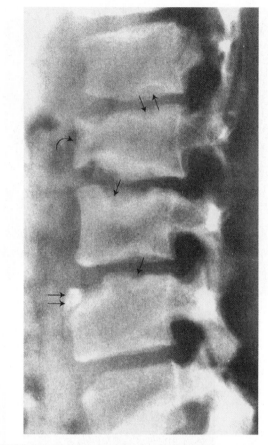

FIGURE 9.45. Nerve block or focal epidural injection. Oblique radiograph during a left L4 temporary nerve block. A needle is placed adjacent to the nerve in the foramen. Radiographic contrast is then injected which flows along the perineural sheath adjacent to the nerve (*arrow*). Some flow will also track proximally into the epidural space. After placement is confirmed, the steroid and possibly anesthetic are injected.

FIGURE 9.47. Lumbar spine lateral radiograph. Scheuermann disease. The involvement of three or more vertebrae by Schmorl nodes (*single straight arrows*) is called Scheuermann disease. Anterior wedging and increased AP diameter of the vertebral bodies (*curved arrow*) may result from this process. There is a limbus vertebra (*double straight arrows*). Note the wavy appearance of the endplates.

FIGURE 9.46. Axial T1-weighted MR image at L5–S1 without **(A)** and with **(B)** intravenous contrast. Scar tissue in a person with recurrent back pain. The *curved arrow* demonstrates an absent portion of lamina from this patient's prior surgery. The *arrow* in **(A)** shows abnormal signal which could be a new disc herniation or scar tissue. **(B)** demonstrates that this area (*arrow*) enhances completely. Disc material does not enhance. The left S1 nerve root (*double arrow*) is displaced and enhances suggesting that it is affected by the scar tissue.

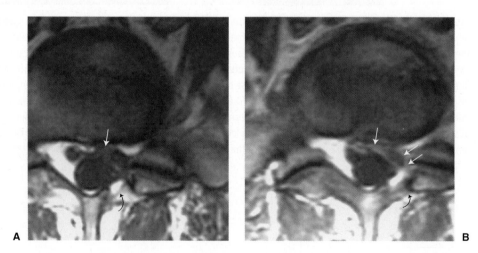

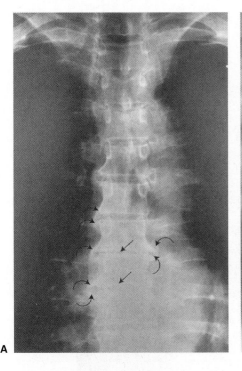

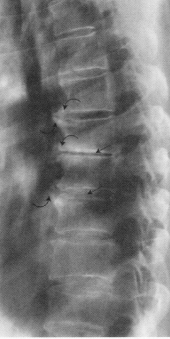

FIGURE 9.48. Thoracic spine AP **(A)** and lateral **(B)** radiographs. Osteoarthritis or degenerative arthritis. Multiple osteophytes (*curved arrows*) are present and multiple disc spaces are narrowed (*straight arrows*) secondary to degenerative disc disease.

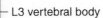

— L3 vertebral body

— L4 vertebral body

— Sacrum

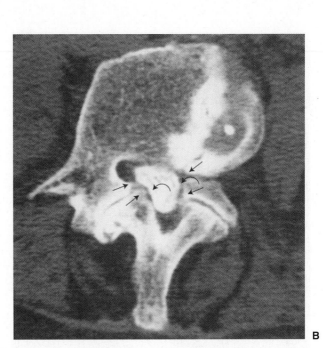

FIGURE 9.49. A: Lumbar myelogram lateral radiographs. Spinal stenosis. The *straight arrows* indicate multiple levels of neural sac compression secondary to spinal canal narrowing that is in turn secondary to degenerative changes in and around the neural canal. The L3–L4 and L4–L5 intervertebral disc spaces are also markedly narrowed (*curved arrows*). **B:** Lumbar spine axial CT image with contrast. Spinal stenosis at the L3–L4 level secondary to hypertrophic facet changes in this 71-year-old man. The *straight arrows* outline the marked narrowing of the spinal canal, and the *curved arrows* indicate the deformity of the thecal sac secondary to the spinal stenosis.

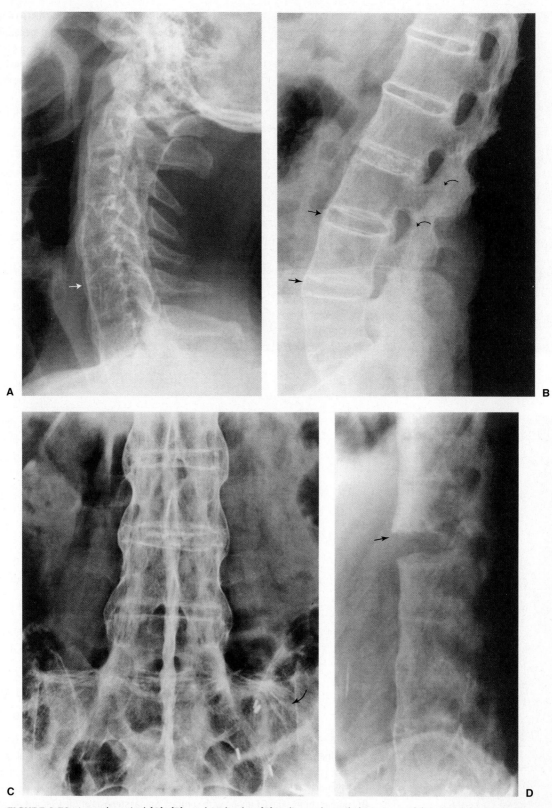

FIGURE 9.50. Lateral cervical **(A), (B),** and AP lumbar **(C)** radiographs. Ankylosing spondylitis. *Straight arrows* demonstrate the syndesmophytes which bridge across disc levels forming a solid "bamboo" spine. The *curved arrows* in **(B)** mark the fused apophyseal joints, while the *curved arrow* in **(C)** is in the expected location of the SI joint, which has fused. **D:** Lateral radiograph in a man with ankylosis spondylitis following a relatively minor fall. There is anterolisthesis of L1 on L2 and a widened L1–L2 disc (*arrow*) due to a fracture through this disc level.

central) of the stenosis. Often, the stenosis is due to a combination of bulging disc, facet arthritis with osteophytes, and thickened ligamentum flavum (see Figs. 9.44C,G and 9.48B).

Ankylosing Spondylitis, Psoriasis, and Reiter Syndrome (Reactive Arthritis)

A group of arthritides which have prominent axial skeleton involvement are collectively known as spondyloarthropathies. The three most frequently discussed are ankylosing spondylitis, psoriasis, and Reiter disease or syndrome, which is now also known as "reactive arthritis."

Ankylosing spondylitis, or Marie–Strumpell disease, is a chronic inflammatory arthritis. It is associated with the HLA-B27 gene and occurs in 1% to 2% of all people positive for that gene. It is most common in young men and most frequently involves the spine and SI joints (Fig. 9.50). Women are affected about one-third as often as men, but they tend to have a milder or even subclinical course of the disease. The SI joints become symmetrically narrowed or completely obliterated. Ankylosing spondylitis in the spine often results in squaring of the vertebral bodies and syndesmophytes, ossification between the outer margin of the vertebral bodies and the disc annulus. These changes radiographically simulate a piece of bamboo and have been termed the "bamboo spine" (Fig. 9.50B,C). Because of the rigidity of the spine and relatively weak fusion across discs, even mild trauma may lead to fractures at the disc levels (Fig. 9.50D). Ankylosing spondylitis may involve other joints, and these joints will have an appearance similar to rheumatoid arthritis.

Psoriasis is probably most known for its characteristic dermatologic manifestations, but its arthritis may coincide or even predate the skin changes. Psoriatic arthritis features both erosions and bony proliferation. When the SI joints are involved, they are asymmetrically involved (Fig. 9.51). Sporadic paravertebral ossification will connect adjacent vertebral bodies.

Reiter syndrome or reactive arthritis consists of a constellation of conjunctivitis, urethritis, and arthritis. The radiographic features are quite similar to psoriasis, but more likely to involve the lower extremity rather than upper extremity joints. The spine and SI joint changes are indistinguishable from psoriasis radiographically.

Rheumatoid Arthritis

There are many synovial joints in the spine, thus rheumatoid arthritis often involves the spine. The severity of rheumatoid arthritis of the spine ranges from mild to severe. There may only be mild narrowing of cervical disc spaces. However, when rheumatoid arthritis involves the odontoid and the atlantoaxial joint, the result can be weakening of the transverse atlantal ligament that holds the odontoid close to the anterior arch of C1. When this ligament becomes involved, subluxation or even dislocation of the atlantoaxial joint may occur (Fig. 9.52). These patients can experience cervical pain either at rest or with head movement. On a lateral radiograph, the normal distance between the anterior border of the odontoid and posterior aspect of the C1 anterior arch is usually less than 2.5 mm in adults. When there is subluxation or dislocation of this joint, the distance becomes greater than 2.5 mm, especially when the cervical spine is flexed.

Flexion and extension lateral cervical spine radiographs may be indicated in rheumatoid arthritis patients when they experience pain with head movement, and before undergoing general anesthesia or any other procedure in which their

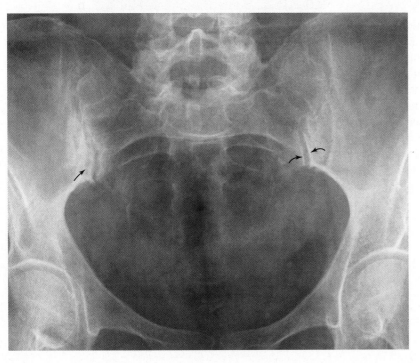

FIGURE 9.51. Pelvis AP radiograph. Psoriasis. There is sclerosis and irregularity of the right SI joint (*straight arrow*) due to sacroiliitis associated with psoriatic arthritis. Compare the appearance to the sharply defined margins of the left SI joint (*curved arrows*).

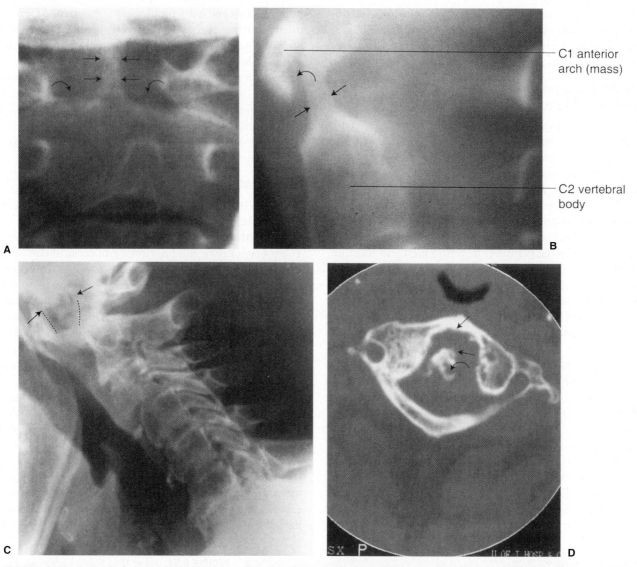

FIGURE 9.52. A: Cervical spine AP open mouth radiograph. Rheumatoid arthritis. The odontoid process (*straight arrows*) is narrowed, osteopenic, and poorly marginated. Note the increased distances between the odontoid process of C2 and the inferior articular processes of C1 (*curved arrows*) due to partial loss of odontoid bone. **B:** Cervical spine lateral tomograph in the same patient. Rheumatoid arthritis. The odontoid (*straight arrows*) is markedly narrowed. The space between the anterior odontoid and the anterior arch of C1 (*curved arrow*) is greater than the normal 2.5 mm or less. This can also occur in ankylosing spondylitis. **C:** Cervical spine lateral flexion radiograph in a different patient than shown in **B.** Rheumatoid arthritis. When the cervical spine is flexed, the space (*straight arrows*) between the anterior surface of the odontoid and the posterior aspect of the anterior arch of C1 (*dotted lines*) is dramatically widened. This widening represents an unstable dislocation of C1 relative to C2. There is grade 1 anterior spondylolisthesis of C2 relative to C3. Note the narrowing of all the cervical disc spaces and the generalized osteopenia. **D:** Cervical spine axial CT image. Rheumatoid arthritis with spinal stenosis in a 55-year-old man. The C1–C2 joint is abnormal with 8-mm distance between the anterior arch of C1 and the odontoid (*between the straight arrows*). There are advanced erosive changes in the odontoid (*curved arrow*).

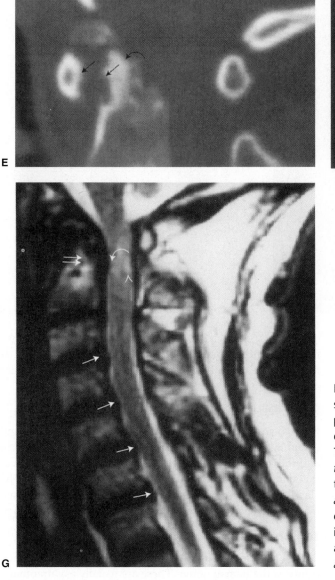

E

F

G

FIGURE 9.52. (*Continued*) Cervical spine CT sagittal reconstruction (**E**) and sagittal CT 3D reconstruction (**F**) in the same patient as shown in **D**. The odontoid is involved with erosive changes and has a distal penciled appearance (*curved arrows*). There is redemonstration of the abnormal C1–C2 joint (*between the straight arrows*). **G:** Cervical spine sagittal T2 MR image in the same patient as shown in (**D**) and (**F**). The odontoid (*double arrows*) is displaced posterior resulting in spinal stenosis and cervical cord compression (*curved arrow*). The increased signal in the compressed cord (*arrowhead*) probably represents edema and/or chronic reaction to the compression. The *single straight arrows* indicate multiple levels of mild spinal stenosis.

head might be hyperflexed or hyperextended. These precautions help to prevent spinal cord injury. As elsewhere, rheumatoid arthritis often is associated with osteopenia and secondary pathologic fractures. The differential diagnosis for osteopenia and vertebral fracture includes osteoporosis, metastatic disease, multiple myeloma, infection, and trauma.

Neuropathic Joints

Charcot joints or neuropathic or neurotrophic joints can occur in the spine as well as the extremities. The joint changes are secondary to lost pain sensation and/or unstable joints found in a variety of neurologic conditions including diabetes mellitus, syringomyelia, and spina bifida with meningocele. The radiographic findings are disc space narrowing, bone destruction and fragmentation, sclerotic subchondral bone, subluxation and dislocation, and marginal bone mass formation. Many of these findings can be found in osteoarthritis and the appearance is that of severe osteoarthritis of the spine.

INFECTION

Osteomyelitis or bone infection is common and has been discussed in Chapter 6. Spine infections are caused by a wide range of organisms, but staphylococcal infections are the most common. As with osteomyelitis elsewhere, patients with spinal osteomyelitis usually have fever and localized pain. The lumbar spine is the most frequently involved, followed by the cervical and then the thoracic spine. The radiographic findings are subtle, and often poor definition of a vertebral endplate is the only finding

FIGURE 9.53. Lower thoracic and upper lumbar spine AP **(A)** and lateral **(B)** radiographs. Osteomyelitis of T11 vertebral body. This 41-year-old patient had back pain and a low-grade fever. There is destruction of the posterior portion of the T11 inferior endplate (*straight arrows*), and the marked narrowing of the T11–T12 intervertebral disc space (*curved arrows*) suggests disc and joint destruction.

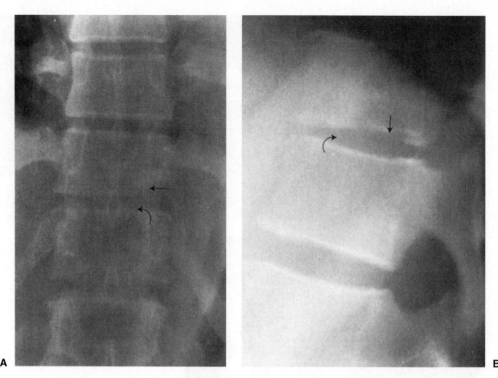

(Fig. 9.53) since the infection usually begins as discitis. With progression, frank bony destruction may be found. Osteomyelitis is in the differential diagnosis of lytic bone lesions. MRI is sensitive to detect osteomyelitis (Fig. 9.54). On T1 MR images, the infections have a decreased signal intensity (they appear dark gray), whereas on T2 images the infections have an increased signal intensity (they appear white). Contrast enhancement is fairly intense and associated abscess may be found, occasionally extending into the epidural space (Fig. 9.54C). The disc is invariably involved, which often helps to differentiate infection from fractures and metastases. CT scans may detect bone and joint destruction that is not visible on radiographs (Fig. 9.54B). CT-guided biopsy (Fig. 9.54B) is a frequent procedure to try to determine the causative organism although an organism will only be identified in approximately 50% of discitis biopsies.

MISCELLANEOUS DISEASES

Diffuse Idiopathic Skeletal Hyperostosis

Diffuse idiopathic skeletal hyperostosis (DISH) or Forestier disease is best demonstrated on a lateral spine radiograph (Fig. 9.55) and is characterized by flowing ossification involving the anterior longitudinal ligament. It is characteristically accompanied by exuberant osteophytes. The overall appearance is similar to the bamboo spine of ankylosing spondylitis; however, ankylosing spondylitis is usually accompanied by obliteration of the SI joints. Spinal stenosis is a significant complication of DISH (Fig. 9.56). As in ankylosing spondylitis, fractures may occur from a relatively minor trauma. Elsewhere in the body, DISH is manifested by prominent bony projections at ligament attachment sites.

Paget Disease

Paget disease is due to an imbalance of osteoclastic and osteoblastic activity that may be metabolic or viral in origin and this has been discussed in Chapter 6. It often involves the spine and, more frequently, the pelvis (Fig. 9.57). The classic spine appearance is the picture frame vertebra caused by increased peripheral vertebra density and central lucency.

Tumors

Benign tumors may involve the spine (Table 9.9). One such tumor is the hemangioma. These are usually asymptomatic

Table 9.9
Some Primary Spine Bone Tumors
Benign
Hemangioma
Osteoid osteoma
Osteoblastoma
Aneurysmal bone cyst
Osteochondroma
Malignant
Multiple myeloma (most common)
Chordoma
Chondrosarcoma
Osteosarcoma
Ewing sarcoma

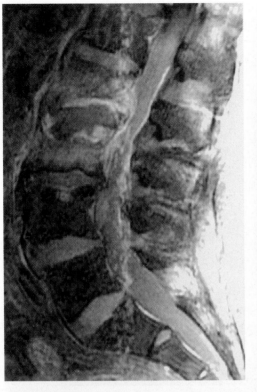

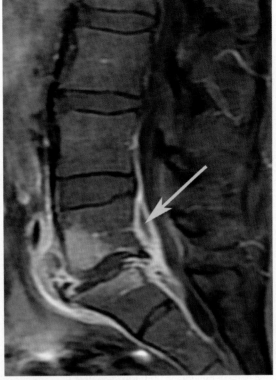

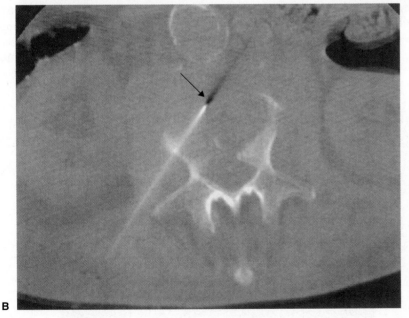

FIGURE 9.54. A: Sagittal T1 MR with intravenous contrast. Discitis. The L2–L3 disc appears enlarged because the adjacent endplates have been destroyed by the infection. There is contrast enhancement (white) surrounding the infected disc and of the involved vertebral bodies. **B:** Axial CT during biopsy in the same patient. The tip of the biopsy needle (*arrow*) is in the infected disc. In only about half of biopsies performed for discitis will an organism be identified. **C:** Sagittal fat-suppressed MR images of the lumbar spine after MR contrast was administered. Discitis is present at L5–S1 with extension of infection to an epidural abscess (*arrow*).

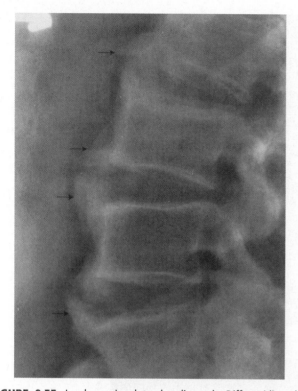

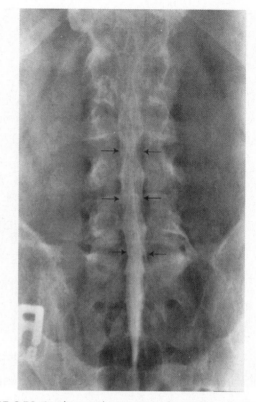

FIGURE 9.55. Lumbar spine lateral radiograph. Diffuse idiopathic skeletal hyperostosis, or DISH. Note the large osteophytes (*arrows*) along the anterior vertebral bodies that extend anteriorly across the disc spaces and ossification of the anterior longitudinal ligament. The intervertebral disc spaces are normal in height.

FIGURE 9.56. Lumbar myelogram PA radiograph in a different patient. Spinal stenosis secondary to diffuse idiopathic skeletal hyperostosis (DISH). The *arrows* indicate multiple levels of spinal stenosis and neural sac compression due to DISH changes in the spinal canal. The overall appearance of the spine is somewhat similar to the bamboo spine of ankylosing spondylitis.

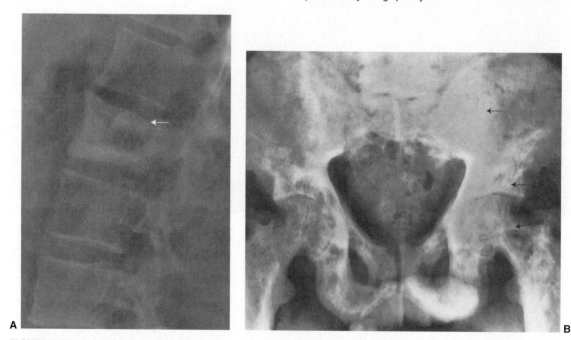

FIGURE 9.57. A: Lumbar spine lateral radiograph. Paget disease L2 vertebra (*arrow*). The L2 vertebra has the classic picture frame appearance secondary to the increased trabecular density in the periphery of the vertebral body. There is mild loss of the L2 vertebral body height compared to the vertical heights of L1 and L3, and this is compatible with a mild compression fracture. The remainder of the lumbar spine is not involved by the Paget disease. **B:** Pelvis AP radiograph. Paget disease. The bone trabeculae are coarse (*arrows*) with an overall increased density and widening or expansion of the bones.

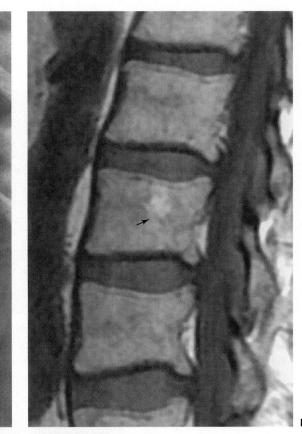

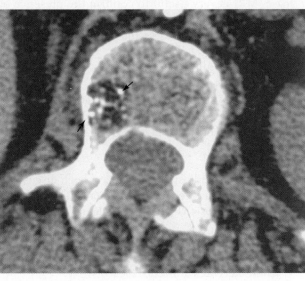

FIGURE 9.58. Hemangiomas in three different patients. **A:** Thoracolumbar spine AP radiograph. T12 vertebral body hemangioma. The prominent vertical trabecular pattern is characteristic of bone hemangioma (*arrow*). Compare the appearance of the T12 vertebral body to those above and below that level. **B:** Sagittal T1 MR of the lumbar spine. The round, focal area of higher signal (*arrow*) is quite characteristic of hemangioma in the spine since it contains a moderate amount of fat. **C:** Axial CT of a thoracic vertebral body demonstrates the punctate appearance of the cross section of coarse trabeculae (*arrows*), similar to that seen in **A.** Note the very low density of the fat within the hemangioma (black).

and an incidental finding in the spine. Hemangiomas in the spine require no therapy unless they become symptomatic. Symptoms may develop when the tumor causes a pathologic fracture or the lesion extends outside the vertebrae and compresses the spinal cord. Hemangiomas (Fig. 9.58; see Fig. 9.44E) can develop in other bones, but in the spine they have a classic appearance with prominent or thickened vertical trabeculae that simulate jail bars or corduroy fabric. The MRI and CT appearances are also quite characteristic and usually do not pose a diagnostic dilemma.

As previously discussed in Chapter 6, *metastatic disease is the most common neoplasm in bone and this includes the spine.* As in other bones, metastatic disease involving the spine can be osteolytic (Fig. 9.59) with and without destruction and/or osteoblastic activity (Fig. 9.60). The primary neoplasms causing osteolytic and osteoblastic bone lesions are listed in Table 9.10.

The importance of visualizing the vertebral pedicles is emphasized in Figure 9.61. When one or both pedicles are missing in patients with known or suspected cancer, the

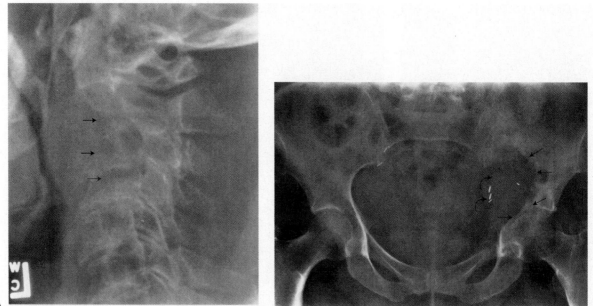

A   B

FIGURE 9.59. **A:** Cervical spine lateral radiograph. Osteolytic metastatic disease of multiple cervical vertebrae. The C2, C3, and C4 vertebral bodies are involved by destructive (lytic) metastatic disease from the lung (*arrows*). **B:** Pelvis AP radiograph. Osteolytic metastatic carcinoma of the cervix involving the left ilium and ischium (*straight arrows*). The extensive involvement of the left ischium has resulted in left acetabular protrusio. There is a large soft tissue metastatic mass in the left pelvis (*curved arrows*).

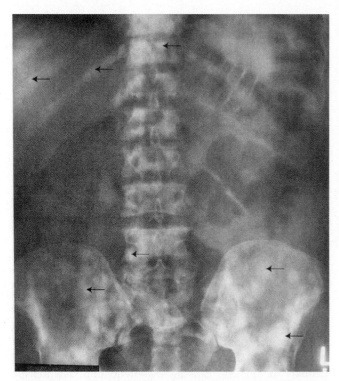

FIGURE 9.60. Abdomen AP radiograph. Osteoblastic metastatic carcinoma of the prostate. The multiple areas of increased density (*arrows*) represent the metastases that involve the pelvis, lumbar spine, dorsal spine, and ribs.

first diagnosis that must come to mind is metastatic disease. MRI is very useful to confirm the presence of metastatic disease in a vertebra with a missing pedicle (see Fig. 9.61C) and to assess the extent and location of the metastases (Fig. 9.62).

Primary tumors of the thecal sac and the spinal cord can mimic bone tumors of the spine. Thus tumors arising from these structures should be considered in the differential diagnosis when dealing with back pain and abnormal radiographs and myelograms.

Others

Osteoporosis and osteomalacia have been discussed in the metabolic disease section of Chapter 6. The typical patient with osteoporosis (Fig. 9.63) is elderly and complains of

Table 9.10
Characteristics of Metastases

Osteoblastic
Prostate
Breast
Lymphoma
Carcinoid
Neuroblastoma (occasional)

Osteolytic
Breast
Lung
Almost all other metastatic tumors

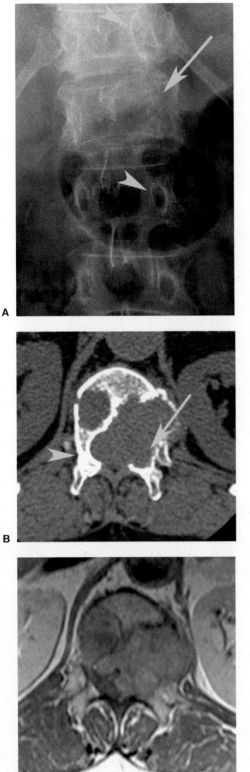

FIGURE 9.61. Absent pedicle sign. **A:** Thoracolumbar spine AP radiograph. The left T12 pedicle is not visualized (*arrow*). Note the normal appearance of the pedicles at adjacent levels (*arrowheads*). **B:** Axial CT image through this level reveals the large amount of bone destruction extending into the region of the pedicle on the left (*arrow*). **C:** Axial T1-weighted MR image also demonstrates the mass and bone destruction. This metastasis was secondary to melanoma. The lesion is not as dark on T1 as some other tumor types.

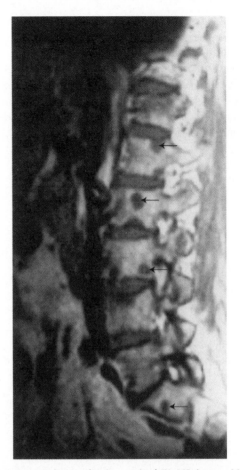

FIGURE 9.62. Lumbosacral spine sagittal T1 MR image. Metastatic carcinoma of the breast. The patient complained of severe back pain, but the radiographs were negative. The *straight arrows* indicate some of the many metastatic lesions present in the lumbar and sacral spine. The metastatic lesions appear black on the T1 MR image but white or gray on T2 images.

back pain, especially if secondary compression fractures are present. Vertebral fractures not only cause back pain, but will also often result in loss of height and kyphosis. A severe kyphosis may decrease thoracic cage and, thus, lung volume. The typical radiographic appearance of osteoporosis in the spine is decreased overall density of the vertebral bodies, and as a result the vertebral endplates appear prominent. As the vertebra become softer than the disc, the endplates can sag, resulting in fish-mouth deformities of the vertebrae. By the time demineralization is seen on radiographs, the osteoporosis is fairly advanced.

Sickle cell anemia is a Mendelian dominant hereditary trait. The disease is variable in severity and characterized by crises that include anemia, fever, severe abdominal and bone pain, and bone infarction. Radiographs may show osteoporosis, bone infarcts, aseptic necrosis, and fish-mouth vertebrae (Fig. 9.64).

Dwarfism and several congenital anomalies have classic or typical appearances of the spine and pelvis, but a discussion is beyond the scope of this introductory text.

FIGURE 9.63. Lumbar spine lateral radiograph. Senile osteoporosis. Note the overall decreased density or osteopenia of the spine. There are multiple compression pathologic fractures secondary to osteoporosis (*straight arrows*). The fractures of L1, L3, L4, and L5 are manifest by a loss of the vertical heights of the involved vertebral bodies. Compare the fractured vertebrae to the normal vertical heights of the T12 and L2 vertebral bodies. Note the multiple fish-mouth deformities (*curved arrows*).

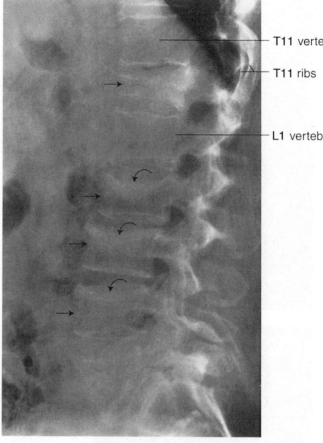

T11 vertebral body

T11 ribs

L1 vertebral body

FIGURE 9.64. Thoracic spine **(A)** and lumbar **(B)** spine lateral radiographs. Sickle cell anemia. There is overall osteopenia and the fish-mouth deformities of the vertebral bodies (*arrows*) are similar to those in senile osteoporosis (see Fig. 9.63). Note the ribs in **A** (*arrowheads*).

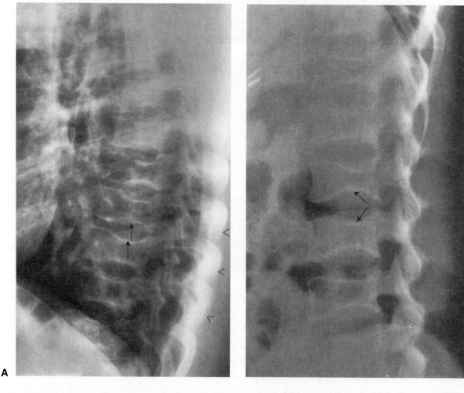

A

B

Approach to Clinical Problems

Initial evaluation of a patient with back pain requires a thorough history and physical examination. If the patient experienced pain 2 or 3 days after playing in the father–son football game, he is more likely to have a muscle strain or delayed onset muscle soreness. Acute pain after lifting a heavy object is more likely a herniated nucleus pulposis. Insidious onset of pain may be related to arthritis, developing osteoporotic compressions, or metastatic disease. The level of clinical suspicion will determine what steps to take next. Most patients will undergo a trial of conservative treatment of rest, physical therapy, and pain medications. If there is no improvement, imaging studies may then be considered. However, if the patient has a known primary neoplasm, MRI or radionuclide bone scan may be the initial study because of a higher clinical suspicion of metastases and the importance of the diagnosis.

Key Points

- Basic observations on spine radiographs should include spinal alignment, the heights of the vertebral bodies and the intervertebral disc spaces, osseous density, presence of the pars interarticularis in the lumbar spine, and presence of the pedicles of each vertebra. An absent pedicle is abnormal and should make you suspicious of a destructive process such as primary and secondary bone neoplasms.
- Spine CT is good for bone detail, localization of fracture fragments and their relationship to the spinal canal and cord, and diagnosis of herniated intervertebral disc disease.
- Cervical spine CT is the appropriate study (instead of radiographs) in the trauma patient.
- Most congenital anomalies of the spine are asymptomatic.
- Spine MRI is good for imaging disease processes that involve the bone marrow fat such as tumor and infection. MRI is also valuable for diagnosis and staging of herniated intervertebral disc disease and evaluating the spinal cord.
- Hyperflexion injuries include teardrop fractures, posterior ligament injury, and facet locking. Locked facets commonly have associated spinal cord injury.
- Odontoid process fractures are frequent in the elderly and result from both hyperflexion and hyperextension injuries.
- A ring is rarely broken in only one location. At least two fractures are usually present in the pelvis.
- Acetabular fractures are evaluated by AP and oblique (Judet) views of the pelvis and CT.
- Following an acetabular fracture, subsequent studies should closely evaluate for the presence of AVN in the femoral head.

FURTHER READINGS

El-Khoury GY. *Essentials of Musculoskeletal Imaging*. New York, NY: Churchill Livingstone, 2003.

Naidich TP, Castillo M, Cha S, et al. *Imaging of the Spine*. Philadelphia, PA: Saunders, 2011.

Renfrew DL. *Atlas of Spine Imaging*. Philadelphia, PA: Saunders, 2003.

QUESTIONS

1. A patient presents to the emergency department with suspected neck trauma, the appropriate imaging study is
   a. lateral radiograph of the cervical spine
   b. four-view series of the cervical spine
   c. CT of the cervical spine
   d. MR of the cervical spine

2. A fracture of the pars interarticularis is called
   a. spondylolysis
   b. spondylolisthesis
   c. limbus vertebra
   d. Scheuermann disease

3. Which term best fits a disc abnormality in which a disc extends beyond expected margin of the annulus by less than 25% circumference and the depth of extension is less than the base of the abnormality?
   a. Sequestration
   b. Extrusion
   c. Protrusion
   d. Bulge

4. The most common cause of scoliosis is
   a. hemivertebra
   b. pedicle bars
   c. radiation in childhood
   d. idiopathic

5. The most common organism causing discitis is
   a. Streptococcus
   b. Staphylococcus
   c. Mycobacterium
   d. Enterococcus

6. In a patient with a cervical spine injury and neurologic symptoms, the primary reason an MRI may be obtained is to
   a. determine the extent of fracture
   b. evaluate the cord for edema or blood
   c. search for additional fractures
   d. assess for ligamentous injury

7. Hip dislocations carry a risk of
   a. osteonecrosis
   b. femoral nerve injury
   c. vascular injury
   d. infection

8. The pain from a disc herniation may be treated by
   a. discogram injection
   b. myelogram injection
   c. epidural injection
   d. contrast injection

9. The following cervical spine fracture is due to a hyperextension injury
   a. facet locking
   b. C5 teardrop fracture
   c. burst fracture
   d. hangman fracture

10. An osteoblastic tumor in the spine is most likely due to which of the following?
    a. Multiple myeloma
    b. Prostate cancer
    c. Hemangioma
    d. Lung cancer

Nuclear Imaging

Thomas A. Farrell

Nuclear medicine uses small amounts of radioactive materials (radiopharmaceuticals) to diagnose and treat disease. The subspecialty is unique, because it provides information about both organ structure and function in patients and the techniques used often identify abnormalities very early in the progress of a disease—often before other diagnostic tests. Because the images generated by nuclear medicine represent a physiologic map revealing less anatomic detail than radiologic studies such as CT or MR, it is necessary to correlate the nuclear medicine images with the corresponding radiologic images.

RADIOPHARMACEUTICALS

When molecules with radionuclide components are prepared for administration to human beings, they are called *radiopharmaceuticals* and they participate in, but do not alter, various physiologic processes. Specific radiopharmaceuticals with particular physiochemical properties are used to study an organ or organ system. The radionuclide portion of the radiopharmaceutical typically emits gamma rays and/or x-rays that can be detected and create a scintigraphic image (often referred to as scan). There are several possible routes of patient administration of radiopharmaceuticals including intravenous, oral, and inhaled.

Over 30 radiopharmaceuticals use technetium-99m (Tc-99m) which has many useful properties as a gamma-emitting tracer nuclide. It is eluted from a Tc-99m generator as the soluble pertechnetate and then either used directly as a soluble salt, or combined with a number of Tc-99m–based radiopharmaceuticals which determine its uptake by various organs. Other radiopharmaceuticals incorporate a radioactive tracer atom into a larger pharmaceutically active molecule, which is localized in the body, after which the radionuclide tracer atom allows it to be detected with a gamma camera. An example is fluorodeoxyglucose (FDG) in which fluorine-18 is incorporated into deoxyglucose to give 18-FDG which is commonly used in positron emission tomography (PET) scanning. Some radioisotopes such as gallium-67 and radioiodine are used directly as soluble ionic salts, without further modification.

The most commonly used nuclear medicine imaging system is a gamma camera which is composed of an array of photomultiplier tubes. Each photomultiplier tube contains a sodium iodide crystal which produces light when struck by gamma or x-rays. The light scintillations are digitized and then processed into an image for physician interpretation. The image is essentially a physiologic map of the radiopharmaceutical distribution within the body. Table 10.1 lists the radiopharmaceuticals and the

Table 10.1

Radiopharmaceuticals Discussed in this Chapter

Radiopharmaceutical	Application
Tc-99m macroaggregated albumin (MAA)	Lung perfusion
Xenon-133, Tc-99m diethylenetriamine pentaacetic acid (DTPA) aerosol	Lung ventilation
Tc-99m iminodiacetic acid (HIDA)	Hepatobiliary dynamics
Tc-99m diphosphonate	Bone
Tc-99m DTPA	Renal glomerular filtration rate
Tc-99m DMSA	Renal masses
Thallium-201, Tc-99m sestamibi, Rb-82	Myocardial perfusion
F-18 fluorodeoxyglucose (FDG)	PET tumor imaging

corresponding imaging procedures that are discussed in this chapter.

Tomography is a basic radiographic technique which improves the visualization of the organ being imaged by blurring or eliminating the adjacent tissue. This technique is widely used in nuclear medicine to improve image quality, for example, single photon emission computed tomography (SPECT) which is an array of gamma cameras mounted on a gantry which rotates around the patient. Resolution of the organ of interest is improved by obtaining images in multiple projections which allows reduction of scatter gamma and x-rays.

SKELETAL IMAGING

Skeletal scintigraphy, more commonly referred to as a bone scan, is a valuable tool for the investigation of a number of disorders of the skeletal system. A Tc-99m–labeled diphosphonate derivative is used in skeletal scintigraphy because this radiolabeled agent is adsorbed onto the

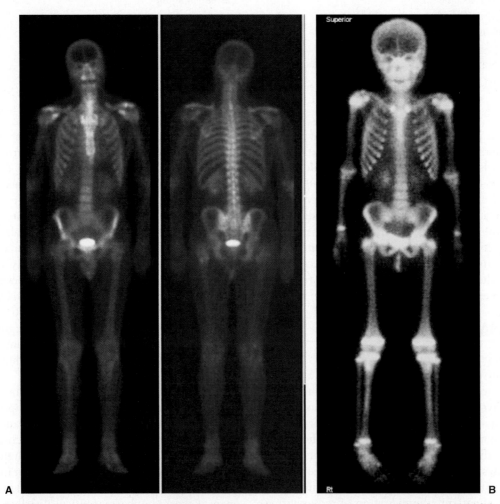

FIGURE 10.1. Normal bone scans. Whole-body images of a normal bone scan in an adult **(A)** and child **(B)**. Note the increased epiphyseal activity on the child's scan.

surface of newly forming hydroxyapatite crystal in the bone. New bone formation occurs in response to almost all skeletal pathology such as fracture, infection, or tumor and therefore scintigraphic images will demonstrate increased gamma-ray activity at the site of increased bone turnover. The normal bone scan appearance in an adult and child are shown in Figure 10.1. Note the multiple areas of increased activity in the child's epiphyses.

A bone scan is very sensitive for detecting metastases and in general will identify a lesion before it is seen in a conventional radiograph. However, it is often not possible to determine whether lesions seen on a bone scan are malignant or benign, and this is particularly true for a single lesion, which often is caused by a benign process such as a fracture or infection. The skeletal system is a common site for metastatic spread of many malignancies such as breast, lung, prostate, and renal carcinomas. Because skeletal metastases usually arise as a result of hematogenous seeding of tumor cells in the bone marrow, most bony metastases are detected in the axial skeleton

Table 10.2
Causes of Nonosseous Uptake on a Bone Scan (False-Positive)

Location	Cause
Head	Stroke
Chest	Myocardial infarct
	Hyperparathyroidism
	Lung metastases (e.g., sarcoma)
Abdomen	Gastric (e.g., hyperparathyroidism)
	Spleen (e.g., sickle cell disease)
Soft tissue	Trauma (e.g., IM injection)
	Myositis

and are seen as numerous foci of increased radionuclide uptake (Fig. 10.2). Well-differentiated thyroid cancer is also prone to disseminate to sites in bone, but these lesions are probably better detected with iodine-131 imaging.

Other skeletal abnormalities are also readily detected with a bone scan. Like metastases, osteomyelitis can be detected earlier with a bone scan than with a plain film (Fig. 10.3). The bone scan may also be useful to detect a fracture which may not be easily seen on plain films. For example, stress fractures (Fig. 10.4) and shin splints (Fig. 10.5) are readily detected on a bone scan but may not be seen on a radiograph. In most cases, a fracture through the full thickness of the bone cortex is readily detected by a plain radiograph. Some full-thickness fractures, such as those in the sacrum, scapula, femoral neck, and small bones of the wrist and ankle, are occasionally difficult to visualize on a radiograph but are detectable by a bone scan (Fig. 10.6). Although regarded as a sensitive test, bone scintigraphy may have false-positive and false-negative results (Tables 10.2 and 10.3).

HEPATOBILIARY IMAGING

Patients with *acute cholecystitis* classically present with right upper quadrant pain/tenderness, fever, and leukocytosis. However, the signs and symptoms of acute cholecystitis often vary and there are a number of conditions that

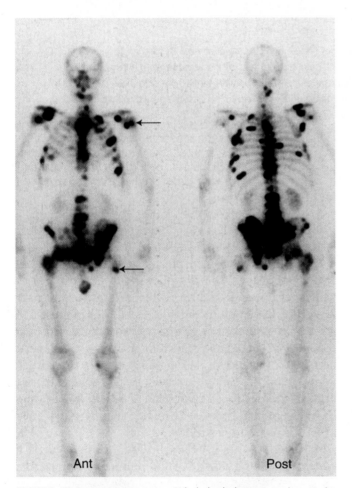

FIGURE 10.2. Bony metastases. Whole-body bone scan in anterior and posterior projections of a 65-year-old man with diffuse skeletal metastases from prostate carcinoma. Images reveal numerous metastatic lesions (black foci), primarily in the axial skeleton and also in the proximal femurs and humeri (*arrows*).

Table 10.3
Causes of Photopenic Bone Lesions (False-Negative Bone Scan)

Multiple myeloma
Avascular necrosis
Postradiation therapy
Rarely metastatic bone disease (e.g., anaplastic, renal cell)
Paravertebral soft tissue lesion invading bone

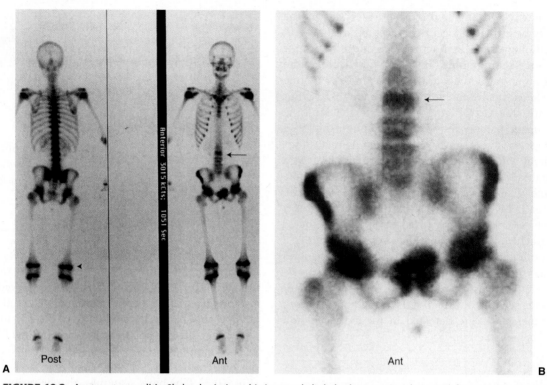

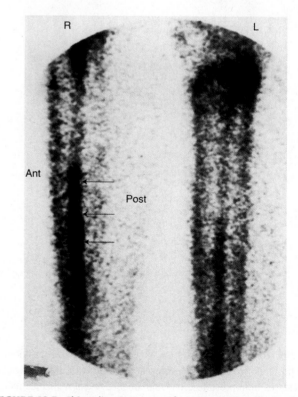

FIGURE 10.3. Acute osteomyelitis. Skeletal scintigraphic images (whole body, **A**; regional view, **B**) from an 18-year-old girl with diabetes who presented with 3 to 4 weeks of low back pain. Radiographs of the vertebra were unremarkable. The images show abnormally increased Tc-99m methylene diphosphonate (MDP) activity in the L3 vertebral body (*arrow*). Biopsy of the site confirmed osteomyelitis. Notice the normal intense uptake of Tc-99m MDP at the growth plates in the lower extremities (*arrowhead*) on the whole-body images.

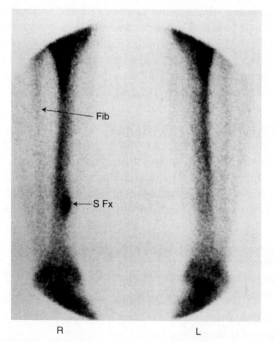

FIGURE 10.4. Stress fracture. A 20-year-old runner with pain in the right calf. Radiographs were normal. Scintigraphic images of the distal lower extremities show focal lesion in the posterior medial aspect of the right distal tibia consistent with a stress fracture (*arrow S Fx*). Notice that the lesion does not involve the full thickness of the tibia. Fibula indicated by *arrow Fib*.

FIGURE 10.5. Shin splint. Bone scan of a patient with calf pain, showing linear pattern of increased uptake (*arrows*) along the posterior aspect of the tibia (enthesopathy).

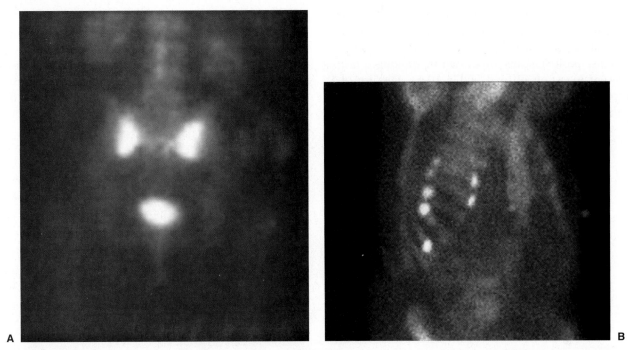

FIGURE 10.6. Bone scans. **A:** Sacral insufficiency fracture. **B:** Multiple rib fractures.

may present in a similar fashion. Consequently, the provisional diagnosis of acute cholecystitis typically requires confirmatory testing with ultrasound and/or hepatobiliary scintigraphy.

Hepatobiliary scintigraphic imaging is performed using a Tc-99m–labeled iminodiacetic acid (HIDA) deriva-

tive that is an analog of bilirubin. This radiopharmaceutical is actively transported into hepatocytes similar to bilirubin and is then excreted unchanged into the biliary tract. Normally HIDA accumulates within the gallbladder within 1 hour of intravenous injection (Fig. 10.7). However, in acute cholecystitis, the gallbladder fails to fill with the

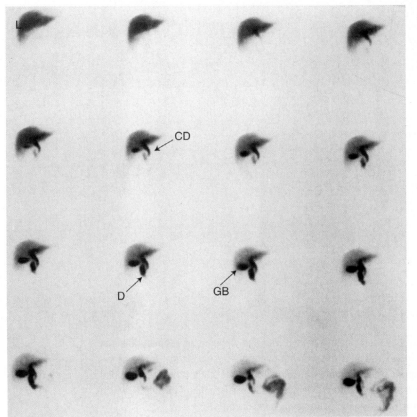

FIGURE 10.7. Normal hepatobiliary (HIDA) study. Images obtained in the anterior view every 2 minutes (moving from left to right and top to bottom) following injection of the hepatobiliary radiotracer show good extraction of the agent by the liver (*L*). The common bile duct (*arrow CD*) is seen along with the duodenum (*arrow D*) and gallbladder (*arrow GB*).

radiotracer because of cystic duct obstruction. This test is extremely sensitive, and a normal result (i.e., visualization of the gallbladder) virtually excludes acute cholecystitis.

False-positive scans are caused by prolonged fasting or recent ingestion of food (Table 10.4). The use of IV morphine has been found helpful in reducing the number of false-positive HIDA scans, thereby improving the speci-

ficity of the test. Morphine causes constriction of the sphincter of Oddi, which augments bile flow through the cystic duct, improving gallbladder visualization (Figs. 10.8 and 10.9). HIDA scanning is also useful in the diagnosis of postoperative bile leaks where accumulation of the radionuclide corresponds to that of extrahepatic bile (Fig. 10.10).

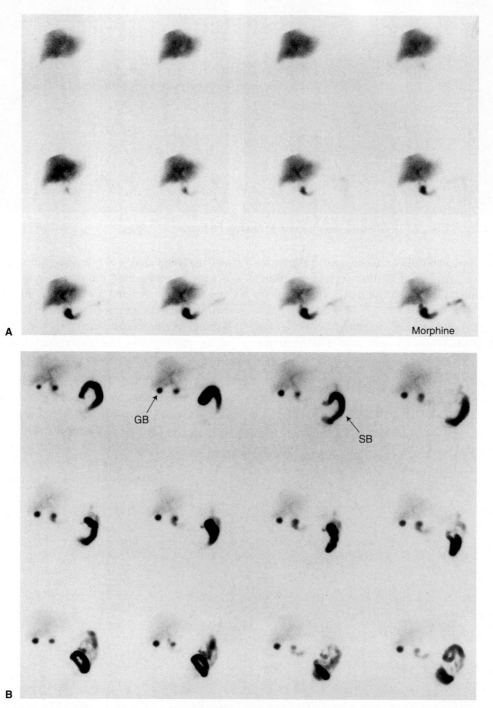

FIGURE 10.8. Normal HIDA study with IV morphine in a patient with right upper quadrant pain. **A:** Initial set of images show normal uptake and excretion by the liver, but over time the gallbladder is not visualized and consequently morphine is given at approximately 40 minutes into the study. **B:** Images obtained immediately following administration of morphine show the gallbladder visualization (*arrow GB*), which effectively rules out acute cholecystitis. Note activity in the small bowel (*arrow SB*).

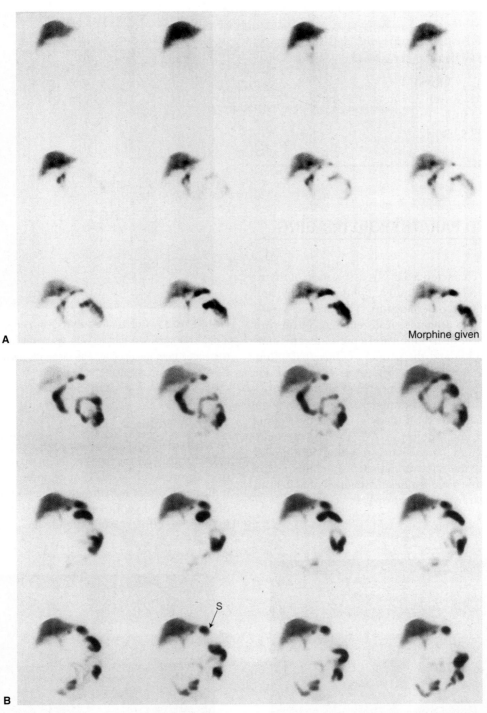

FIGURE 10.9. Acute cholecystitis. Hepatobiliary study in a patient with fever and right upper quadrant pain. **A:** Initial set of images show normal uptake and excretion by the liver, but the gallbladder is not visualized and consequently morphine is given at approximately the time of the image at bottom right. **B:** Images obtained immediately following injection of morphine continue to show absence of gallbladder activity, indicating cystic duct obstruction and acute cholecystitis. Note the reflux of radioactive bile into the stomach (*arrow S*).

Table 10.4

Causes of False-Positive Results with Hepatobiliary Imaging in the Evaluation of Acute Cholecystitis

Prolonged fasting (3 days)
Ingestion of food within 2 hours of the study
Chronic cholecystitis
Chronic alcohol abuse
Pancreatitis

THYROID AND PARATHYROID IMAGING

Graves Disease

Graves disease is characterized by the association of thyrotoxicosis, diffuse goiter, infiltrative ophthalmopathy, and occasionally infiltrative dermopathy. The thyroid scintigram typically shows a symmetrically enlarged gland with homogeneous tracer distribution and a prominent pyramidal lobe (Fig. 10.11) and the patient's radioactive iodine uptake (RAIU) is increased. While there is no cure for Graves disease, the goal of treatment is to reduce the thyroid's ability to produce hormones. Three treatment options are available: Medical therapy, radioactive iodine (I-131) therapy, and surgery. I-131 therapy partially destroys the thyroid parenchyma resulting in fibrosis. Studies evaluating the safety of radioactive iodine therapy have failed to show any significant carcinogenic effect in doses used to treat hyperthyroidism.

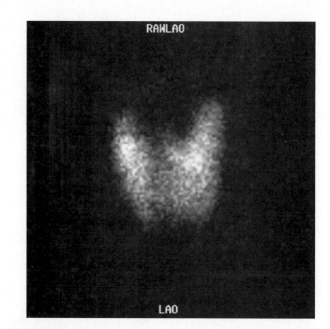

FIGURE 10.11. Graves disease. Tc-99m pertechnetate scan shows a diffusely increased uptake with visualization of a pyramidal lobe (superiorly from the midline). The diagnosis must be confirmed by an elevated radioactive iodine uptake.

Thyroid Nodules

Nuclear imaging can be used to describe a thyroid nodule as hot or cold on the basis of its relative uptake of radioactive isotope such as Tc-99m or Iodine-123. Hot nodules indicate autonomously functioning nodules and cold nodules indicate hypofunctional or nonfunctional thyroid tissue (Fig. 10.12). Radionuclide imaging is unreliable in

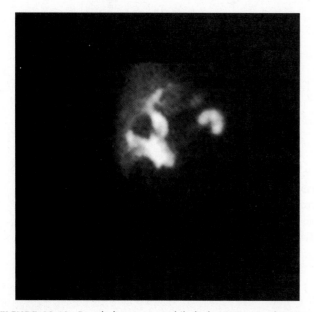

FIGURE 10.10. Postcholecystectomy bile leak. HIDA scan shows extravasation and accumulation of radiopharmaceutical in the gallbladder bed.

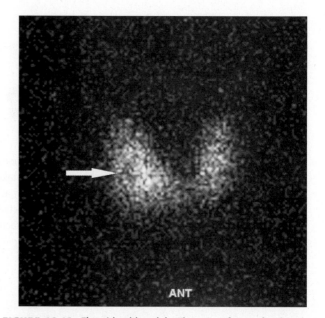

FIGURE 10.12. Thyroid cold nodule. There is a focus of reduced uptake in the mid right thyroid lobe (*arrow*).

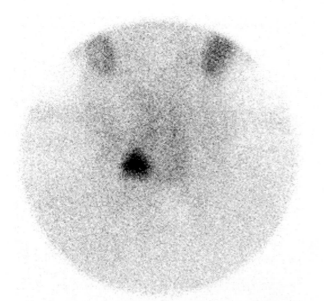

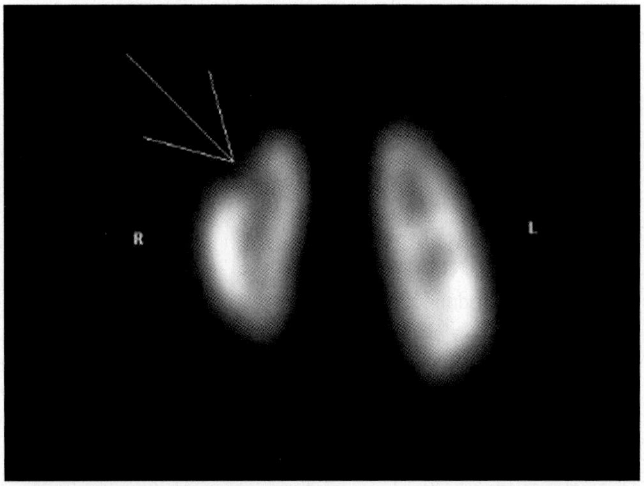

FIGURE 10.14. Renal DMSA scan shows upper pole cortical loss in the right kidney (*arrowhead*).

FIGURE 10.13. Parathyroid adenoma in a patient with hypercalcemia. Delayed imaging after Tc-99m sestamibi injection shows increased uptake in the right neck consistent with a parathyroid adenoma.

diagnosing thyroid cancer as 4% of hot nodules are shown to contain tumor, compared with 16% of cold nodules. This technique has largely been replaced by ultrasound and ultrasound-guided biopsy in the diagnostic workup of thyroid nodules. See Thyroid Biopsy in Chapter 12.

Parathyroid Imaging

Tc-99m sestamibi is absorbed more quickly by a hyperfunctioning parathyroid gland than by a normal gland. Over 60% of parathyroid adenomas may be successfully imaged using this technique. Chief cell parathyroid adenomas in particular have a very high avidity for sestamibi, in contrast to oxyphil/clear cell parathyroid adenomas which have almost no avidity. Images of the neck and chest are obtained immediately and 2 hours postinjection of Tc-99m sestamibi (Fig. 10.13). Smaller-volume parathyroid adenomas, those glands in the upper position, and patients with multiglandular disease are all less likely to be reliably imaged with sestamibi scans.

RENAL IMAGING

Tc-99m dimercaptosuccinic acid (DMSA) localizes in the proximal and distal convoluted renal tubules and is the tracer of choice for renal parenchymal and anatomical evaluations (Fig. 10.14). It is not suitable for dynamic perfusion studies. On the other hand, Tc-99m diethylenetriamine pentaacetic acid (DTPA) is the tracer of choice for dynamic renal perfusion and the detection of renal and ureteral obstructions. About 95% of the dose is filtered through the glomeruli with a normal mean renal transit time of 3 minutes. At 2 hours there is less than 10% renal retention.

Angiotensin-Converting Enzyme Inhibitor Renal Scintigraphic Imaging for Renal Artery Stenosis

Scintigraphic imaging of glomerular filtration combined with administration of an angiotensin-converting enzyme (ACE) inhibitor, such as captopril, is used to identify patients with hypertension caused by renal artery stenosis.

In patients with renal vascular hypertension, renin secretion is increased secondary to the hemodynamic effects of a functionally significant stenosis in the renal artery. Decreased perfusion pressure as a result of the stenosis causes the juxtaglomerular cells to increase secretion of renin. Renin acts on angiotensinogen to form angiotensin I. Angiotensin I is converted to angiotensin II by ACE. Angiotensin II stimulates release of aldosterone and also acts as a potent vasoconstrictor of the peripheral vasculature, including vasoconstriction of the efferent renal arterioles distal to the glomerulus in the underperfused kidney with the stenosis. The efferent vasoconstriction acts to preserve the transglomerular pressure gradient and therefore, helps preserve the glomerular filtration rate (GFR) in the affected kidney. If an ACE inhibitor such as captopril is administered to a patient with renal artery stenosis, angiotensin II levels will drop and the efferent arterioles will dilate, leading to a fall in GFR (Fig. 10.15). In contrast, patients with essential hypertension will have no effect from captopril on the renal scintigraphic images.

VENTILATION AND PERFUSION LUNG IMAGING FOR THE DIAGNOSIS OF PULMONARY EMBOLISM

Pulmonary embolism (PE) is the third most common cause of cardiovascular mortality in the US. The clinical diagnosis of PE is often difficult as symptoms and signs

FIGURE 10.15. Captopril renogram positive for renal artery stenosis. **A:** Scintigraphic images of the kidneys in the posterior projection, 1 to 3 minutes and 3 to 5 minutes following intravenous injection of a Tc-99m–labeled agent that is filtered by the glomerulus. **B:** Repeat images following administration of captopril show a significant decrease in the concentration of this agent (and, therefore, decrease in GFR) in the left kidney compared to the precaptopril study. This finding indicates renal artery stenosis causing renal vascular hypertension.

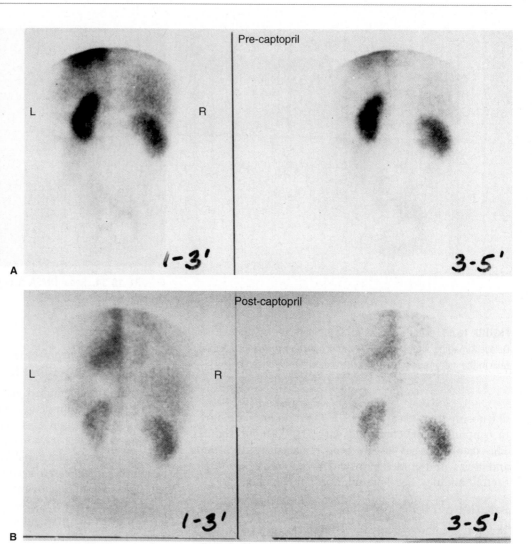

such as dyspnea, chest pain, tachypnea, and tachycardia are nonspecific. A chest radiograph should be obtained in all patients suspected of having PE to exclude other causes of the patient's symptoms such as pneumonia, pneumothorax, and heart failure. However, a normal chest radiograph does not exclude PE and even if the chest radiograph is abnormal and consistent with PE, this alone is rarely sufficient to make an accurate diagnosis necessitating further testing.

Ventilation–perfusion (V/Q, Q is the physiologic symbol for flow rate) lung imaging is highly sensitive for diagnosing PE. Images of regional pulmonary perfusion are obtained by intravenously injecting several hundred thousand tiny particles of macroaggregated human albumin that are radiolabeled with Tc-99m. These albumin particles measure between 10 and 40 μm and because the diameter of pulmonary capillaries and precapillary arterioles is less than 10 μm, the radioactive particles lodge in these vessels throughout the lung fields in concentrations that are directly proportional to the regional pulmonary blood flow. Because less than 0.1% of the total cross

section of the pulmonary vasculature is occluded by the injected radiolabeled particles, complications are extremely rare. Figure 10.16 shows a normal lung perfusion scan.

Pulmonary emboli are often large enough to occlude the segmental pulmonary arteries, and hence the flow defects on the images will often appear segmental in configuration (Fig. 10.17A). However, occlusion of smaller arteries may occur, and the perfusion pattern may; therefore, reveal defects that are somewhat smaller (subsegmental).

Lung perfusion defects are also seen in pneumonia, chronic obstructive pulmonary disease (COPD), and atelectasis due to localized reflex vasoconstriction. So a perfusion defect alone is not diagnostic of PE and for this reason scintigraphic ventilation imaging of the lungs is combined with the perfusion study. Images of regional pulmonary ventilation are obtained by having the patient inhale either radioactive xenon gas or an aerosolized form of Tc-99m DTPA. The combination of ventilation and perfusion scans improves the specificity of the test for the diagnosis of PE. Ventilation is usually normal in regions of the lung that show perfusion defects caused by PE giving a mismatched

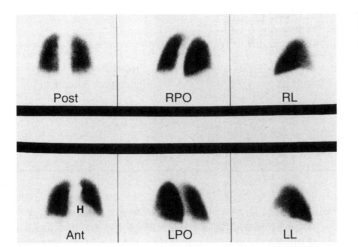

FIGURE 10.16. Normal lung perfusion images in six projections. *Ant,* anterior; *Post,* posterior; *LPO,* left posterior oblique; *RPO,* right posterior oblique; *LL,* left lateral; *RL,* right lateral. *H* designates area of absent activity due to the heart.

Table 10.5
Causes of Matched Ventilation/Perfusion Defects with an Abnormal Chest Film
Pneumonia
Chronic obstructive lung disease
Atelectasis
Asthma

defect (Figs. 10.17 and 10.18). In contrast, matched defects characterized by abnormal regional perfusion and corresponding abnormal regional ventilation are found in other lung diseases (Fig. 10.19 and Table 10.5).

Typically, results from the ventilation/perfusion scan are used to estimate the probability that acute PE has occurred. A normal perfusion scan indicates virtually no chance that the patient has a PE while multiple perfusion

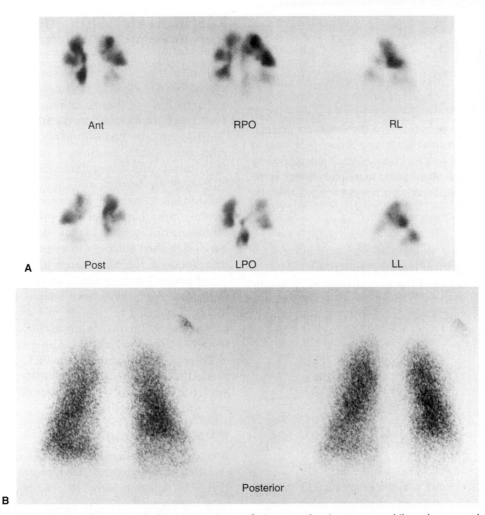

FIGURE 10.17. Pulmonary embolism. **A:** Six-view perfusion scan showing numerous bilateral segmental defects. **B:** Single-breath ventilation images showing normal ventilation. This mismatch pattern is essentially diagnostic for PE.

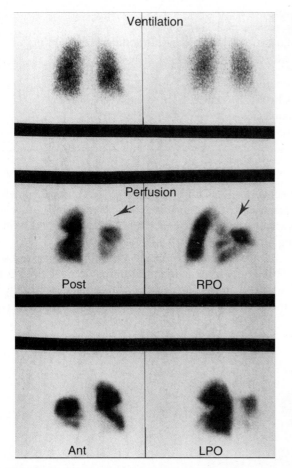

FIGURE 10.18. Pulmonary embolism. Top two images are posterior ventilation images with xenon-133 showing uniform ventilation to both lungs. Bottom four images are from the perfusion study showing multiple segmental defects. *Arrow* points to perfusion defects in the right upper lobe. This mismatch pattern indicates a high probability for PE.

defects with a normal ventilation scan indicate a high probability that the patient has PE (Table 10.6).

CT is now considered the examination of choice in patients with suspected PE. The standard chest CT protocol is modified so the patient is scanned when the contrast

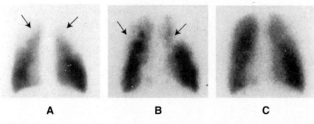

FIGURE 10.19. COPD. Patient with chronic obstructive pulmonary disease showing matching ventilation and perfusion defects in upper lobes (*arrows*). **A:** Posterior perfusion image. **B:** Posterior initial breath-hold ventilation image. **C:** Later equilibrium ventilation image showing eventual filling of defects seen on the initial ventilation image.

Table 10.6

Interpretation of Ventilation/Perfusion Scans

Result	Probability of Pulmonary Embolism
Normal	0%
Low probability	<20%
Intermediate probability	20–80%
High probability	>80%

bolus maximally opacifies the pulmonary arteries (PE protocol) and this test has a sensitivity of 95% for the diagnosis of PE. V/Q scans are still performed in patients who are allergic to intravenous contrast, in the presence of renal failure and in women of childbearing age. The last of these indications is important because the absorbed radiation dose to the breast is 100 times greater in women undergoing chest CT for PE than those having a V/Q scan.

POSITRON EMISSION TOMOGRAPHY AND PET/CT

PET differs from the more conventional nuclear medicine procedures described so far because the radioisotopes that are used emit positrons rather than gamma or x-rays. Positrons have a higher energy (0.5 MeV vs. 140 keV for Tc-99m) and the PET scanner is consequently designed differently. After a positron is emitted, it travels a very short distance (a few millimeters) in body tissue, combines with an electron, and the mass of the positron and electron are converted into energy in the form of two gamma rays that travel in opposite directions. These "simultaneous" gamma rays are detected by the PET scanner, which then creates a three-dimensional image of the distribution of the radioisotope in the body.

Positron-emitting radioisotopes include C-11, N-13, O-15, and F-18. They have a short half-life and can in theory be labeled to virtually any organic molecule normally used by the body such as glucose (or glucose analogues), water, or ammonia, or into molecules that bind to receptors. Currently, the main PET radiopharmaceutical used clinically is F-18–labeled FDG which is a glucose analogue, imaging of which depicts the distribution of glucose metabolism in the body.

Oncologic Imaging

Because many malignant tumors demonstrate enhanced metabolism of glucose relative to normal organs, whole-body PET imaging with FDG can be used to detect and stage malignancy. PET images of a patient with metastatic nonsmall cell lung cancer (NSCLC) are shown in Figure 10.20. Although the absolute level of tumor glucose metabolism can be quantified on PET, in practice this

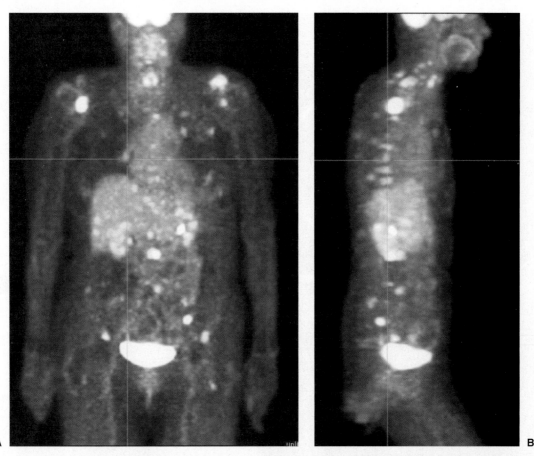

FIGURE 10.20. Lung carcinoma with widespread metastases. Frontal and lateral projections of a whole-body FDG-PET scan showing numerous foci of increased uptake (including the spine) consistent with metastatic disease.

is time-consuming and requires arterial blood sampling of FDG levels. An alternative semiquantitative measurement is used and referred to as the Standardized Uptake Value (SUV), which is directly related to glucose metabolism and much simpler to determine from PET images. The SUV serves as a normalized target-to-background measure and in general, lesions with an SUV of 2.5 or greater are likely to be malignant, whereas values below 2.5 are more likely to be physiologic in origin or caused by benign lesions. One hour after intravenous administration, high FDG activity is normally present in the brain, heart, and urinary tract (excretory route). Sites of variable physiologic tracer uptake include the digestive tract, thyroid, and skeletal muscle. Elsewhere in the body, tracer activity is typically low.

To further improve localization of lesions detected on PET, patients are commonly scanned on combined PET/CT scanners. These scans improve both the sensitivity and the specificity for malignant tumor detection. Tumor types commonly referred for PET/CT evaluation in clinical practice include NSCLC, head and neck cancers, lymphomas, colon cancer, breast cancer, and melanoma. There are many clinical applications including initial staging, detection of recurrent tumor,

and evaluation of response to chemotherapy (Figs. 10.21 and 10.22).

Limitations of PET

Some malignancies are known to be "not PET avid." These include prostate carcinoma, neuroendocrine tumors, and sarcoma metastases. The reasons for the lack of uptake include low glucose metabolism, such as seen in well-differentiated tumors, low proliferation rates, high mucin content, and necrosis. PET is not useful within 2 months of surgical resection due to a high false-positive rate, which may be the result of inflammation or granulation tissue. Furthermore when performed within 4 weeks of chemotherapy, PET has a false-negative rate of over 80% and surgical decisions should not be based on the results of PET without further investigation. Other limitations to the widespread use of PET arise from the high costs of cyclotrons needed to produce the short-lived radionuclides and the need for on-site equipment to produce the radiopharmaceuticals after radioisotope preparation. In addition, the radiation dose from the PET radionuclide is usually around 5 to 7 mSv and when combined with a CT scan (the current standard of practice), the radiation exposure may be substantial—up to 25 mSv for an adult. Future

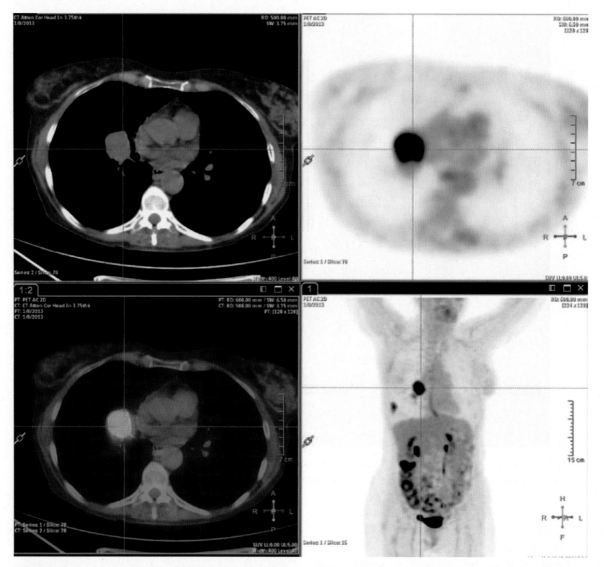

FIGURE 10.21. Lung carcinoma with hilar metastasis. PET/CT images clockwise from top left. **A:** Axial CT shows a right hilar mass. **B:** Axial PET showing increased uptake in the mass. **C:** Coronal PET showing increased uptake in a smaller peripheral right lower lobe mass. **D:** Fusion of PET/CT images **A** and **B**.

developments may include the use of a PET/MR combination which may produce as good anatomic images with less radiation exposure.

CARDIAC IMAGING

Cardiac imaging accounts for nearly 50% of all nuclear medicine tests. The two main areas of interest are cardiac function, specifically left ventricular function, and myocardial perfusion imaging (MPI) in patients with known or suspected coronary artery disease (CAD).

Ventricular Function Imaging

Radionuclide ventriculogram (or multigated scan—MUGA) may be used to assess ventricular function and can be performed in two ways. A first pass technique involves scanning a rapid bolus of a Tc-99m radiotracer as it passes through the heart chambers—this is more accurate for right ventricular evaluation as there is no chamber overlap. The second and more commonly used technique is called equilibrium scanning as it requires Tc-99m RBC imaging, gated to the ECG over several cardiac cycles. Ventricular function is evaluated by calculating the ejection fraction (EF), which is the volumetric fraction of blood pumped out of the ventricle during the cardiac cycle. The normal EF range is 55% to 70%. Common causes of poor ventricular function are ischemia, aortic and mitral valve diseases, and toxins such as chemotherapy (doxorubicin), viral infections, and alcohol. In patients receiving doxorubicin, a decline of 10% or more in absolute left ventricular EF to a value of 50% or less is a recommendation to discontinue the drug. Ventricular function may also be measured using echocardiography and MRI. Cardiac arrhythmias during

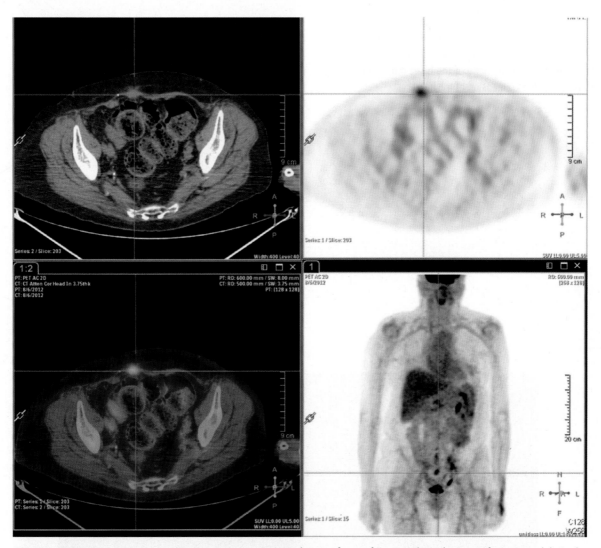

FIGURE 10.22. Postoperative carcinoma recurrence. PET/CT shows a focus of increased uptake in a soft tissue nodule in the anterior abdominal wall of a patient who had a hemicolectomy for colonic carcinoma. Biopsy confirmed recurrence.

image acquisition can limit reproducible assessment of ventricular function.

Myocardial Perfusion Imaging

MPI is usually done using intravenously injected thallium-201 chloride (^{201}Tl) or Tc-99m–labeled agents such as sestamibi or tetrofosmin. Thallium is a potassium analogue (indicator of cell membrane integrity) and is the only SPECT radionuclide that assesses myocardial redistribution and viability. SPECT imaging is used to obtain perfusion images of the heart using one of these agents. The heart is imaged in a 180-degree arc and data acquired which are formatted to give a three-dimensional image. Short-axis (Fig. 10.23) and long-axis views are used for interpretation. A normal cardiac SPECT thallium-201 study shows uniform perfusion throughout the myocardium.

Stress testing improves the sensitivity of MPI for the detection of CAD and can be performed during either exercise or IV injection of adenosine or dipyridamole. Arterioles distal to a normal coronary artery will dilate substantially in response to either exercise or pharmacologic stimulation. As a result, perfusion (and, therefore, radiotracer concentration) will increase considerably in the myocardium supplied by a normal artery whereas myocardial perfusion will change little if at all distal to a significant arterial stenosis. Therefore, significant CAD will cause a perfusion defect on the cardiac images immediately following stress. Perfusion defects seen on the stress images that become less severe or normalize on delayed images are referred to as *reversible* and almost always contain viable myocardium (Fig. 10.24). Reversible defects typically also have wall motion at rest. Defects that do not change from stress to the delayed images are called *fixed* and usually contain scar tissue (Fig. 10.25). However, in some instances fixed defects may still contain viable tissue.

FIGURE 10.23. Normal myocardial single photon emission computed tomography (SPECT) views. SPECT short-axis cross section of the left ventricle. The short-axis cross-sectional view is obtained by slicing the three-dimensional image of the heart muscle in planes perpendicular to the long dimension of the heart.

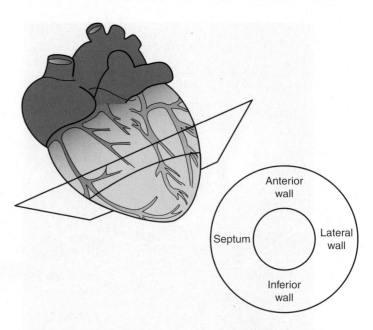

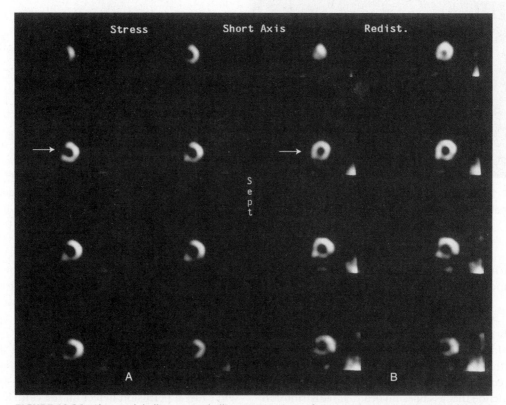

FIGURE 10.24. Abnormal thallium scan. Thallium SPECT images from a patient with a stenosis of the left anterior descending coronary artery; short-axis stress images column **(A)** showing a severe perfusion defect in the septum, which is reversible on rest/redistribution images column **(B)**.

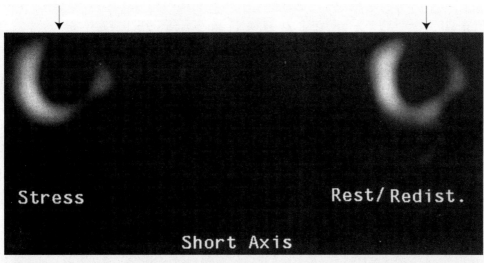

FIGURE 10.25. Abnormal thallium scan. Thallium SPECT images from a patient with previous anterior myocardial infarction. Short-axis images show severe defects in the anterior (*arrows*) and lateral walls, both of which are fixed (unchanged from stress to rest/redistribution images). These findings are consistent with scarring.

The major limitation of using Tl-201 scintigraphy alone is the high false-positive rate which is attributed predominantly to image attenuation artifacts that are interpreted as perfusion defects. Although quantification of ^{201}Tl images improves specificity, the false-positive rate remains problematic, particularly in women where breast attenuation may be mistaken for perfusion abnormalities secondary to anterolateral ischemia or in situations involving obesity where inferior perfusion defects may be seen. The presence of a left bundle branch block can also lead to a false-positive stress test anteriorly during exercise, in which case pharmacologic agents such as adenosine or regadenoson should be used.

The Tc-99m–labeled perfusion agents enhance the specificity of SPECT and provide information regarding regional and global left ventricular systolic function via ECG gating of images. Because of the more favorable physical characteristics of Tc-99m imaging with a gamma camera, there is less gamma-ray scatter and attenuation than with ^{201}Tl, which results in fewer false-positive artifacts and a lower radiation dose. These agents also allow better-gated acquisition, permitting the simultaneous evaluation of regional systolic thickening, global left ventricular function, and myocardial perfusion.

Performing the stress phase of the examination first followed by a resting phase allows identification and characterization of myocardial perfusion defects due to ischemia. Typically a combination of Tl-201 and Tc-99m perfusion agents are used at rest and stress, for example, same day Tl-201 at rest and Tc-99m agent at stress (Fig. 10.26). Alternatively low and high doses of a Tc-99m agent can be given at rest and during stress respectively (Fig. 10.27).

Historically, it was believed that ischemic LV dysfunction was due to a combination of repetitive ischemia, myocardial stunning and hibernation and was therefore potentially reversible in patients undergoing revascularization. This generated the concept of viable myocardium; that is, the distinction between reversible dysfunction and irreversible dysfunction due to myocardial necrosis. Several imaging techniques evaluating myocardial viability including those already described were developed with the aim of selecting patients in whom recovery of LV function and improvement of prognosis would outweigh the risk of surgical revascularization. The STICH Trial did not confirm an impact of viability on the outcome of patients undergoing revascularization or medical therapy, and cautioned against relying on the concept of viability alone in the management of patients with LV dysfunction. The study concluded that we should not use viability studies such as SPECT thallium or dobutamine echo to exclude patients from surgical revascularization.

As PET/CT scanners become more prevalent, myocardial PET perfusion imaging is being used in patients with known or suspected CAD in place of SPECT (Thallium, Tc sestamibi). Certain patient groups that are difficult to image with conventional SPECT imaging are particularly likely to benefit from PET imaging, such as obese patients, women, patients with previous nondiagnostic tests, and patients with poor left ventricular function attributable to CAD considered for revascularization. The radioisotope rubidium-82 (Rb-82) acts physiologically just like thallium in the heart yet unlike thallium or technetium it emits a positron giving superior image resolution compared to SPECT (Fig. 10.28). The use of Rb-82 may reduce the radiation dose to the patient by a factor of 10 compared to Tc-99m. In addition to viability imaging, cardiac PET imaging allows quantification of resting and stress blood flow, coronary flow reserve,

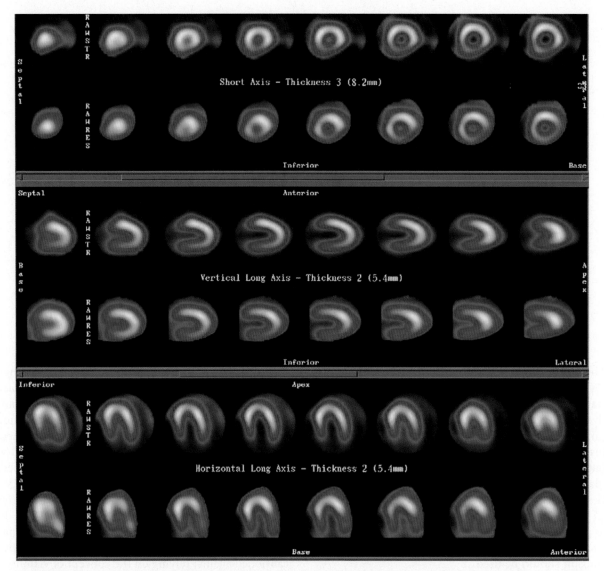

FIGURE 10.26. Normal stress rest thallium-Tc scan. Rest myocardial perfusion images were obtained after thallium was given IV (second, fourth, and sixth rows). Stress images were obtained after Tc-99m tetrofosmin was given IV (first, third, and fifth rows).

and subclinical microvascular abnormalities in response to pharmacologic stress. Integrated CT angiography and Rb-82 PET perfusion imaging on hybrid PET/CT systems is an exciting new prospect in the study of the structure and function of the heart.

There is consensus across national and international guidelines in favor of MPI as a noninvasive diagnostic tool for the detection of obstructive CAD in patients with intermediate pretest probability of disease. The American College of Cardiology (ACC) and the American Heart Association (AHA) support the exercise ECG as the initial test but recommend stress imaging in subgroups including women with diabetes and those in whom a poor exercise performance is anticipated. ACC/AHA guidelines rely on the size and magnitude of stress induced nuclear perfusion defects in order to determine "appropriateness" of revas-

cularization therapy. As a secondary test, MPI is indicated in patients with nondiagnostic or unexpected exercise ECG results; that is, patients with a low or high pretest likelihood of CAD and an abnormal or normal exercise ECG, respectively.

RADIONUCLIDE THERAPY

Although a detailed discussion of the therapeutic applications of administered radionuclides is beyond the scope of this chapter, it is important to recognize this aspect of nuclear medicine (Table 10.7). Generally, the radioactive isotopes being used for therapy emit beta particles, and in the future alpha particle emitters may also be used. Currently, the most common radioisotope used in therapy is I-131 to treat thyroid disorders such as Graves

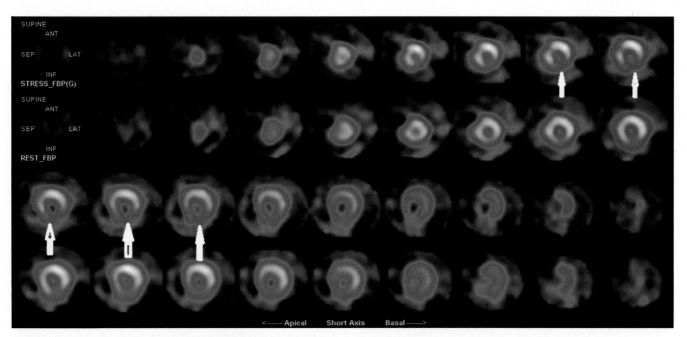

FIGURE 10.27. **Short axis views of abnormal stress nuclear imaging (Tc-99m Tetrofosmin).** The first and third rows are of stress images demonstrating an inferolateral defect (white arrows). The second and fourth rows are of rest images demonstrating normal inferolateral perfusion at rest. The "reversible" stress induced defect is consistent with viable myocardium in the inferolateral wall.

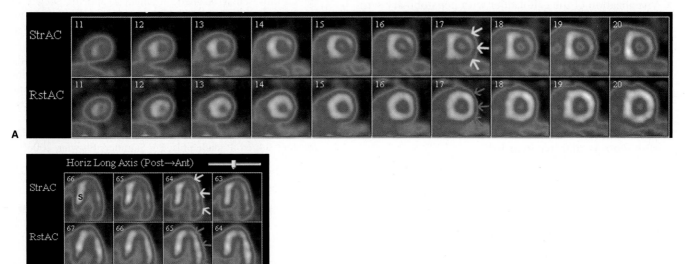

FIGURE 10.28. Myocardial rubidium imaging **A, B:** Rb-82 cardiac PET images from a patient with chest pain ultimately found to have a high-grade stenosis of the circumflex artery which supplies the lateral wall of the left ventricle. **A:** The short-axis stress images reveal decreased perfusion (*white arrows* on one of the slices) to the lateral wall of the left ventricle (LV) in the top row, which then appears "reversible" (the signal improves) on rest images in the bottom row (*light gray arrows*). **B:** The horizontal long-axis images from same patient demonstrate the same defect in perfusion by revealing much diminished rubidium signal coming from the lateral wall (*white arrows* on one of the images) in the stress images which again shows significant improvement on the rest images (reversibility) as depicted by light gray *arrows*. *S,* septum; *StrAC,* stress attenuation corrected; *RstAC,* rest attenuation corrected.

Table 10.7	
Therapeutic Radiopharmaceuticals	
Radioisotope	**Disease**
Yttrium-90	Liver tumors
Phosphorus-32	Polycythemia vera
Iodine-131	Thyroid cancer, Graves disease

disease and thyroid cancer. Because the iodine is trapped by the abnormal thyroid cells, the radiation effect is limited to the thyroid gland. Intra-arterial radioembolization with microspheres containing yttrium-90, a beta emitter, has become a widely accepted treatment for primary and some secondary hepatic tumors.

Key Points

- Nuclear imaging is performed using radiolabeled molecules which are injected or inhaled creating a physiologic or functional image.
- Abnormalities are usually described as increased or reduced uptake.
- CT is the current standard technique for diagnosing PE.
- Ventilation–perfusion lung imaging may play a role in the workup of certain patients with suspected PE; for example, women under 50 years.
- Visualization of the gallbladder with hepatobiliary scintigraphy almost always rules out the diagnosis of acute cholecystitis.
- Bone scintigraphy is a sensitive test for detecting skeletal metastases, osteomyelitis, and fractures.
- Patients with multiple myeloma may have a negative bone scan.
- Captopril renal imaging accurately detects hemodynamically significant renal artery stenosis in patients with renovascular hypertension.

- Fusion PET/CT imaging can detect and stage many malignant tumors.
- Myocardial stress perfusion imaging is an accurate technique for detecting CAD and can be performed with either SPECT or PET.
- Rubidium-82 is a promising myocardial PET perfusion agent.

ACKNOWLEDGMENTS

The author thanks Brian Clarke, CNMT, for his original drawings of Figure 10.23 (short axis), and Dr. Parvez Shirazi for supplying the images for Figure 10.15 (captopril scan). Drs Michael Salinger and David Najman reviewed the cardiology section.

FURTHER READINGS

Bonow RO, Maurer G, STICH Trial Investigators, et al. Myocardial viability and survival in ischemic left ventricular dysfunction. *N Engl J Med.* 2011;364(17):1617–1625.

Hendel RC, Berman DS, Di Carli MF, et al. Appropriate use criteria for cardiac radionuclide imaging: A report of the American College of Cardiology Foundation Appropriate Use Criteria Task Force, the American Society of Nuclear Cardiology, the American College of Radiology, the American Heart Association, the American Society of Echocardiography, the Society of Cardiovascular Computed Tomography, the Society for Cardiovascular Magnetic Resonance, and the Society of Nuclear Medicine. *J Am Coll Cardiol.* 2009;53(23):2201–2229.

Husain S. Myocardial perfusion imaging protocols: Is there an ideal protocol? *J Nucl Med Technol.* 2007;35:3–9.

McArdle BA, Dowsley TF, deKemp RA, et al. Does rubidium-82 PET have superior accuracy to SPECT perfusion imaging for the diagnosis of obstructive coronary disease? A systematic review and meta-analysis. *J Am Coll Cardiol.* 2012;60(18):1828–1837.

Mettler FA, Gilberteau M, eds. *Essentials of Nuclear Medicine Imaging.* 5th ed. Philadelphia, PA: Saunders Elsevier, 2006.

QUESTIONS

1. Which of the following is false regarding a "superscan"?
   a. May show increased uptake in bones and soft tissue
   b. May be caused by metastatic disease
   c. May be caused by metabolic disease
   d. May show reduced or absent uptake in the distal appendicular skeleton

2. Which of the following is true regarding the imaging of shin splints?
   a. They are typically hot on the blood flow phase
   b. Increased uptake is seen at the cortical level

   c. They occur on the posterolateral surface of the mid tibia
   d. They have characteristic plain film findings

3. A patient has thyrotoxicosis and a low radioactive iodine uptake at 24 hours. The differential diagnosis includes all the following except:
   a. Graves disease
   b. Subacute thyroiditis
   c. Amiodarone intake
   d. Thyrotoxicosis factitia

4. A diabetic has a nonhealing foot ulcer. The following are true of a three-phase bone scan in this patient except:
   a. Osteomyelitis may be indistinguishable from a neuropathic joint
   b. Osteomyelitis may be distinguished from cellulitis
   c. A fourth phase image may be helpful in patients with peripheral vascular disease
   d. A negative bone scan excludes the diagnosis of osteomyelitis

5. Regarding ventilation perfusion scanning for pulmonary embolism, the following are true except:
   a. Most PEs do not cause pulmonary infarcts
   b. The perfusion abnormality should be smaller than the corresponding chest film abnormality
   c. Most matched perfusion defects are due to vasoconstriction associated with an airway abnormality
   d. Up to 80% of patients with an intermediate probability V/Q scan have pulmonary embolism

6. A bone scan on an 8-month-old baby shows multiple foci of increased uptake. The differential diagnosis includes:
   1. Nonaccidental injury
   2. Multifocal osteomyelitis
   3. Osteogenesis imperfecta
   4. Metastatic neuroblastoma
   a. a
   b. a, b, c
   c. a, c
   d. a, b, c, d

7. The following tumors are usually not FDG avid on PET scan except:
   a. Mucinous colon carcinoma
   b. Bronchoalveolar carcinoma
   c. Neuroendocrine
   d. Small cell lung carcinoma

8. When performing a V/Q scan for suspected pulmonary embolism, radionuclide dose modification is recommended for patients who have/are:
   a. Contrast allergy
   b. Azotemia
   c. Pulmonary AV shunt
   d. Women of childbearing age

9. Regarding thyroid scintigraphy, which is true?
   a. Most cold spots are malignant
   b. It is a good screening test for thyroid disease
   c. Uptake in the pyramidal lobe is seen in thyroiditis
   d. I-123 is the preferred agent for suspected retrosternal goiter

10. Patient instructions prior to a PET/CT for malignancy include all except:
    a. Nothing by mouth within 6 hours
    b. High carbohydrate diet within 24 hours
    c. May take artificial sweeteners
    d. No exercise within 24 hours

11. The following features are regarded as advantages of Tc-99m sestamibi over thallium for cardiac imaging except:
    a. Shorter half-life means a higher dose can be given
    b. Higher myocardial extraction fraction
    c. Higher count rate
    d. Optimal energy for use with standard gamma camera

Breast Imaging

Laurie L. Fajardo • Limin Yang

Approximately one in eight women in the United States will develop cancer of the breast during her lifetime, and this incidence appears to be increasing. Unfortunately, there is no known cause of most breast cancers, and therefore the best way to prevent mortality is early detection of the nonpalpable and potentially curable disease using mammography. It is generally believed that the earlier breast cancer is diagnosed, the smaller the chance of metastases and the better the long-term prognosis. Consequently, mammography is widely used for the screening of breast cancer in the general asymptomatic female population. *Screening mammography should be used in conjunction with regular breast self-examination and an annual clinical breast examination performed by a physician* (Table 11.1). Diagnostic mammography is also a key tool in the evaluation of patients with known or suspected breast disease. There is little doubt that mammograms are best interpreted by qualified radiologists. In addition, a radiologist may perform image-guided breast biopsy allowing an accurate and cost-effective diagnosis of nonpalpable breast lesions. Given the prevalence of breast disease, all physicians should be aware of the clinical applications and limitations of breast imaging. The purpose of this chapter is to review the importance of screening mammography for early cancer detection and the use of diagnostic mammography, ultrasound (US), and magnetic resonance imaging (MRI) in the management of breast disease.

SCREENING MAMMOGRAPHY

The mortality rate for breast carcinoma has fallen by almost 30% over the past 20 years. Several large reputable studies have linked this reduction in mortality with earlier detection of breast carcinoma due to screening mammography. Critics of routine screening argue that women may go through unnecessary treatment such as surgery, radiotherapy, and chemotherapy for cancers that would not have posed a risk as some cancers will be diagnosed and treated that would never have caused any harm. In the United Kingdom, it is estimated that screening prevents about 1,300 deaths per year, but it also may result in about 4,000 women receiving treatment for a condition that would not have been threatening.

In 2009 the U.S. Preventive Services Task Force (USPSTF) revised their recommendations for screening mammography for women aged 40 to 49 years, because there was only moderate certainty that the net benefits for this age group were small. Previously routine screening mammography was recommended every 1 to 2 years starting at age 40. Their current recommendations are for biennial rather than annual screening in women aged 50 to 74 years. No recommendation was made for women over age 74, citing insufficient evidence. The Society of Breast Imaging (SBI) and The American College of Radiology (ACR) strongly criticized the USPSTF recommendations,

Table 11.1
General Screening Mammography Guidelines

1. Yearly mammograms are recommended starting at age 40; high risk, begin by age 30, but not before 25, or 10 years earlier than the age of diagnosis of the youngest affective relative, whichever is later; and 8 years after chest radiation therapy. The age at which screening should cease depends on the potential risks and benefits of screening in the context of overall health status and longevity.
2. Clinical breast examination should be part of a periodic health examination about every 3 years for women in their 20s and 30s and every year for women aged 40 and older.
3. Women should know how their breasts normally feel and report any breast change promptly to their healthcare providers. Breast self-examination is suggested for women starting in their 20s.

Table 11.2
ACR/SBI Recommendations for Age at Which Annual Screening Mammography Should Start

Age 40
- Women at average risk

Younger than Age 40
- *BRCA1* or *BRCA2* mutation carriers: By age 30, but not before age 25
- Women with mother or sister with premenopausal breast cancer: By age 30 but not before age 25, or 10 years earlier than the age of diagnosis of relative, whichever is later
- Women with 20% lifetime risk for breast cancer on the basis of family history (both maternal and paternal): Yearly starting by age 30 but not before age 25, or 10 years earlier than the age of diagnosis of the youngest affected relative, whichever is later
- Women with histories of mantle radiation received between the ages of 10 and 30: Beginning 8 years after the radiation therapy but not before age 25
- Women with biopsy-proven lobular neoplasia, ADH, DCIS, invasive breast cancer, or ovarian cancer regardless of age

From: Lee CH, Dershaw DD, Kopans D, et al. Breast cancer screening with imaging: Recommendations from the Society of Breast Imaging and the ACR on the use of mammography, breast MRI, breast ultrasound, and other technologies for the detection of clinically occult breast cancer. *J Am Coll Radiol.* 2010;7(1):18–27; copyright © 2010 Elsevier.

and they have jointly published their own recommendations for screening mammography (Table 11.2). These recommendations are on the basis of evidence-based medicine where available. Where evidence is lacking, the recommendations are based on consensus opinions. The ACR and SBI firmly stand behind their recommendation that screening mammography should be performed annually beginning at age 40 for women at average risk for breast cancer.

As can be seen from these recommendations, several risk factors influence the onset and type of screening. One of these risk factors is a *BRCA* gene mutation which is associated with a rare hereditary breast–ovarian carcinoma syndrome. As many as two-thirds of women born with a deleterious mutation in *BRCA1* will develop breast cancer by age 70, and one-third will develop ovarian cancer by age 70. Approximately one-half of women with a deleterious mutation in *BRCA2* will develop breast cancer by age 70, and up to one-quarter will develop ovarian cancer by age 70. The ACR/SBI recommendations include annual screening mammograms and also cover the role of MR of women with BRCA mutations.

Technique for Screening and Diagnostic Mammography

The importance of a well-performed mammogram cannot be overemphasized. A standard screening mammogram consists of two views: A *mediolateral oblique* (MLO) view with the central x-ray beam traversing the breast obliquely in a medial to lateral direction (Fig. 11.1A) and a *craniocaudal* (CC) view (Fig. 11.1B) with the central x-ray beam traversing the breast in a head to foot direction. It is necessary to compress the breast during the examination to

visualize all the breast tissue and to minimize radiation dose, and patients should be warned that compression may be uncomfortable. As with other forms of imaging, mammography has limitations and adjunct screening using US and MRI is becoming more widely accepted. A diagnostic workup may require specific mammographic views including microfocus magnification compression views for microcalcifications and focal (spot) compression views for mass or focal asymmetry and possibly the need for US and/or MRI. For women under 30 years who present with a breast mass, US is the best initial examination to perform.

Diagnostic mammography is performed most commonly when a breast mass is palpated, or a radiologist finds an abnormality on a screening mammogram. The vast majority of screening and diagnostic mammograms performed in the United States use digital technology which has replaced film-screen mammography. The advantages of digital mammography include the ability to use image-processing techniques to enhance the images, the use of computer-assisted diagnostic techniques (CAD) in lesion detection and characterization, and the electronic transmission and storage of images. Compared

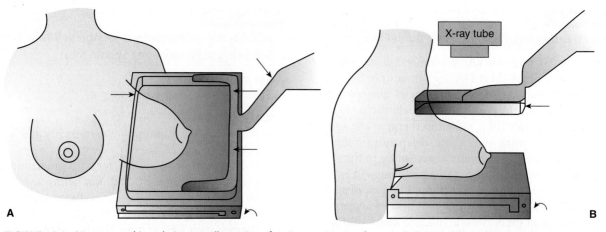

FIGURE 11.1. Mammographic technique. **A:** Illustration of patient positioning for a mediolateral oblique (MLO) mammogram. The x-ray beam passes obliquely through the breast in a medial to lateral direction. The breast is routinely compressed between the compression device (*straight arrows*) and the radiographic cassette (*curved arrow*). The cassette contains a radiographic film on which the image will be recorded. Compression improves the diagnostic quality of the images by reducing the breast to a more uniform thickness. **B:** Illustration of patient positioning for a craniocaudal (CC) mammogram. The x-ray beam passes through the breast in a head to foot or cephalad to caudad direction. The compression device (*straight arrow*) is more easily visualized in this illustration. Again, the image will be recorded on the film in the radiographic cassette (*curved arrow*).

with film-screen mammography, digital mammography has been shown to be superior in detecting breast cancer in women younger than 50 years, pre- or perimenopausal women, and those with dense breasts.

It is important that the mammographer (technologist) be properly trained and qualified and that the federally mandated mammography quality controls are met.

WHAT WE SHOULD SEE ON A MAMMOGRAM

In general, breast tissue is composed predominately of fibroglandular tissue in younger women and gradually replaced with adipose tissue in older women. Correspondingly, normal mammograms show a mixture of fat and fibroglandular tissue. Normal MLO and CC views of the breast are shown in Figure 11.2. Notice that breast images are a combination of fat (black) and soft tissues (gray to white). This background of black and gray, especially the black, enhances visualization of masses and calcifications.

Approximately 85% of breast carcinomas are of ductal origin and are discrete by imaging modalities.

The two most important mammographic findings suspicious for malignancy are masses and microcalcifications. Other suspicious abnormalities include focal asymmetry, architectural distortion, and skin or nipple deformity. Any structural changes over time require attention and further workup, unless otherwise explained such as surgical scar.

The Breast Imaging Reporting and Data System (BI-RADS) initiative was instituted by the ACR in the late 1980s to address a lack of standardization and uniformity

in mammography practice reporting. An important component of this system is the lexicon, a dictionary of descriptors of specific imaging features which historically have been shown to be predictive of benign and malignant disease. Use of the BI-RADS lexicon promotes communication, quality assurance, research, and improved patient care. Initially, BI-RADS was developed for mammographic findings, but it now includes US and MRI findings (Table 11.3). This system is continuously revised on the basis of experts' opinions and evidence-based findings.

Masses

Using BI-RADS terminology, a mass is a space-occupying lesion seen on two different mammographic projections. Masses are described in terms of their shape, border (margin), density, location, size, and associated findings such as microcalcifications and architectural distortion.

Table 11.3	
BI-RADS Classification	
BI-RADS Category	
0	Incomplete
1	Negative
2	Benign finding(s)
3	Probably benign
4	Suspicious abnormality
5	Highly suggestive of malignancy
6	Known biopsy-proven malignancy

BI-RADS Category 4 or 5 warrants biopsy.

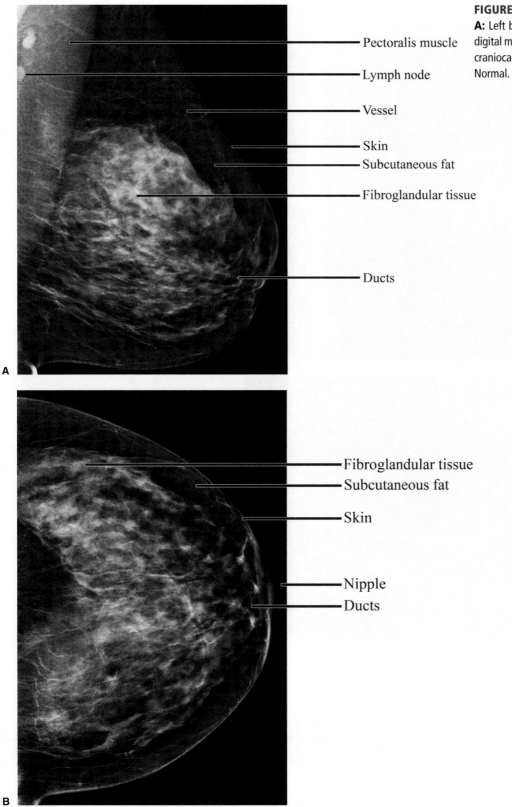

Pectoralis muscle

Lymph node

Vessel

Skin
Subcutaneous fat

Fibroglandular tissue

Ducts

A

Fibroglandular tissue
Subcutaneous fat

Skin

Nipple
Ducts

B

FIGURE 11.2. Normal mammogram. **A:** Left breast mediolateral oblique (MLO) digital mammogram. Normal. **B:** Left breast craniocaudal (CC) digital mammogram. Normal.

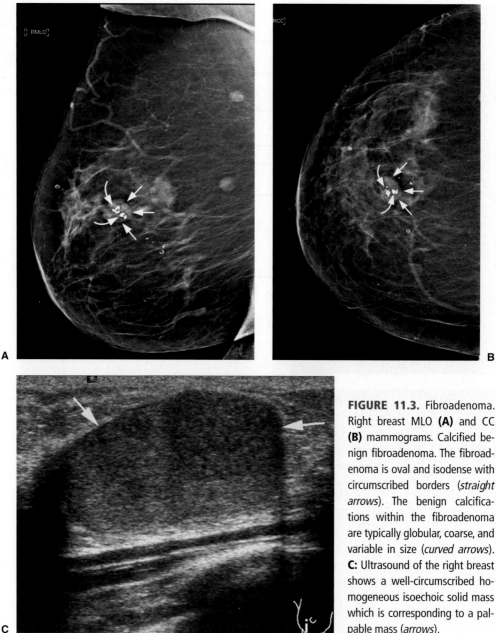

FIGURE 11.3. Fibroadenoma. Right breast MLO **(A)** and CC **(B)** mammograms. Calcified benign fibroadenoma. The fibroadenoma is oval and isodense with circumscribed borders (*straight arrows*). The benign calcifications within the fibroadenoma are typically globular, coarse, and variable in size (*curved arrows*). **C:** Ultrasound of the right breast shows a well-circumscribed homogeneous isoechoic solid mass which is corresponding to a palpable mass (*arrows*).

Benign Masses

Benign breast disease (Table 11.4) may or may not be symptomatic or have associated masses. A fibroadenoma (Fig. 11.3) is a common benign mass that generally occurs in young women and may be single or multiple. On physical examination, fibroadenomas are often movable. The mammographic appearance is an oval circumscribed mass sometimes associated with coarse "popcorn" calcifications. On sonography, fibroadenomas will usually appear isoechoic.

Table 11.4
Common Causes of Benign Breast Disease

- Cystic disease
- Mastitis, abscess
- Fibroadenoma, benign phyllodes tumor
- Lipoma, hamartoma
- Sclerosing adenosis, fibrocystic changes
- Fat necrosis

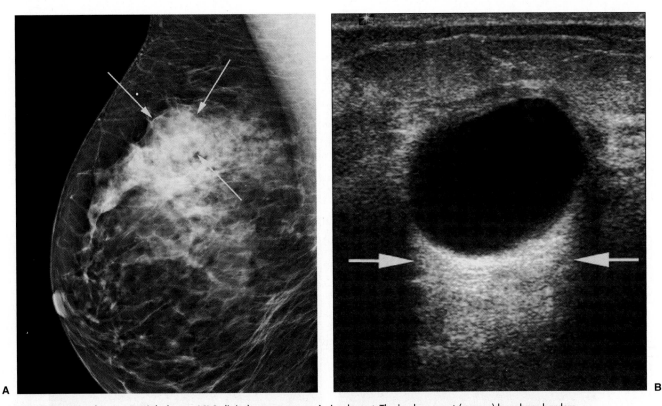

FIGURE 11.4. Simple cyst. **A:** Right breast MLO digital mammogram. A simple cyst. The isodense cyst (*arrows*) has sharp borders and no calcifications. Note the difference between the smooth sharp borders of this benign cyst compared to the irregular and poorly defined borders of the carcinoma in Figure 11.7. **B:** Right breast ultrasound of the lesion **(A)**. This is the classic appearance of a benign simple cyst. The cyst is a round well-circumscribed anechoic mass with very thin cyst–parenchymal transition. Posterior acoustic enhancement (*arrows*) is commonly found immediately posterior to a cyst.

Benign cystic disease is another common clinical entity which may present as a tender or nontender palpable mass or as an incidental nonpalpable mammographic finding. The mammographic appearance of a cyst is usually an isodense mass with well-defined borders (Fig. 11.4A). Although a cyst is usually rounder and more circumscribed than a solid mass on a mammogram, mammography cannot differentiate a solid mass from a cyst and US is needed to make this distinction. US of a breast cyst (Fig. 11.4B) usually shows a well-defined anechoic mass with characteristic posterior acoustic enhancement. Cysts may be treated with US-guided needle aspiration. Some benign lesions, such as breast hamartoma, are easily diagnosed on mammography without any additional imaging or intervention needed (Fig. 11.5).

When breast implants are placed for augmentation implant displaced views are required to visualize the breast tissue surrounding the implant. When implants are placed following mastectomy, routine screening mammography is not required for the postmastectomy breast. Implants may vary in appearance from less dense (saline) to dense (silicone) and in their location—either posterior (retropectoral or subpectoral) (Fig. 11.6) or anterior (prepectoral) to the pectoralis muscle. MR is useful in evaluating implant integrity.

Malignant Masses

Common mammographic and ultrasonographic findings of malignancy are listed in Table 11.5. Malignant masses are usually irregularly shaped and of high density with ill-defined or spiculated borders (Fig. 11.7). Microcalcifications are frequently associated within and/or outside of the mass. When suspicious findings are present, it is important to evaluate the extent of the disease such as multifocality/multicentricity on the imaging studies. Multifocality means that there are other disease foci in the same breast quadrant. Multicentricity means that there are other disease foci in a different breast quadrant. Asymmetric densities and architectural distortions are also suspicious for malignancy, especially if they are new.

Microcalcifications

Microcalcifications may be the first indicator of malignancy, especially if they are new, pleomorphic, or branching (Fig. 11.8A). However, it should be emphasized that most breast calcifications are benign. Benign microcalcifications are homogeneous in size and shape (usually punctate, round, or coarse) and more diffusely scattered (Fig. 11.8B). Malignant microcalcifications are more heterogeneous in

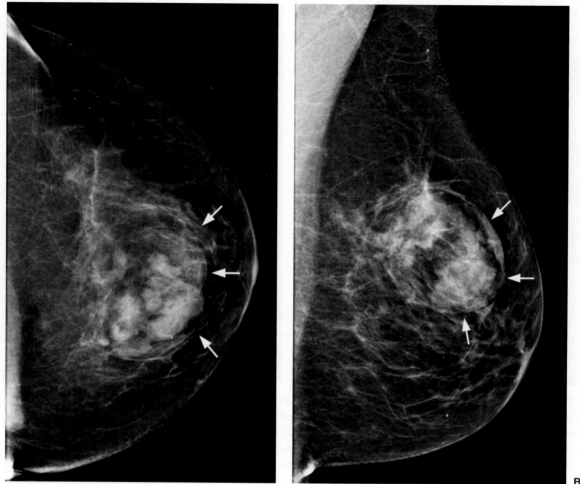

FIGURE 11.5. Hamartoma (fibroadenolipoma). The CC **(A)** and MLO **(B)** views of the left breast show a well-defined mass with heterogeneous internal density which is not different from the surrounding normal breast tissue except it is confined within a thin wall in the upper inner left breast (*arrows*). This benign mass is usually impalpable due to its soft nature. This mammographic appearance is diagnostic.

<table>
<tr><td colspan="2">

Table 11.5

Mammographic/Ultrasonographic Findings Suspicious for Malignancy

1. A mass on a mammogram with
   a. ill-defined or spiculated borders
   b. malignant calcifications
   c. high radiopaque density
   d. skin retraction or thickening
2. Microcalcifications that are (with or without a mass)
   a. pleomorphic
   b. fine linear branching or segmental
   c. clusters
3. Architectural distortion or focal asymmetry
4. Irregular hypoechoic solid mass on ultrasound with ill-defined/spiculated border, thick boundary echogenicity, and/or surrounding architectural distortion

</td></tr>
</table>

shape and size (pleomorphic), more clustered in a small area, and linearly or segmentally distributed (see Fig. 11.8A). Some calcifications are so small (100 to 200 microns) that magnification is needed when viewing mammograms. The description of microcalcifications using BI-RADS terminology includes the shape, distribution, location, and associated findings such as a mass.

LIMITATIONS OF MAMMOGRAPHY

Overall, about 40% of women who have mammograms have dense breast tissue which may mask small breast carcinomas. US and MRI can also find tumors that mammograms miss, but they produce even more false-positive examinations. If all women with dense breasts had US, more early cancers would be found, but thousands of unnecessary biopsies would also be performed. A concern is that while the significance of breast tissue density is uncertain, reporting it may alarm women and lead to an avalanche of needless screening tests and biopsies.

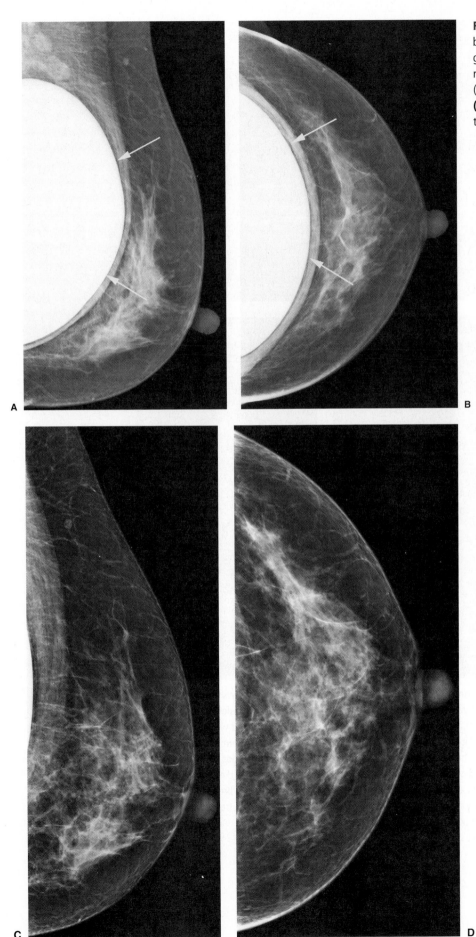

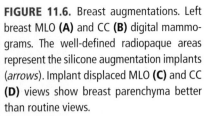

FIGURE 11.6. Breast augmentations. Left breast MLO **(A)** and CC **(B)** digital mammograms. The well-defined radiopaque areas represent the silicone augmentation implants (*arrows*). Implant displaced MLO **(C)** and CC **(D)** views show breast parenchyma better than routine views.

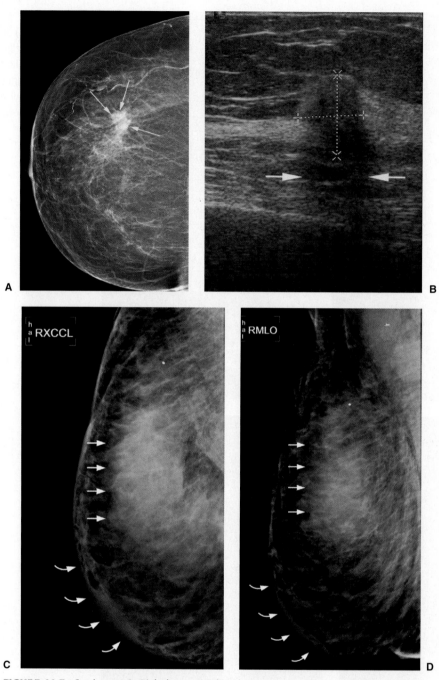

FIGURE 11.7. Carcinoma. **A:** Right breast CC digital mammogram shows an infiltrating ductal carcinoma in an 84-year-old woman. The high-density malignant mass lesion (*arrows*) has spiculated and poorly defined borders which are in contrast to the sharp and well-defined border of the benign cyst in Figure 11.4A. **B:** Ultrasound image of the same patient shows an ill-defined hypoechoic mass which is taller than wide. Note that there is posterior acoustic shadowing (*arrows*). The *X*s and *crosses* are electronic caliper marks that measure the dimensions of the mass. **C,D:** Inflammatory carcinoma. MLO **(C)** and XCCL **(D)** views of the left breast show a large ill-defined high-density mass (*straight arrows*) with surrounding thickened trabeculation. Note the markedly thickened skin (*curved arrows*).

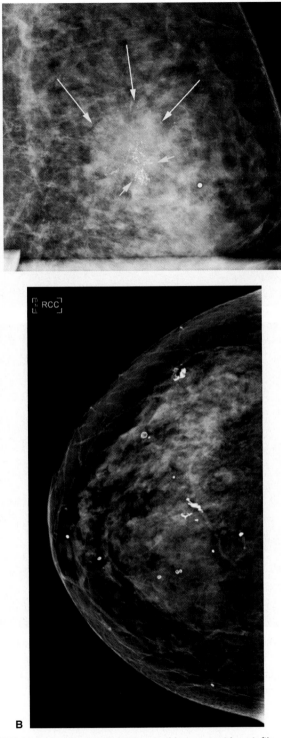

FIGURE 11.8. Carcinoma. **A:** A 38-year-old woman with an infiltrating ductal carcinoma. Left breast digital MLO magnification compression view demonstrates the classical appearance of malignant calcifications (*short arrows*) in the mass (*long arrows*). Note the difference between the coarse benign calcifications in Figure 11.3 and these pleomorphic malignant calcifications. Also, the high-density and poorly defined borders of the associated mass are more obvious in this magnification compression view. A skin marker (*white dot*) indicates that this mass is palpable. **B:** CC digital mammogram of the right breast shows scattered, diffuse calcifications that are round in shape. These calcification are benign and do not require biopsy.

INDICATIONS FOR BREAST ULTRASOUND AND MAGNETIC RESONANCE

US is an essential imaging modality for breast diseases as it allows distinction between cystic and solid breast masses. Advances in technology now allow tissue characterization using harmonic imaging, compound imaging, elastography, and three-dimensional (3D) image acquisition. US is also used for percutaneous core biopsy, preoperative wire lesion localization and cyst/abscess drainage and has the advantage of real-time visualization of the procedure. The ultrasonographic description of a mass using BI-RADS terminology includes its shape, orientation, margin, boundary with adjacent tissue, internal echo pattern, and posterior acoustic features. Characteristics suggesting benignity include circumscribed round/oval shape, parallel orientation with the ductal structures ("being wider than tall"), thin capsule, and gentle lobulation. Characteristics suggesting malignancy include an irregular shape, spiculated/angular/microlobulated border, antiparallel orientation to the ductal structures ("being taller than wide"), and surrounding architectural distortion (Fig. 11.7B).

MR is also increasingly used to evaluate the extent of disease in women diagnosed with breast cancer, especially those with dense breast tissue which is not well imaged by mammography (Table 11.6). For women at high risk for breast cancer, MR is used in addition to (not as a replacement for) screening mammography. Breast US has also been used as a supplemental screening test, but has not been shown to be better than MR. Although US is less costly than MR, it has a higher false-positive rate. Advantages of MR include better evaluation of the 3D extent of the disease, using intravenous contrast (Fig. 11.9A), diagnosis of otherwise occult malignancies in the same or opposite breast (Fig. 11.9B), differentiation between scar and recurrent cancer, and presurgical planning in a known cancer patient (Fig. 11.9C) and evaluation of response to chemotherapy (Fig. 11.10).

Table 11.6
Indications for Breast MR

1. High-risk screening: Recommended for women with an approximately 20–25% or greater lifetime risk of breast cancer, including women with a strong family history of breast or ovarian cancer and women who are 8 years post chest radiation therapy. BRCA mutations, or 8 years after chest radiation therapy
2. Positive axillary lymph nodes with negative mammogram
3. Presurgical planning, extent of the disease
4. Monitor effect of chemotherapy
5. Evaluation of residual disease
6. Silicone implant rupture

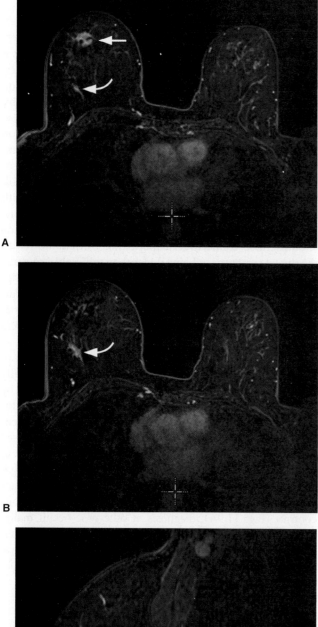

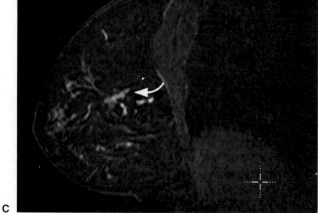

FIGURE 11.9. MRI of breast carcinoma. Postcontrast subtraction MRI demonstrate an irregular enhancing mass (*straight arrow* **(A)**) near 12 o'clock position of the right breast, which was a newly diagnosed invasive ductal carcinoma with internal nonenhancing component representing postbiopsy changes. **B,C:** A clumped linear nonmass-like enhancement in the upper outer right breast (*curved arrows*) was biopsied under MRI guidance which confirmed ductal carcinoma in situ.

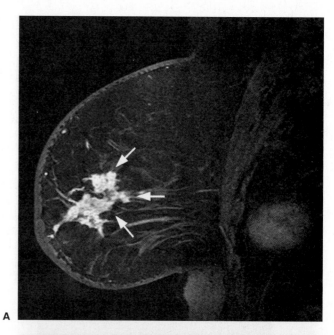

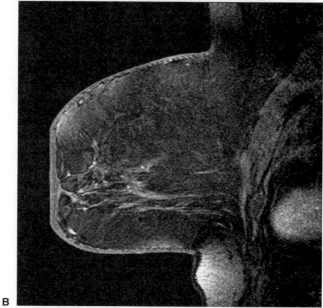

FIGURE 11.10. MRI post-treatment. Contrast-enhanced subtraction breast MR images before **(A)** and after **(B)** 3 months of neoadjuvant chemotherapy show a marked decrease in contrast uptake, indicating that the tumor (*arrows*) is responding to treatment.

BREAST BIOPSY

Biopsy of a breast lesion is essential for diagnosis and treatment planning. Several options are available for image guidance (US and stereotactic) and types of biopsy needle (fine and core). The choice of a biopsy technique should depend on the clinical and radiographic features of the lesion and the experience of the physician. In general, more biopsy tissue is preferred because of the additional testing required to determine hormone sensitivity etc.

A fine-needle aspirate (FNA) biopsy is used to evaluate axillary lymph nodes when core biopsy of a suspicious breast lesion is performed and it can also be used for aspiration of symptomatic (painful) or indeterminate cystic breast lesions. Analysis by an experienced cytologist is critical for accurate interpretation of FNA biopsy results. However, FNA biopsy does not distinguish between invasive and in situ breast cancer and the false-negative rate for identifying breast malignancy is as high as 40%. This technique is particularly useful in the evaluation of cystic lesions detected by ultrasonography.

Core-needle biopsy uses a bigger needle (9G to 14G) to remove a narrow cylinder of tissue in contrast to a collection of cells obtained with FNA. The larger sample permits more detailed pathologic analysis and determination of hormone receptor levels. A type of core needle commonly used is a vacuum-assisted biopsy needle, characterized by a single core needle insertion, with acquisition of contiguous and larger tissue samples. Because most of the lesions detected during screening are impalpable, subsequent needle biopsy must be image guided. Ultrasonography-guided biopsy is usually the most straightforward approach, but some lesions particularly

microcalcifications, are better seen on mammography and require stereotactic needle biopsy.

As well as sampling nonpalpable breast lesions, stereotactic biopsy is used primarily for calcifications and other lesions not visible on US. The stereotactic technique uses radiographic imaging performed in at least two planes to localize and guide the core biopsy needle to target a lesion in 3D space. A minimum of five to six passes is required when sampling microcalcifications to minimize sampling error. Specimen radiography is also required to ensure that representative calcifications are obtained. Once the biopsy is complete, an inert metallic clip is deployed into the biopsy site through the trocar as a marker for future reference in case it can no longer be visualized after biopsy.

Excisional Breast Biopsy

This biopsy is usually done surgically. A finding of atypical ductal hyperplasia on core-needle biopsy is an indication for open biopsy which may reveal ductal carcinoma in situ (DCIS) in as many as 50% of patients. Radial scars diagnosed by core biopsy should also be regarded as high-risk lesions requiring excision biopsy.

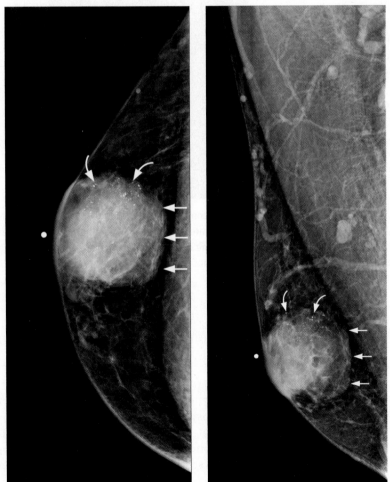

FIGURE 11.11. Male breast carcinoma. Left male breast CC **(A)** and MLO **(B)** digital mammograms. The *straight arrows* indicate the large round high density mass with ill-defined margins and associated pleomorphic microcalcifications (*curved arrows*) in the subareolar left breast.

A   B

Sentinel Node Biopsy

One of the most important prognostic factors in women with early stage breast cancer is the status of the axillary lymph nodes. Axillary lymph node dissection (ALND) which has been considered a routine staging surgical procedure, may result in lymphedema and nerve injury. For those patients with clinically negative axillary nodes, sentinel lymph node biopsy (SLNB) is the preferred method of staging disease in the axilla because of less morbidity than ALND. Injection of a Technetium-99m–labeled colloid and/or blue dye around the tumor or subareolar skin permits identification of an SLN which is then biopsied. Approximately 40% of patients with a positive sentinel lymph node will have residual disease in the axilla. The false-positive rate for SLNB is less than 5%.

DISEASES OF THE MALE BREAST

All of the diseases that occur in the female breast can potentially occur in the male breast. The incidence of male breast carcinoma was approximately 2,190 cases in 2012 in the United States accounting for 1% of all breast cancers. Men tend to be diagnosed at an advanced stage and thus have poorer survival. Mammography and clinical breast examination have no role for screening of breast cancer in males. The indications for male diagnostic mammography and the images obtained are similar to those for females. Male breast carcinomas are similar in appearance to female breast carcinomas. They most commonly present as irregular or ill-defined solid masses (Fig. 11.11). Pathologically, invasive lobular carcinomas are less common in men than in women due to less developed lobular structures in men.

Gynecomastia is a benign enlargement of the male breast tissue due to proliferation of the glandular component, and may be confused with breast cancer. The causes for gynecomastia are listed in Table 11.7. Usually, men present with a tender subareolar breast mass, which may be unilateral or bilateral. On mammography, there is breast tissue in the subareolar zone that may contain calcification (Fig. 11.12). The need for biopsy will be determined by a combination of symptoms, physical and mammographic or ultrasonographic findings. There is no association

Table 11.7
Causes of Gynecomastia
Physiologic (neonatal, pubertal, elderly) Adult men • An increase in the ratio of estrogen to androgen (e.g., liver cirrhosis, testicular tumor, chronic renal disease) • Drugs (spironolactone, digitalis, steroids)

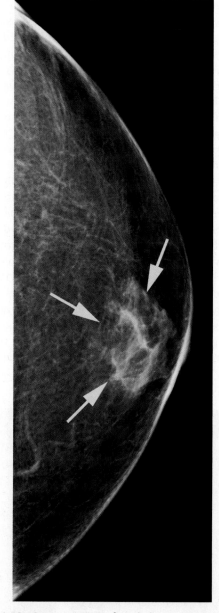

FIGURE 11.12. Gynecomastia. Left male breast CC digital mammogram. The *arrows* indicate the typically increased but normal appearing subareolar fibroglandular tissue without calcification. Normal male mammograms should not show any fibroglandular tissue.

between gynecomastia and the subsequent development of breast carcinoma.

OTHER IMAGING TECHNOLOGIES

Digital breast tomosynthesis (DBT) (3D mammography) is a modification of the standard two-dimensional (2D) digital mammography to yield a 3D image by using tomography which allows better visualization/characterization

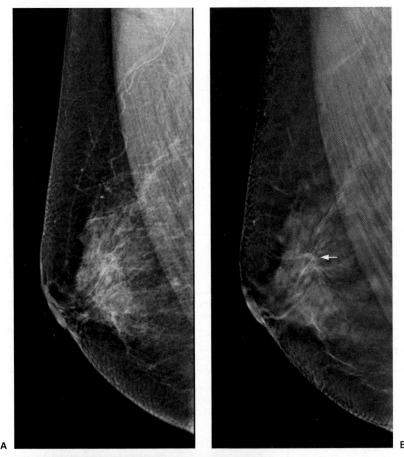

A

B

FIGURE 11.13. Digital breast tomosynthesis. Conventional 2D MLO digital mammogram **(A)** and single image from a 3D digital breast tomosynthesis (DBT) scan **(B)** depicting a small irregular/spiculated mass (*arrow*) just above the nipple in the middle one-third of the breast. Note that the conspicuity of the mass is significantly better on the DBT image.

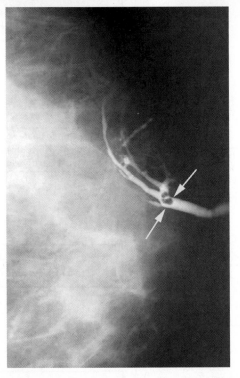

FIGURE 11.14. Galactography. A 48-year-old woman with intraductal papilloma in the left breast. Left CC view shows a small rounded filling defect (*arrows*) in the contrast-filled duct in left subareolar area.

of lesions by removing overlapping structures present in the planes other than the plane in which the lesion is located (Fig. 11.13).

PET scanning with fluorodeoxyglucose (FDG) is complementary to conventional staging procedures and should not be a replacement for either bone scintigraphy or diagnostic CT. PET and PET/CT have been shown to be particularly useful in the restaging of breast cancer, in evaluation of response to therapy.

Galactography is a technique which opacifies the intraductal system and related abnormalities by injecting contrast material. Active nipple discharge is necessary to perform this examination because the diseased duct must be identified prior to cannulation and contrast injection. An intraductal abnormality is seen as a "filling defect" in a contrast-filled duct or as abrupt cutoff of the visualized duct (Fig. 11.14). Extraductal abnormality may be seen causing external compression. Galactography has been largely replaced by improved US imaging techniques.

Suggested Workup of Common Clinical Problems

Suggested algorithms for the workup of two common clinical scenarios are shown in Figure 11.15.

FIGURE 11.15. Clinical algorithms. **A:** Screening for breast carcinoma. **B:** Workup of a palpable breast mass.

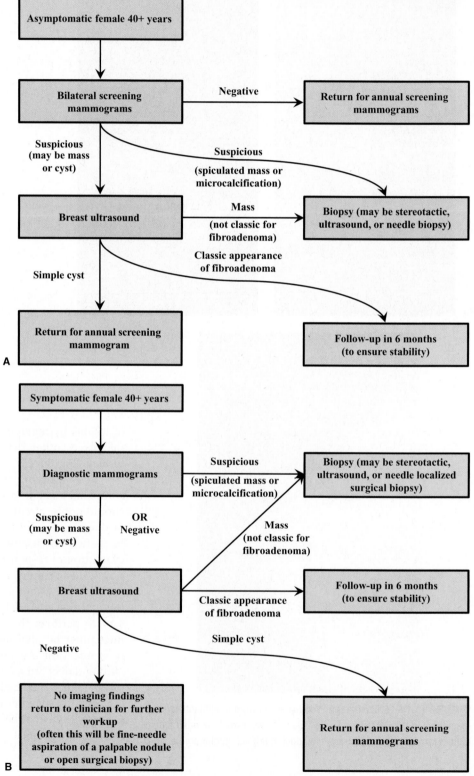

Key Points

- Approximately one in eight females in the United States will develop carcinoma of the breast.
- Mammograms should be interpreted by qualified radiologists and high-quality mammography is imperative in the early detection of breast cancer.
- A screening mammogram consists of MLO and CC views.
- Screening mammography must be combined with regular breast examinations.
- Mammographic findings suspicious for malignancy include an irregularly shaped mass, pleomorphic microcalcifications, skin retraction or thickening, architectural distortion, or focal asymmetry (asymmetric compared to opposite breast).
- Calcifications that are suspicious for malignancy include new calcifications, pleomorphic calcifications, and fine linear branching/segmental calcifications.
- Ultrasonography is useful in differentiating solid from cystic breast masses.

MRI is useful in evaluating the extent of known breast cancer, differentiating between scar and recurrent cancer, implant rupture, and screening high-risk patients as a supplemental test to screening mammography.

FURTHER READINGS

Berg WA, Birdwell RL, Gombos E, et al. *Diagnostic Imaging: Breast*. Altona: AMIRSYS, 2006.

Berg WA, Zhang Z, Lehrer D, et al. Detection of breast cancer with addition of annual screening ultrasound or a single screening MRI to mammography in women with elevated breast cancer risk. *JAMA*. 2012;307(13):1394–1404.

Cardenosa G. *Breast Imaging Companion*. Philadelphia, PA: Lippincott Williams and Wilkins, 2007.

Lee CH, Dershaw DD, Kopans D, et al. Breast cancer screening with imaging: Recommendations from the Society of Breast Imaging and the ACR on the use of mammography, breast MRI, breast ultrasound, and other technologies for the detection of clinically occult breast cancer. *J Am Coll Radiol*. 2010;7(1): 18–27.

Conant E, Brennecke C. *Breast Imaging: Case Review Series (Case Review)*. Philadelphia, PA: Mosby, 2006.

D'Orsi CJ, Bassett LW, Berg WA, et al. Mammography. In: D'Orsi CJ, Mendelson EB, Ikeda DM, eds. *Breast Imaging Reporting and Data System (BI-RADS)*. 4th ed. Reston, VA: American College of Radiology, 2003.

Independent UK Panel on Breast Cancer Screening. The benefits and harms of breast cancer screening: An independent review. *Lancet*. 380(9855):1778–1786.

Pisano ED, Gatsonis C, Hendrick E, et al. Diagnostic performance of digital versus film mammography for breast-cancer screening. *N Engl J Med*. 2005;353(17):1773–1783.

Saslow D, Boetes C, Burke W, et al. American cancer society guidelines for breast screening with MRI as an adjunct to mammography. *CA Cancer J Clin*. 2007;57(2):75–89.

U.S. Preventive Services Task Force. Screening for breast cancer: U.S. Preventive services task force recommendation statement. *Ann Intern Med*. 2009;151(10):716–726.

QUESTIONS

1. Which is the best choice for the indications of screening mammogram?
   a. Asymptomatic women without high-risk factors starting at age 30 annually
   b. Asymptomatic women without high-risk factors starting at age 40 annually
   c. Asymptomatic women without high-risk factors starting at age 50 biannually
   d. Women with 1-week breast pain

2. The advantage of digital mammogram versus film-screen mammogram includes the followings except
   a. use computer-assisted diagnostic techniques (CAD) to aid in detecting abnormalities
   b. better detecting breast cancer in pre- or perimenopausal women
   c. rapid transmission of the imaging to another location and storage of the images electronically
   d. better detecting breast cancer in women with fatty breast

3. Indications for diagnostic mammogram include the following except
   a. recent lumpectomy new baseline
   b. 40-year-old women with bloody nipple discharge
   c. 50-year-old women with history of benign breast biopsy
   d. 50-year-old women with recent unilateral skin indentation

4. Which one of the following calcifications is most suspicious for ductal carcinoma in situ?
   a. Round and punctate microcalcifications
   b. Dystrophic calcifications
   c. Amorphous microcalcifications
   d. Clustered pleomorphic microcalcifications

5. The differential diagnosis of the circumscribed solid mass on ultrasound are the following except
   a. fibroadenoma
   b. phyllodes tumor
   c. simple cyst
   d. medullary carcinoma

6. Which one of the following statement about male gynecomastia is true?
   a. It carries increased risk for malignancy
   b. It has to be bilateral
   c. It can be due to certain medications, liver disease, or testicular tumor
   d. Only in elderly

7. Indications for breast MRI are the following except
   a. women with dense breast tissue
   b. evaluation of extent of the disease with recently diagnosed breast cancer
   c. silicone implant rupture
   d. BRCA mutations

8. Which one of the following is more suggestive malignancy?
   a. Circumscribed low-density oval mass on mammogram
   b. Circumscribed isoechoic oval mass on ultrasound
   c. Irregular high density mass with spiculated borders on mammogram
   d. Lobulated anechoic mass with septations and posterior enhancement on ultrasound

9. The indications for high-risk screening mammogram prior to age 40 are the following except
   a. mother diagnosed with postmenopausal breast cancer
   b. BRCA mutations
   c. mother diagnosed with premenopausal breast cancer
   d. history of lymphoma at young age 8 years post chest radiation therapy

10. What is the best initial imaging modality for 29-year-old women with breast lump?
    a. Diagnostic mammogram
    b. Breast MRI
    c. Tomosynthesis
    d. Breast ultrasound

Interventional Radiology

Thomas A. Farrell

Interventional radiology (IR) is a diverse practice of patient care using minimally invasive image-guided procedures to diagnose and treat disease nonoperatively. Percutaneous diagnostic and therapeutic procedures are performed using fluoroscopy, ultrasound, computed tomography (CT), or magnetic resonance (MR) imaging for guidance. These procedures, which may be categorized as vascular (i.e., arteriography, venography) and nonvascular (e.g., drainage of abscesses, obstructed kidneys and bile ducts), are performed in an IR suite and are often done on an outpatient basis. Many procedures that were previously performed surgically are now accomplished by an interventional radiologist with less morbidity and a shorter hospital stay.

Since 1953, when Dr. Sven-Ivar Seldinger described a method of percutaneous arterial access using a hollow-core needle, guidewire, and catheter, IR has continued to evolve, as new techniques and devices are developed to enhance patient care. Technical advances have led to significant improvements in patient safety and procedural diversity. As these rapid changes in endovascular technologies continue to expand, so will the possibilities of image-guided, minimally invasive procedures.

Because IR is procedural, interventional radiologists become more involved in patient care. Many IR practices offer an active inpatient and outpatient consult service and also employ specially trained nurse practitioners and physician's assistants as physician extenders. Patients are routinely worked up by the IR service and are subsequently followed up postprocedure. The preprocedure workup consists of patient assessment as well as evaluation of previous imaging studies (Table 12.1). Postprocedure follow-up is essential to determine whether the procedure has been successful and free of complications. This all-inclusive clinical service underlines that there is more to IR than simply doing procedures. Because procedures performed by interventional radiologists are invasive, the risk of complications is ever present. It is important that the patient be aware of these risks so that an informed consent can be made by weighing the possible risks of a procedure against its potential benefits. A physician should never place a patient in a position of risk unless the risks, benefits, and alternatives of the planned procedure have been discussed, understood, and consented to before the procedure. It is in the physician's best interest to be honest and forthright

Table 12.1

Interventional Radiology Preprocedure Checklist

Indication for procedure/question(s) to be answered
  from procedure
Contraindications for procedure
Review prior imaging and noninvasive studies
Check for contrast allergy
Written informed consent
Check coagulation parameters and serum creatinine
Need for prophylactic antibiotics
Patient should be fasting and well hydrated
Discontinue heparin infusion

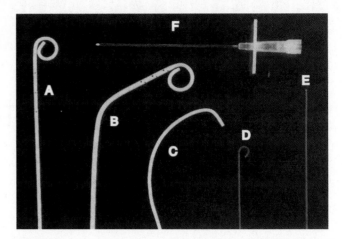

FIGURE 12.1. Tools of the trade. **A:** Pigtail catheter. **B:** Angled pigtail catheter. **C:** Cobra catheter. **D:** J-tipped guidewire. **E:** Straight (Bentson) guidewire. **F:** An 18G needle for vessel puncture.

when dealing with patients and their expectations about the outcomes of a procedure.

The aim of this chapter is to explain the background, indications, and basic techniques of the procedures commonly performed in IR so that the reader will gain an understanding of how this subspecialty contributes to patient care.

INSTRUMENTS AND TOOLS OF THE TRADE

IR procedures are performed in imaging suites with fluoroscopy and digital subtraction angiography (DSA). Ultrasound, CT, and MR imaging are also utilized by the interventional radiologist.

Endoluminal and endovascular procedures require administration of a contrast agent for improved visualization. Nonionic iodinated contrast is most frequently used to delineate, radiographically, the lumen of an artery, vein, and biliary duct, gastrointestinal (GI) or urinary tract. Alternatively carbon dioxide gas or gadolinium can be used in patients with renal insufficiency or allergy to radiographic contrast agents.

There is a variety of commercially available catheters, sheaths, guidewires, angioplasty catheters, vascular stents, and caval filters and familiarity with these and their use requires training and experience. There are numerous preformed shapes and types of angiographic catheters, most of which are made from flexible plastic material such as polyethylene or polyurethane. Wire braiding may be incorporated into the catheter shaft to increase stiffness and improve its torque. Catheter diameters are measured in French (F) size, where 3F = 1 mm (outside diameter). Most angiographic catheters are in the 4F to 7F range. Aortic angiography is performed with pigtail catheters that have several side holes proximal to the tip allowing rapid flow of a contrast bolus while the pigtail loop stabilizes the catheter preventing recoil (Fig. 12.1A,B). Selective angiography (renal, celiac, and superior mesenteric arteries) is performed with a curved end-hole catheter such as a Cobra C2 (Fig. 12.1C). A variety of catheters and guidewires may be necessary during a procedure, and placement of a vascular sheath with a

hemostatic valve at the site of access reduces vessel trauma and facilitates rapid catheter and guidewire exchange.

Catheters used in the drainage of abscesses, obstructed kidneys (percutaneous nephrostomy), and bile ducts are made of polyurethane and are of greater diameter (8F to 22F) than angiographic catheters. These drainage catheters are usually placed using the Seldinger technique after which they are secured in position by deploying a locking pigtail mechanism formed by pulling on a suture that runs in the catheter shaft and is attached to its tip. The pigtail loop itself contains large side holes for drainage purposes. The smaller diameter catheters occlude more easily with debris and should be routinely changed over a guidewire every 6 to 8 weeks when continued drainage is required.

Guidewires increase the ease and safety of catheter placement. The outer shell of a guidewire consists of a very tightly wound but flexible metal spring coil. A stiff central core provides rigidity over a variable length of the guidewire. The balance between these two components dictates the handling characteristics of the guidewire. For example, the distal 15 cm of a Bentson guidewire is floppy, allowing easy coiling (Fig. 12.1E), whereas a J-tipped guidewire reduces the risk of damaging the vessel wall because of its blunt tip (Fig. 12.1D). Guidewires usually range in diameter from 18 thousandths of an inch (0.018″) to 38 thousandths of an inch (0.038″). The standard length for most wires is 145 cm, while longer guidewires (260 cm) are available to facilitate catheter exchange.

Needles used in arteriography vary in size from a 21G needle through which a 0.018-inch guidewire will pass to an 18G needle that accepts a 0.035-inch guidewire (Fig. 12.1F).

ANGIOGRAPHY

Angiography is a technique of imaging blood vessels, usually by injecting contrast material via an intraluminally placed catheter. Blood vessels may also be visualized noninvasively using computed tomography angiography (CTA) or magnetic resonance angiography (MRA), which takes advantage of the inherent contrast between flowing blood and stationary tissue.

Catheter Arteriography

Diagnostic arteriography begins by catheterizing an artery (usually common femoral or brachial) using the Seldinger technique (Fig. 12.2). After placing a hollow-core needle into the artery, a guidewire is inserted through the needle and advanced into the artery. The needle is exchanged for a vascular catheter or sheath. Subsequent catheter movement and exchange is performed over a guidewire. Sonographic and fluoroscopic guidance is often necessary using this technique. Large vessel arteriography is performed using flush catheters (pigtail). Smaller arteries are selectively cannulated using catheters of various shapes and sizes. Microcatheters are used for sub- or superselective arteriography.

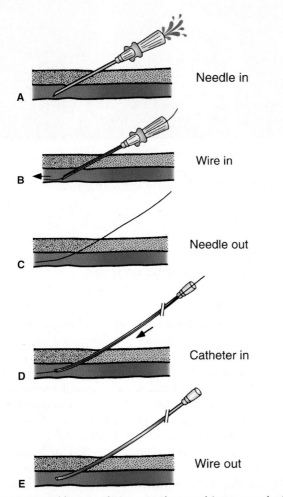

FIGURE 12.2. Seldinger technique. **A:** The vessel is punctured with the needle. **B:** A guidewire is advanced through the needle into the vessel. **C:** The needle is removed leaving the guidewire in place. **D:** A catheter is advanced over the guidewire into the vessel. **E:** The guidewire is removed and the catheter flushed.

After the catheter is safely positioned in the artery of choice, the guidewire is removed and contrast injected through the catheter during image acquisition usually with DSA which involves the acquisition of several mask images before injection of contrast, allowing for subsequent subtraction of nonvascular structures from the next set of images which are acquired as the contrast agent flows through the lumen of the vessel producing the arteriogram. The catheter can be exchanged or repositioned for additional imaging. After completion of the procedure, the catheter is removed from the artery and hemostasis obtained at the arteriotomy site using manual compression or a percutaneous closure device such as a nitinol clip which grasps the arterial wall externally in a purse-string fashion and closes the arteriotomy with minimal impact on the vessel diameter. Post procedure recovery time for the patient is 2 to 6 hours.

Noninvasive angiography (MRA/CTA) is gradually replacing diagnostic catheter arteriography, except where intervention is expected or other examinations are inconclusive. Pulmonary arteriography, formerly considered the gold standard in the diagnosis of pulmonary embolism (PE) has largely been replaced by CT, which has a high specificity and sensitivity (see Figure 3.50C). Both CTA and MRA are widely used in the evaluation of aortic, visceral, renal, and peripheral arterial disease (PAD) (Fig. 12.3). However, the administration of gadolinium commonly used in MRA, is associated with a higher incidence of nephrogenic systemic sclerosis in patients with renal impairment.

Peripheral Arterial Disease

Generally, the diagnosis of peripheral arterial disease (PAD) has already been made by the time an arteriogram is requested. The initial evaluation includes an assessment of the patient's symptoms (intermittent claudication, rest pain, nonhealing ulcer), physical examination, and a review of the noninvasive imaging tests, such as CT, MR, duplex ultrasonography, and segmental limb pressures before proceeding to angiography. Rather than being an end point, the angiogram helps formulate a comprehensive plan in the patient's subsequent management as it evaluates the extent and severity of disease and provides a road map for intervention (balloon angioplasty, stenting, surgery, etc.). Patients with diabetes may present with a more advanced stage of ischemia as they are prone to developing peripheral neuropathy that may mask the above symptoms. Diabetics also tend to have a greater prevalence of small vessel (infrageniculate) disease, which is more difficult to treat surgically and contributes to a less favorable long-term prognosis compared to other causes of PAD.

Arteriographic examination of patients with PAD may be divided into three anatomic regions: Aortoiliac, infrainguinal, and infrageniculate. Abdominal aortic aneurysms (AAA) occur most commonly below the level of the renal arteries. The number of renal arteries should also be noted,

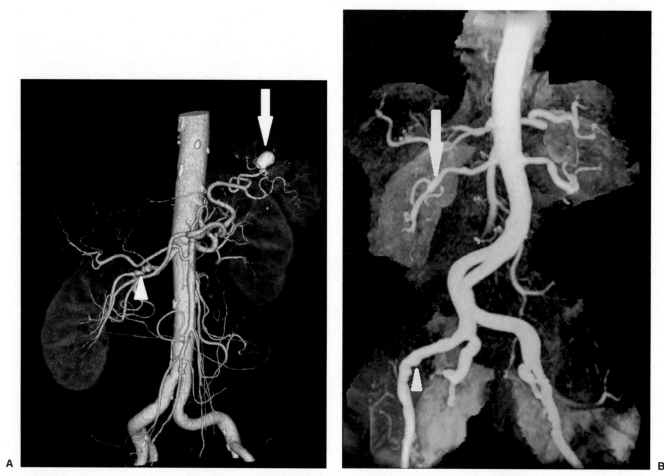

FIGURE 12.3. A: CTA of Abdomen. Volume rendered images of the abdomen show the abdominal aorta and its branches. There are multiple stenoses in the mid right renal artery consistent with fibromuscular dysplasia (*arrowhead*). There is also a calcified splenic artery aneurysm (*arrow*). **B:** *MR angiography* of the abdomen and pelvis shows multiple stenoses of both renal (*arrow*) and external iliac arteries (*arrowhead*) consistent with fibromuscular dysplasia.

as should the presence of stenoses in these vessels. Bilateral oblique views of the pelvis should be obtained during the arteriogram, as hemodynamically significant stenoses can be missed if only a frontal view is performed.

In general, arterial stenoses are not regarded as significant unless they reduce the lumen diameter by 50% angiographically. Measurement of a pressure gradient across it can more accurately assess the significance of a arterial stenosis, with a 10-mm Hg gradient or greater being regarded as significant and worthy of further treatment such as angioplasty or stenting. If the gradient is less than 10 mm Hg, a vasodilator such as nitroglycerin may be given intra-arterially to simulate exercise and possibly unmask a significant stenosis. Common sites for endovascular intervention include the carotid, renal, aortoiliac, and femoropopliteal arteries.

In the absence of satisfactory femoral pulses bilaterally, either the brachial or radial arteries can be used for percutaneous access.

VASCULAR INTERVENTIONS

Thrombolysis

Thrombolysis is the process of dissolving blood clot in order to re-establish patency of an occluded (thrombosed) vessel, using drugs such as urokinase and tissue plasminogen activator (t-PA). These drugs are infused directly into the thrombosed grafts and vessels via catheters to ensure a very high local concentration of the drug. Contraindications for thrombolysis include internal bleeding, recent intracranial hemorrhage, or surgery (Table 12.2).

Complications of thrombolysis include bleeding and distal embolization of thrombus. The cumulative probability of major complications increases with duration of infusion, rising from less than 10% after 16 hours to more than 30% at 40 hours. Once thrombolysis is complete, angioplasty, stenting, or surgery can be used to treat any underlying vessel stenoses that contributed to the occlusion. Treatment of an acute native arterial occlusion is

Table 12.2

Contraindications for Arterial Thrombolysis

Absolute

Active gastrointestinal (GI) or genitourinary (GU)
    bleeding
Recent (<12 mo) cerebral hemorrhage/infarct/surgery
Irreversible limb ischemia

Relative

History of GI or GU bleeding
Recent thoracic/abdominal surgery
Recent trauma
Severe uncontrolled hypertension

better done mechanically, either surgical embolectomy or catheter-directed aspiration.

Balloon Angioplasty

Percutaneous transluminal balloon angioplasty (PTA) has become an established technique in the treatment of vascular stenoses due to atherosclerotic plaque and fibromuscular dysplasia. The precise pathophysiologic mechanism of PTA in atherosclerotic plaque is controversial. However, most agree that PTA results in a controlled plaque and intimal fracture with localized dissection into the underlying media thereby increasing the intraluminal diameter. The plaque, intima, and media are subsequently remodeled to give a smoother endoluminal surface. The appropriate angioplasty balloon catheter should be chosen so that its inflated diameter is the same size or slightly larger than the adjacent nondiseased vessel. Initially, the

stenosis is crossed with a guidewire that is left across the lesion until the procedure is finished. Heparin and nitroglycerin may be given intra-arterially to prevent thrombosis and vessel spasm, respectively. The angioplasty balloon is advanced across the stenosis, inflated, and deflated slowly under fluoroscopic guidance. Repeat angiography and pressure measurements should be obtained to evaluate the results of angioplasty. Suboptimal angioplasty results may require placement of an endovascular stent.

Iliac artery angioplasty improves inflow to the lower limb and requires balloons that are 7 to 10 mm in diameter. Again, a guidewire is left across the stenosis during the procedure, the success of which is judged on angiographic and hemodynamic criteria. Stent placement should be considered if the postangioplasty pressure gradient is greater than 10 mm Hg, there is residual stenosis of greater than 30%, or if a flow-limiting dissection is present (Fig. 12.4). Simultaneous PTA of both common iliac arteries, known as the kissing balloon technique, is effective in treating bilateral proximal common iliac artery stenoses.

Infrainguinal angioplasty (superficial femoral and popliteal arteries) is gaining clinical acceptance as patency outcomes for PTA and stenting rivals outcomes of surgical bypass procedures. Infrageniculate angioplasty (anterior/posterior tibial and peroneal arteries) is usually performed for limb salvage or to reduce the extent of an impending below-the-knee or forefoot amputation for ischemia. This technique requires a fine diameter guidewire (0.010″ to 0.018″) and angioplasty balloon (2 to 3 mm in diameter) because of the smaller vessel size (Fig. 12.5).

Renal artery angioplasty is usually performed with a 5- to 7-mm diameter balloon. Atheromatous disease usually involves the proximal or ostial portion of the vessel in

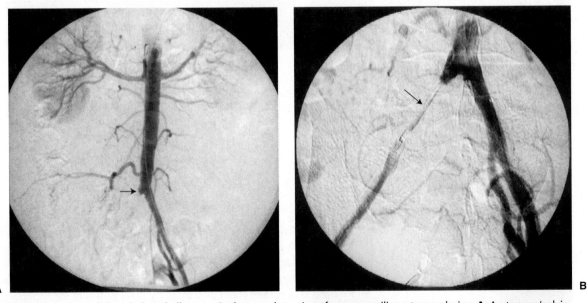

FIGURE 12.4. Arterial thrombolysis, balloon angioplasty, and stenting of a common iliac artery occlusion. **A:** Aortogram/pelvic angiogram shows occlusion of the right common iliac artery (*arrow*). **B:** Partial recanalization of the right common iliac artery following thrombolysis performed via an infusion catheter (*arrow*). (*continued*)

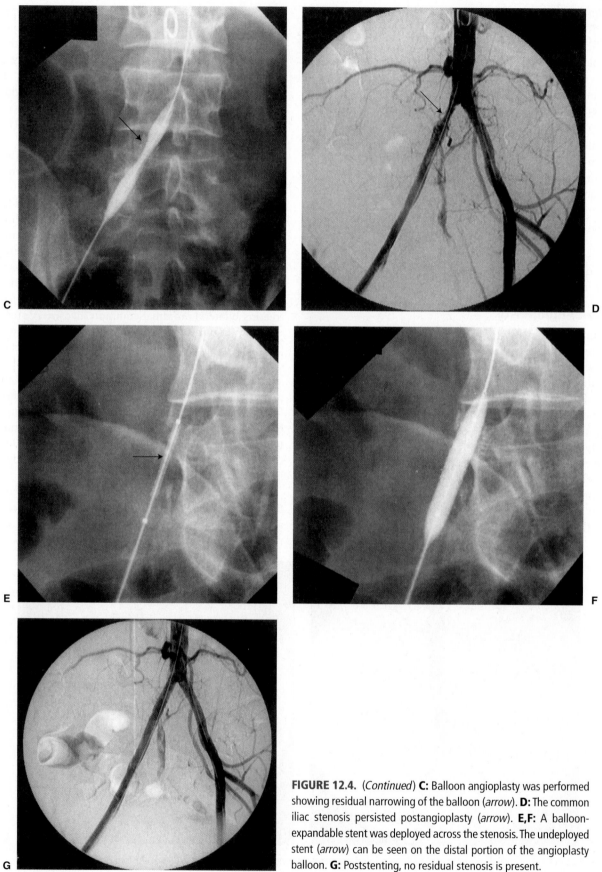

FIGURE 12.4. (*Continued*) **C:** Balloon angioplasty was performed showing residual narrowing of the balloon (*arrow*). **D:** The common iliac stenosis persisted postangioplasty (*arrow*). **E,F:** A balloon-expandable stent was deployed across the stenosis. The undeployed stent (*arrow*) can be seen on the distal portion of the angioplasty balloon. **G:** Poststenting, no residual stenosis is present.

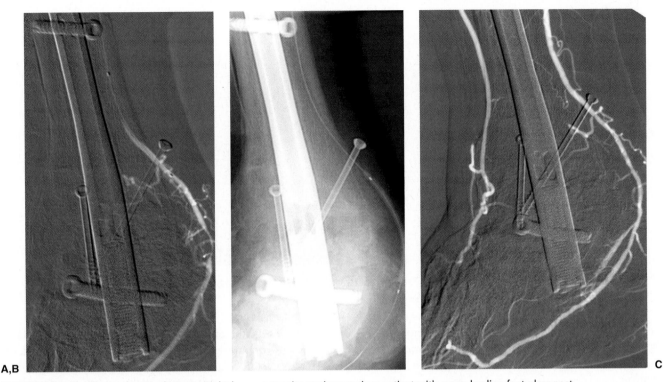

FIGURE 12.5. Small vessel angioplasty. **A:** Right lower extremity angiogram, in a patient with a non healing foot ulcer post internal fixation of an ankle fracture, which shows a focal stenosis in the distal posterior tibial artery. **B:** The stenosis was traversed and balloon dilated with a 2-mm diameter angioplasty balloon. **C:** Follow up angiography showed improved flow which resulted in prompt healing of the ulcer.

contrast to fibromuscular dysplasia that usually affects the midportion of the vessel. The improvement in renal function and hypertension following renal artery angioplasty is equivalent to that obtained after surgical revascularization (Fig. 12.6). Renal artery stenting is performed if there is a residual stenosis or significant dissection postangioplasty (Fig. 12.7). Ostial renal artery stenoses are often stented primarily, without balloon predilatation. It has been noted that improvement in hypertension and renal function is not universal postangioplasty/stent. Cardiovascular Outcomes in Renal Atherosclerotic Lesions (CORAL) is an ongoing multicenter study funded by the National

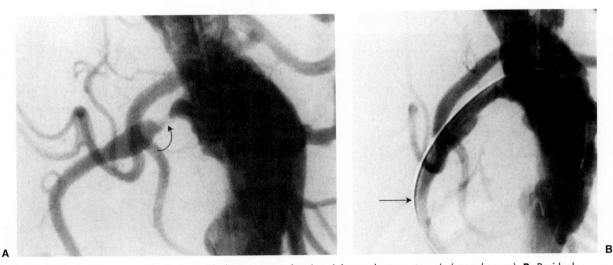

FIGURE 12.6. Renal artery angioplasty. **A:** Flush aortogram showing right renal artery stenosis (*curved arrow*). **B:** Residual stenosis persists postballoon angioplasty. Note that the guidewire (*arrow*) is left across the stenosis.

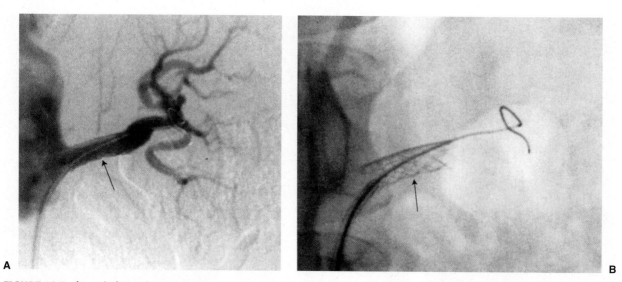

FIGURE 12.7. (A and **B)** Renal artery stenting. Palmaz stent (*arrow*) has been placed across a left renal artery stenosis.

Institutes of Health, which has randomized more than 900 patients with greater than 60% stenosis to optimal medical therapy alone or optimal medical therapy plus renal artery stenting.

Endovascular Stents

Peripheral Endovascular Stents

There are two main indications for endovascular stent placement: (a) A residual pressure gradient of more than 10 mm Hg postangioplasty, which is regarded as an indication for either repeat angioplasty or stent placement and (b) postangioplasty flow-limiting dissection, in which the goal of stent placement is to appose the dissected flap against the wall and improve flow. The balloon–stent combination is placed across the stenosis and the balloon is inflated, thus opening and deploying the stent. The balloon is then deflated and removed (Fig. 12.8). There are two general types of metallic endovascular stents, balloon-expandable and self-expanding. Deployment of the balloon-expandable stent is described above. Deployment of the self-expanding stent, which does not require delivery on an angioplasty balloon, involves withdrawal of a covering sheath, after which the stent expands. Postdilatation with an angioplasty balloon may be necessary. Self-expanding stents are usually more flexible than balloon-mounted stents, which is an advantage when stenting tortuous vessels (Fig. 12.9). Covered (polytetrafluoroethylene [PTFE], Dacron) stents are available for treatment of vascular injury resulting in pseudoaneurysm, hemorrhage, or arteriovenous (AV) fistula. Drug-eluting stents are increasingly being used in the treatment of superficial femoral artery stenoses. These stents are coated with drugs which

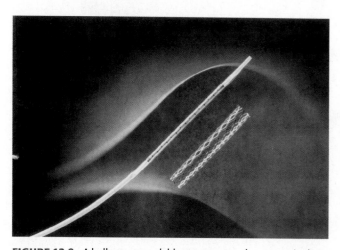

FIGURE 12.8. A balloon-expandable stent mounted on an angioplasty balloon and in its expanded form. (Courtesy of Cordis Corporation.)

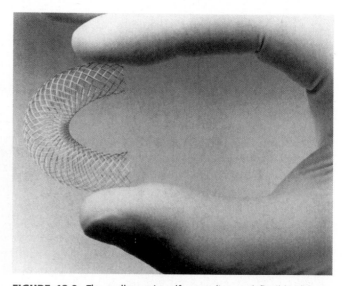

FIGURE 12.9. The wallstent is self-expanding and flexible. (Photograph courtesy of Boston Scientific.)

prevent cellular proliferation and are designed to reduce restenosis which develops inside the stent.

Aortic Stent Grafts

Stent grafts have revolutionized the treatment of AAA, reducing the severity and duration of the procedure and postprocedure morbidity and hospital stay. The majority of patients are discharged within 48 hours of the procedure, which is usually done in the operating room or combined operative/fluoroscopy suite, under general or epidural anesthesia. Preprocedural imaging such as a CT scan of the abdominal and pelvis is essential for precise vessel measurement and localization of arterial branches Through bilateral common femoral artery surgical cutdowns, the various components of the aortic stent graft are introduced and deployed in the abdominal aorta and iliac arteries, under fluoroscopic guidance. The device, which is composed of woven polyester on a wire exoskeleton frame, is deployed in the infrarenal aorta and extends down to the common or external iliac arteries (Fig. 12.10). Postprocedure follow-up with CT scans initially every 6 months is important for the detection of an endoleak, which is a leak into the aneurysm sac which may cause the sac to enlarge. In the absence of such endoleak, the aneurysm sac should reduce in size (Fig. 12.11).

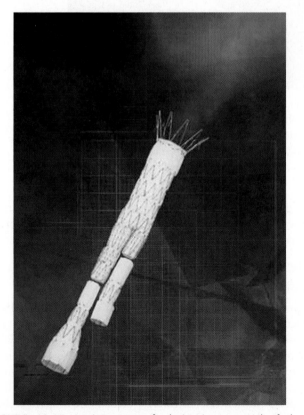

FIGURE 12.10. Aortic stent graft device is composed of three components—a main body and two iliac extensions—which can be custom made to suit each patient. The components are placed through femoral artery cutdowns. (Courtesy of Cook Medical, Inc.)

Complications of Angiography

Complications of angiography are rare and the main ones are listed in Table 12.3. Risk factors for these complications include hypertension and obesity and their prevention includes meticulous techniques including common femoral artery puncture over the femoral head and constant manual pressure directly over the puncture site after removal of the catheter until hemostasis is achieved. The post angiogram hematoma may extend into the retroperitoneum when the puncture site is above the inguinal ligament (Fig. 12.12A). Incomplete or intermittent compression over the puncture site may also result in the formation of a pseudoaneurysm (Fig. 12.12B). Dissection of vessel wall may occur if the needle/wire or catheter is introduced subinitmally (Fig. 12.12C), and distal embolization of mural plaque or thrombus is a risk following any endovascular manipulation (Fig. 12.12D). Complications following brachial or axillary arterial puncture are more common than with femoral artery puncture because of the smaller vessel size and the close proximity of the vessels to nerves within a common sheath in the arm. Dissection or thrombosis, of the access artery may require endovascular intervention or surgical repair. Pseudoaneurysms may be treated with direct injection of thrombin under US guidance.

Contrast-induced nephropathy usually results in transient renal insufficiency, and occasionally, permanent renal failure. In most patients this complication is usually mild and self-limiting, with serum creatinine levels peaking by 3 to 5 days and returning to normal within 2 weeks. The pathophysiology of this complication is thought to be due to a combination of vasoconstriction and direct toxicity of contrast on the renal tubules. Patients with diabetes and patients with preexisting renal impairment (serum creatinine greater than 1.6 mg%) are at increased risk for developing contrast-induced renal failure. Clinical judgment, adequate hydration, iso-osmolar or low-osmolar iodinated contrast, or alternative contrast agents (CO_2, gadolinium) should be used in high-risk patients (elderly, creatinine (Cr) >1.6, DM).

Systemic allergic or anaphylactoid reactions to radiographic contrast media are rare, with their severity depending on the type, dose, route, and rate of contrast delivery. Allergic reactions may be categorized as mild, moderate, or severe (Table 12.4). The prevalence of most allergic reactions to iodinated contrast is greater with the intravenous route. Many studies suggest a lower incidence of severe reactions when nonionic iodinated contrast is used. The mortality rate, which is equivalent for high and lower osmolar contrast agents, is approximately 1 per 45,000 examinations. Moderate contrast reactions characterized by hypertension, hypotension, wheezing, and laryngospasm occur in 1% to 2% of contrast administrations. Allergic reactions are usually mild (nausea, cough, hives, and flushing), are even more common, and can be treated symptomatically. Allergy to seafood is not a predisposition

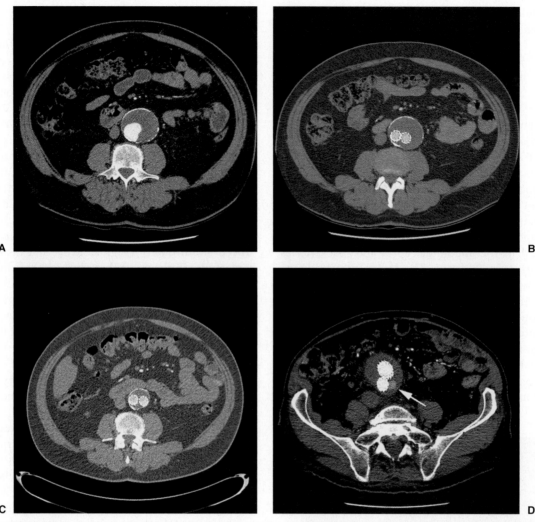

FIGURE 12.11. Aortic endograft follow-up. Serial CT studies show an infrarenal abdominal aortic aneurysm (AAA) measuring 4.5 cm in diameter **(A)**. Six months post-AAA endograft placement, the excluded aneurysm sac now measures 4 cm **(B)** and at 18 months postendograft, it has further reduced to a diameter of 3.2 cm **(C)**. CT abdomen in a patient post-AAA endograft shows contrast within the aneurysm sac but outside the endograft (*arrow*) **(D)**. This is an endoleak which occurs because of persistent blood flow into the aneurysm which in this patient is due to retrograde flow from a lumbar artery.

Table 12.3
Complications of Angiography

Systemic
    Allergic contrast reaction
    Renal failure
Local
    Puncture site
        Hematoma
        Pseudoaneurysm
        Arteriovenous fistula
Intraluminal
    Subintimal dissection
    Thrombosis
    Distal embolization

to developing an allergic reaction to iodinated contrast. The standard of care is premedication with steroids prior to contrast administration.

Therapeutic Embolization

Gastrointestinal Hemorrhage

Selective angiography and therapeutic embolization have become important techniques in the management of patients with acute upper and lower GI bleeding. Initially, a nuclear medicine study using radiolabeled red cells is helpful to confirm the presence and anatomic location of the bleeding vessel. Selective angiography of the celiac, superior mesenteric, or inferior mesenteric arteries is then performed. Once a bleeding site has been demonstrated, the catheter can be used to control bleeding by embolization such as gelatin sponge pledgets or coils to mechanically occlude flow (Fig. 12.13).

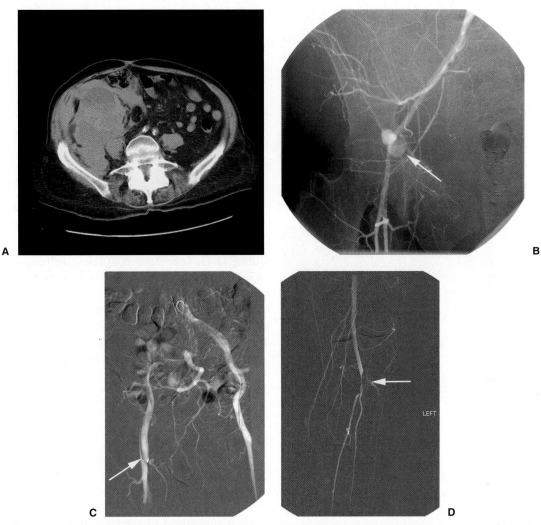

FIGURE 12.12. Complications of arterial interventions. **A:** This CT scan shows a hematoma occupying most of the right hemipelvis. The retroperitoneal hematoma could be traced down to the right external iliac artery where the physician performing an angiogram had made the initial arterial puncture. **B:** The well-defined focal bulge (*arrow*) is a pseudoaneurysm which has formed at the site of a previous common femoral arterial puncture. **C:** The vertically oriented well-defined curvilinear filling defect (*arrow*) in the right external iliac is a dissection flap. **D:** The well-defined intraluminal filling defect in the distal popliteal artery (*arrow*) is an embolus which migrated there after balloon angioplasty of a stenosis containing atherosclerotic plaque upstream in the superficial femoral artery.

Table 12.4			
Allergic Contrast Reactions			
Type	**Mild**	**Moderate**	**Severe**
Incidence (%)	5–15	1–2	0.1
Clinical features	Nausea	Bronchospasm	Laryngospasm
	Vomiting	Dyspnea	Facial edema
	Urticaria	Vasovagal reaction	Cardiorespiratory arrest
		Hypertension	Seizures
Treatment	Monitor vital signs	Oxygen	Oxygen/IV fluids
	Observe for clinical deterioration	β^2 agonist	Epinephrine SC or IV
			β^2 agonist
			Diazepam

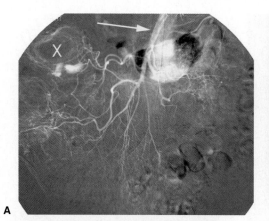

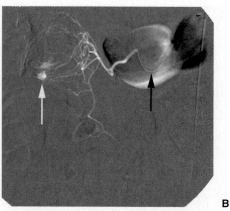

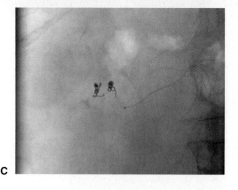

FIGURE 12.13. Embolization of a GI bleed. **A:** This superior mesenteric angiogram (*arrow*) shows extravasation of contrast, which represents hemorrhage into the colon at the hepatic flexure (*X*). **B:** This extravasation (*white arrow*) is confirmed on selective angiography of the right colic artery performed with a microcatheter (*black arrow*). **C:** Several stainless steel coils 2 to 3 mm in diameter were deployed through the microcatheter occluding the right colic branch at the bleeding site.

Hemoptysis

Patients with massive hemoptysis may be successfully treated by embolizing the appropriate bronchial arteries, which arise directly from the thoracic aorta or from intercostal branches, with particles measuring 300 to 500 μm in diameter. Great care should be taken to avoid embolization of the arterial supply to the spinal cord which may result in paralysis.

Uterine Fibroid Embolization

Fibroids are the most common benign tumors in females and may present as pain, menorrhagia, anemia or pressure symptoms related to mass effect. Traditionally, patients were treated with hysterectomy or myomectomy. Uterine fibroid embolization offers an effective and less invasive treatment option. After bilateral selective catheterization of the uterine arteries, inert particles up to 900 microns (0.9 mm) in size are injected, infarcting the fibroids, eventually reducing their size and improving symptoms. The fibroid size reduces by 60% at 6 months after treatment and up to 90% of patients notice an improvement in their pain, menorrhagia, or pressure symptoms.

Tumor Embolization

Arterial embolization is also utilized for regional cancer therapy. Bland embolization of primary or metastatic tumors is performed to decrease blood flow to a tumor, depriving it of nutrients. Bland embolization is usually performed for vascular tumors, bleeding from tumor or adjacent invaded organs, and for palliation. In the case of renal cell carcinoma, the kidney or metastatic lesion is often embolized prior to surgery to decrease bleeding during nephrectomy or resection (Fig. 12.14).

The liver has a dual blood supply (hepatic arterial and portal venous) and liver tumors depend largely on the arterial supply for growth. Chemoembolization is performed in patients with primary or metastatic liver cancer, subselectively embolizing the arterial supply of the tumor with chemotherapeutic drugs and inert particles. Chemoembolization has the advantage of prolonging the tumor exposure to a high concentration of drug(s) while also infarcting the tumor (Fig. 12.15). Radioembolization is another form of liver embolization in which numerous 10 to 50 micron glass or resin beads, containing Yttrium-90 are injected intra-arterially permitting a highly concentrated dose of radiation which is confined to the liver. The maximum range of emission is 11 mm and 94% of the radiation dose is delivered in 11 days.

Trauma

The interventional radiologist has an important role in the management of trauma patients. Most emergent trauma procedures referred to IR involve bleeding or injury to the vascular system. Vessel injury with bleeding, intimal injury, pseudoaneurysm, or fistula can be diagnosed and immediately treated in the angiography suite, often using

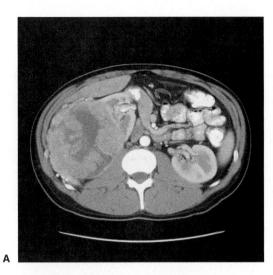

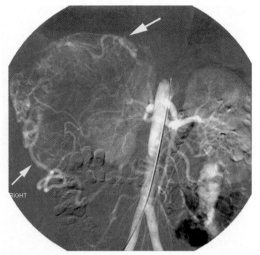

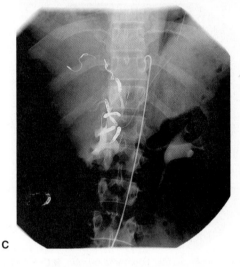

FIGURE 12.14. Preoperative embolization of a renal carcinoma. **A:** The CT scan shows a large hypervascular right renal carcinoma. **B:** Abdominal aortography confirms it hypervascular nature (*arrows*). **C:** Postembolization of the renal artery branches and nonrenal branches (lumbar and inferior phrenic arteries) with stainless steel coils. The prophylactic embolization reduced the operative morbidity and blood loss as the surgeon was operating in a "bloodless" field. (Courtesy of Dr. D. Warner.)

covered stents or embolization techniques (Figs. 12.16 and 12.17).

Hemorrhage Associated with Pelvic Fracture

Prior to the introduction of external fixation devices, much of the early mortality associated with pelvic fractures was due to internal hemorrhage. At present, up to 20% of patients with pelvic fractures require the services of IR for the diagnosis and treatment of hemorrhage. In general, surgery is not a satisfactory treatment option for this problem as exploration will decompress the pelvic hematoma, reduce the tamponade effect, and lead to further blood loss. A diagnostic pelvic angiogram is performed with a pigtail catheter placed above the aortic bifurcation. Active hemorrhage is diagnosed by extravasation of contrast. The bleeding vessel may then be embolized with either a metal coil or gelfoam, both of which can be placed through a selective 5F angiographic catheter. Gelfoam results in temporary vascular occlusion that recanalizes within 2 to 3 weeks, whereas a metal coil usually results in a permanent occlusion. Pelvic ischemia following selective arterial embolization is unusual due to the extensive collateral blood supply.

Traumatic Aortic Injury

Eighty percent of those who sustain a laceration to the thoracic aorta following blunt trauma die at the scene of the accident, en route to the hospital, or shortly after arriving in hospital. The cause of death in most cases is exsanguination from aortic transection. The precise mechanism of aortic transection is uncertain. It may be due to sudden deceleration where the mobile descending aorta shears from the relatively fixed aortic arch, as the most common site for aortic transection is just distal to the origin of the left subclavian artery. As in all trauma patients, rapid clinical evaluation is important, but up to 50% of patients surviving accidents with blunt aortic injuries have no external physical signs of injury. Multidetector CT of the chest has replaced catheter aortography as the gold standard for diagnosing aortic arch injury (see Figure 3.85). One should be aware of a normal anatomic variant in the aortic arch that may be misdiagnosed as traumatic aortic injury—the so-called ductus bump, which lies proximally on the inferior surface of the aortic arch and represents the site of attachment of the ductus arteriosus (Fig. 12.18). Emergent deployment of a

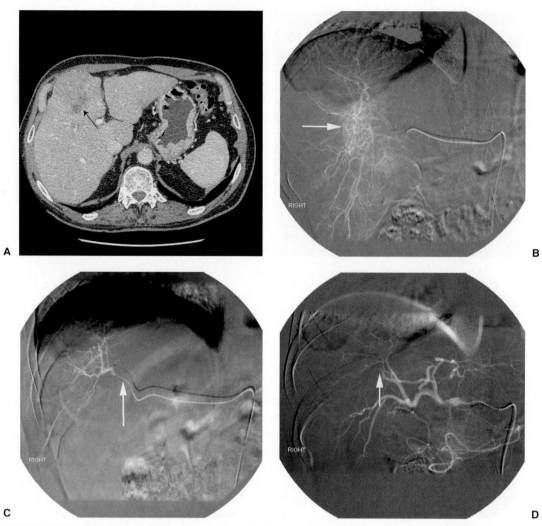

FIGURE 12.15. Chemoembolization of a hepatoma. **A:** CT shows a hypervascular hepatoma (*arrow*). **B,C:** Selective hepatic angiography confirms the tumor's hypervascularity (*arrow*) and more clearly defines its arterial supply. **D:** Angiography postchemoembolization of the hepatoma confirms occlusion (*arrow*) of its main hepatic arterial branch.

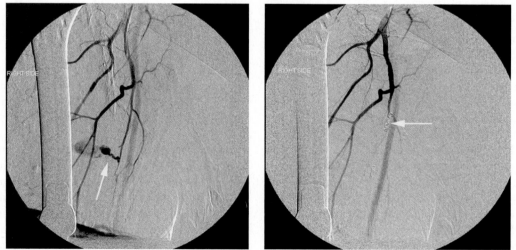

FIGURE 12.16. Embolization of a leaking pseudoaneurysm. This patient presented with a rapidly expanding thigh hematoma after hip replacement surgery. **A:** A thigh angiogram shows a pseudoaneurysm (*arrow*) in the distal profunda femoris artery. **B:** Several stainless steel coils were deployed through the angiographic catheter occluding the arterial branch proximal to the pseudoaneurysm.

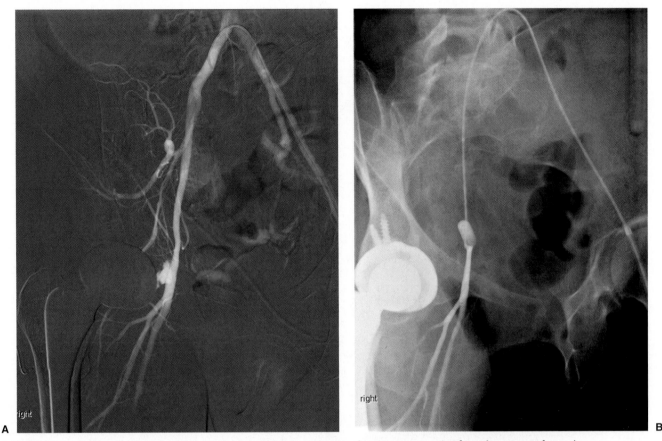

A   B

FIGURE 12.17. Balloon tamponade above arterial tear. **A:** Pelvic angiogram showing extravasation from the common femoral artery following inadvertent puncture during hip replacement. **B:** Balloon occlusion of external iliac artery proximal to common femoral laceration shows no extravasation. This allowed patient transfer to the OR for surgical repair of the laceration.

thoracic stent graft is being increasingly used with success in the treatment of acute aortic transection.

Venous Imaging and Interventions

Diagnostic venography is performed in all extremities, as well as centrally, for surgical planning or evaluation of deep venous thrombosis (DVT) when vascular ultrasound is indeterminate. Most venography is performed in conjunction with interventional procedures (placement of central venous catheters, caval filters, and adrenal vein sampling).

Central Venous Access

Central venous catheters are placed for a variety of indications including administration of antibiotics, chemotherapy, and hemodialysis (HD). There are essentially two types of catheters: Tunneled and nontunneled. Tunneling refers to the creation of a subcutaneous tract in which the catheter lies before it enters the vein. The tunnel acts as a physical barrier reducing the incidence of catheter-related infection and also enhancing catheter security. A fibrous cuff is present on tunneled catheters causing a localized fibrotic reaction, stabilizing it within the subcutaneous tissues. The optimal position for placement of the catheter tip is between the mid superior vena cava (SVC) and the right atrium. The right internal jugular vein is the preferred site for these catheters. Use of either subclavian vein as venous access site is not considered appropriate because of the risk of long-term venous stenosis and occlusion. Another type of tunneled venous access is a port device consisting of a subcutaneously implanted reservoir in the chest wall or upper arm to which the catheter is connected. Ports should only be accessed percutaneously with a noncoring needle (Fig. 12.19).

For short-term venous access (less than 90 days) a nontunneled catheter, such as a peripherally inserted central catheter (PICC) is appropriate. A PICC is inserted by direct percutaneous puncture of either arm or forearm veins and advanced under fluoroscopic guidance until the tip lies in the SVC.

Inferior Vena Cava Filters

The purpose of an inferior vena cava (IVC) filter is to prevent PE by trapping clot. Filter placement is indicated

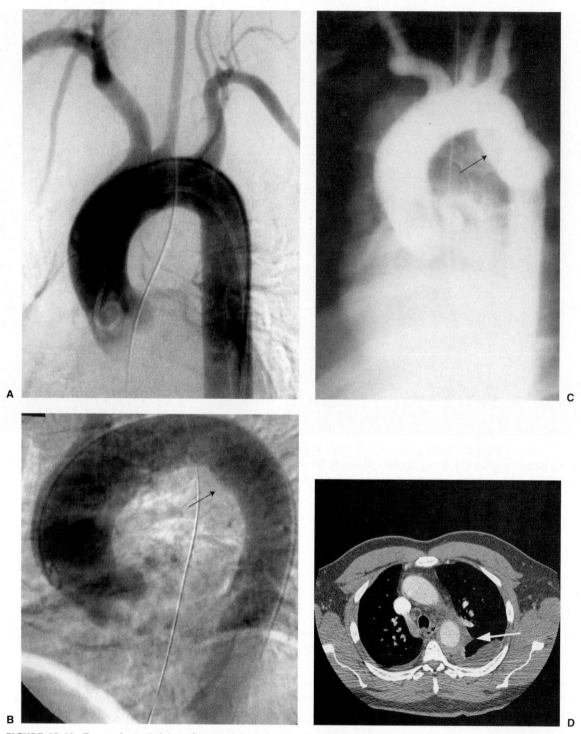

FIGURE 12.18. Traumatic aortic injury. Thoracic aortograms are performed in the left anterior oblique (LAO) view for optimal visualization of the aortic arch. **A:** Normal aortic arch. **B:** Ductus bump, normal variant (*arrow*). **C:** Aortic transection distal to the origin of the left subclavian artery. **D:** This CT scan of the chest shows an intramural hematoma (*arrow*) of the aortic arch consistent with aortic transection.

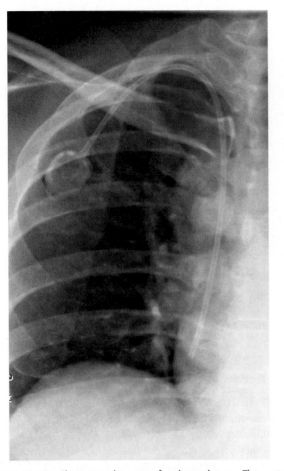

FIGURE 12.19. *Chest port* placement for chemotherapy. The port reservoir is in the infraclavicular subcutaneous tissue. The catheter passes subcutaneously to the right internal jugular vein on its way to the right atrium.

in patients in whom anticoagulation for DVT/PE is contraindicated or ineffective. Currently, there are several types of permanent filters available (Fig. 12.20), all of which are made from either stainless steel or nitinol, an alloy of nickel and titanium, and which are introduced percutaneously through the common femoral or internal jugular vein. The filter depends primarily on its legs to trap clot in the infrarenal IVC reducing the risk of renal vein thrombosis. Retrievable IVC filters may be placed in trauma patients or others at short-term risk of PE. The design of retrievable filters differs from permanent filters in that their legs or struts are more likely to perforate the IVC wall. They also have a hook at the top to facilitate retrieval with a loop snare (Fig. 12.21). These filters should be retrieved as soon as possible after placement in the IVC because of an increased risk of caval perforation and subsequent inability to retrieve them safely (Fig. 12.22). If the indication for filter placement remains at the end of this time then the filter may either be exchanged or replaced with a permanent filter.

Venous Thrombolysis

Deep venous thrombosis can be treated using catheter-directed thrombolysis in a manner similar to arterial thrombolysis. Complete thrombolysis may take several days of continuous thrombolytic infusion. An underlying venous stenosis can be subsequently treated with balloon angioplasty and stent placement (Fig. 12.23).

Hemodialysis Access Interventions

At the end of 2009, almost 400,000 End Stage Renal Disease (ESRD) patients were being treated with some form

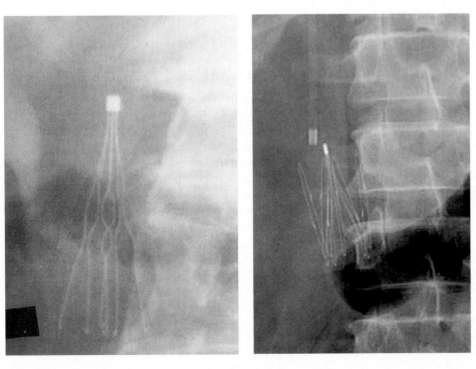

FIGURE 12.20. Permanent inferior vena cava filters. **A:** Greenfield filter. **B:** Braun Venatech filter (which has side struts to prevent tilt).

A

B

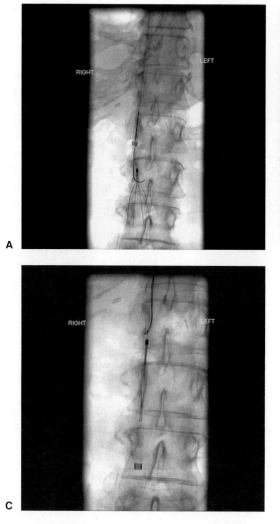

FIGURE 12.21. IVC filter retrieval. **A:** Under fluoroscopy a retrieval snare has been advanced from the right internal jugular vein to the retrievable IVC filter. **B:** The snare is then used to retrieve the filter by its hook and the filter is collapsed by advancing a sheath (*arrow at tip of sheath*) down over it. **C:** The snared filter and sheath are then removed from the internal jugular vein access site.

of dialysis in the United States, the vast majority of whom were getting HD. Vascular access is a generic description where blood is removed from and returned to the body during HD. A vascular access may be an AV fistula (56% of patients on HD), an AV graft (36%), or a catheter (18%). An AV fistula is the preferred type of vascular access because it is associated with fewer complications such as infection and clotting. Catheters have the highest rate of infection compared with other access types. The Fistula First Breakthrough Initiative is dedicated to improving care for people with chronic kidney disease by increasing AV fistula placement and use in suitable HD patients. Surgically created AV fistulae should be 6 mm in diameter, less than 6-mm deep, have flow rates of 600 mL/min at 6 weeks (rule of 6's). However, 25% of all AV fistulae fail to mature, mostly because of stenosis and competing accessory veins which may successfully be treated with balloon angioplasty and coil embolization respectively.

Using the percutaneous skills described above, including thrombolysis, angioplasty, and stent placement, HD access (AV) fistulae and grafts are declotted and maintained, preserving graft function and longevity. Proper

graft or fistula maintenance can add many years to the life of an HD-dependent patient.

NONVASCULAR INTERVENTION

Image-Guided Biopsy

Biopsy allows the retrieval of cells or tissue for a pathologic diagnosis and usually involves the percutaneous introduction of a needle under image guidance (usually ultrasound or CT). Image guidance ensures a safe needle trajectory and sufficient material for analysis. As with all percutaneous interventions, bleeding is a risk, so the patient should discontinue their anticoagulants and have a platelet count above 50,000. There are two types of biopsy needles, Fine and Core. As its name suggests a fine needle has a narrow diameter (23G or 25G) and most often yields an aspirate, suitable for cytology (Fig. 12.24A). Core needles are bigger and acquire their sample using a spring-loaded cutting mechanism yielding a core of tissue, for example, liver (Fig. 12.24B).

Thyroid

Thyroid nodules occur in almost 50% of adults and the majority of these are benign but this determination can

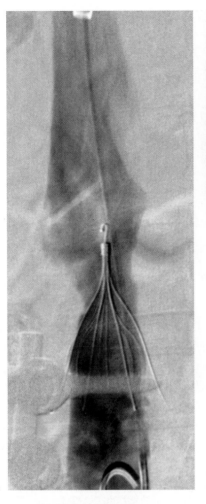

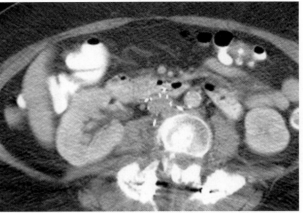

FIGURE 12.22. Complication of temporary IVC filter. **A:** Inferior vena cavography shows perforation of the IVC wall by legs of a temporary IVC filter. **B:** CT abdomen confirms perforation of the IVC.

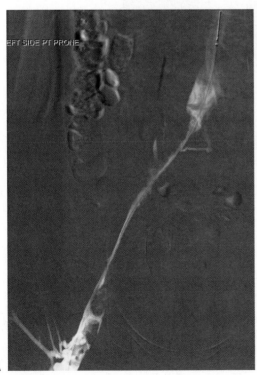

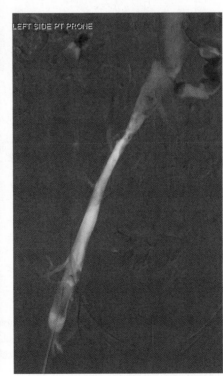

FIGURE 12.23. Venous thrombolysis in a patient May–Thurner syndrome. **A:** Pelvic venogram with the patient in the prone position shows extensive thrombosis of the left iliofemoral venous system across which an infusion catheter has been placed for thrombolysis. **B:** Follow-up venography after 24 hours shows partial resolution of the clot. (*continued*)

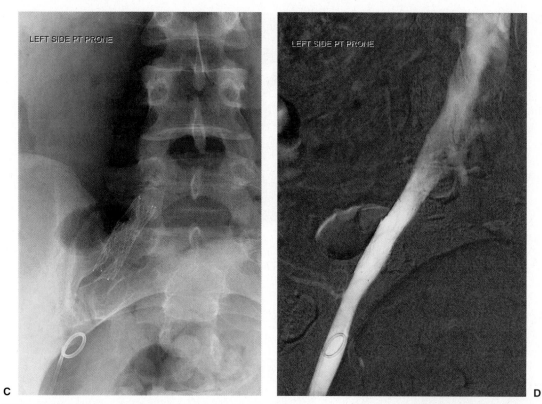

C

D

FIGURE 12.23. (*Continued*) **C,D:** At 48 hours there is complete resolution of the iliofemoral clot and a self-expanding stent has been placed to treat the underlying venous stenosis which was due to external compression of the left common iliac vein by the common iliac artery.

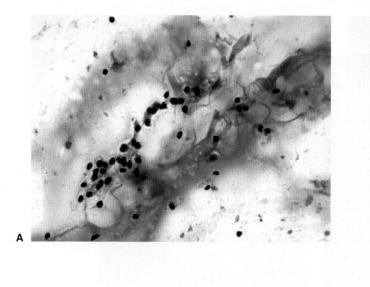

A

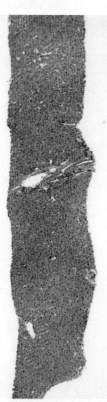

FIGURE 12.24. Biopsy specimens. **A:** Cytology specimen obtained using a fine needle. Note details of the individual cells are visible. **B:** Core liver biopsy specimen shows tissue rather than individual cells.

B

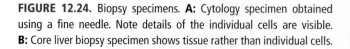

<table>
<tr><td>Table 12.5</td></tr>
</table>

Patients with a High Risk of Thyroid Carcinoma*ª*

History of thyroid cancer in one or more first-degree
relatives

History of external beam radiation as a child

Exposure to ionizing radiation in childhood or
adolescence

Prior hemithyroidectomy with discovery of thyroid
cancer

^{18}FDG avidity on PET scanning

*ª*Biopsy is indicated in any patient with a 5-mm or greater thyroid
nodule and a high-risk history (American Thyroid Association).

only be made pathologically by reviewing cells aspirated
using a fine needle (23G or 25G) inserted into the nodule
under US guidance. Generally US-guided biopsy is not
indicated in nodules less than 10 mm unless there is a
history of high risk of thyroid carcinoma (Table 12.5).

Lung

Biopsy may be done under CT or less commonly US guided
if adjacent to the pleura. There is a 10% to 15% risk of
pneumothorax. A fine needle aspirate (FNA) is usually sufficient to distinguish small cell from nonsmall cell carcinoma (NSLC). However, with the advent of biologic chemotherapeutic agents such as tyrosine-kinase inhibitors,
measurement of biomarkers requires more tissue and this
is best achieved with a core biopsy. Transbronchial biopsy
is used to obtain random parenchymal tissue samples and
is helpful in confirming the diagnosis of sarcoid.

Liver

The two main reasons for liver biopsy are diffuse parenchymal diseases such as Hepatitis and Cirrhosis and focal
abnormalities such as malignancy which may be primary
(hepatoma) or secondary (metastases). A core biopsy is
necessary for evaluation of the parenchyma and this is usually done percutaneously. The presence of ascites, low platelet count, or prolonged Prothrombin Time (which are all
features of chronic liver disease) increases the risk of bleeding with percutaneous liver biopsy. An alternative biopsy
technique involves advancing a long-core biopsy needle to
the right hepatic vein from the right internal jugular vein
and via the right atrium. After the liver tissue adjacent to the
right hepatic vein is biopsied using this transjugular technique, any bleeding that occurs will be intravascular
(hepatic vein) reducing the risk of significant complication.

Kidney

Similar to liver biopsies, core biopsies are used in the diagnosis of parenchymal renal diseases such as glomerulone-
phritis. FNA may be sufficient for lesions such as carcinoma or metastases. The main risk associated with core
biopsy is bleeding (Fig. 12.25).

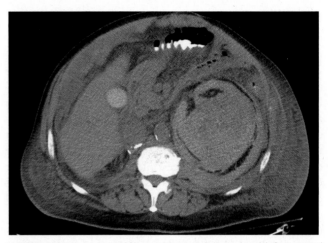

FIGURE 12.25. Post renal biopsy. CT scan shows a large left perirenal
hematoma following core needle renal biopsy.

Lymphoma or metastatic carcinoma may present as
retroperitoneal adenopathy. CT-guided biopsy of these
nodes may be done with the patient in the prone position
(Fig. 12.26). The technique is well tolerated and risk of
bleeding is low.

Urologic Interventions

Percutaneous nephrostomy is a valuable tool in the treatment of urinary obstruction, which is most commonly
caused by calculi, neoplasms, or benign strictures. With
the patient in the prone position, the obstructed renal pelvis is accessed using the Seldinger technique during which
an 8F or 10F pigtail drainage catheter is passed over a
guidewire and the loop formed and secured in the renal
pelvis. Further intervention such as ureteral stenting or
stone removal (nephrolithotomy) may be performed
through this percutaneous renal access. Mild hematuria is
not uncommon after percutaneous nephrostomy and usually resolves within 72 hours.

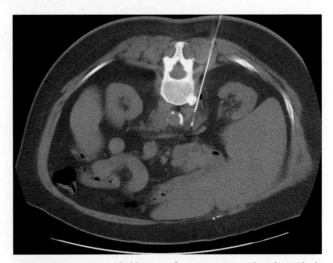

FIGURE 12.26. CT-guided biopsy of a retroperitoneal node. With the
patient in the prone position, a right paraspinal approach is used to
advance a core biopsy needle in to a right para-aortic lymph node. The
diagnosis was lymphoma.

Percutaneous Biliary Drainage and Stenting

Obstructive jaundice may be further evaluated by a percutaneous transhepatic cholangiogram (PTC) whereby a long 22G needle is advanced through the liver parenchyma from a site in the eleventh intercostal space in the right midaxillary line or through the left lobe, using a subxiphoid approach and ultrasound guidance. The needle is then slowly withdrawn while injecting contrast to opacify any bile ducts that may have been traversed. Successful PTC is more likely if the ductal system is dilated. Once a bile duct is opacified, a larger (21G or 18G) needle is then used to percutaneously access one of the opacified ducts peripherally. The tract is dilated over a guidewire and an attempt to traverse the biliary obstruction is made, followed by placement of an internal–external biliary drainage catheter to decompress the ductal system. Permanent self-expanding metallic stents may be placed percutaneously or endoscopically when internalized biliary drainage is desired, as in the case of a malignant obstruction. Alternatively, temporary short plastic stents may be placed in the common duct when surgery is planned or in patients with benign strictures.

Percutaneous cholecystostomy (external gallbladder drainage) has become an accepted interim treatment for patients with acute cholecystitis. The gallbladder is accessed percutaneously and the tract dilated over a guidewire, over which a pigtail drainage tube is advanced into the gallbladder and connected to gravity drainage. A tube check after 5 to 7 days may reveal a patent cystic and common duct, at which time the tube is capped pending cholecystectomy after a further 5 to 7 weeks.

Percutaneous Feeding Tubes

Radiologically guided placement of percutaneous gastrostomy and gastrojejunostomy tubes for enteral nutrition has gained widespread acceptance in the management of patients who cannot eat or swallow because of stroke, head injury, and head and neck tumors. The stomach is accessed percutaneously under fluoroscopic guidance using the Seldinger technique and the tract dilated over a guidewire. A 12F or 14F self-retaining pigtail feeding tube is placed over a guidewire and secured within the stomach (Fig. 12.27). If delivery of liquid feeds directly into the small bowel rather than the stomach is preferred, then a gastrojejunostomy tube can be placed in a transgastric fashion as described above and the tip directed through the pylorus to the proximal jejunum.

Regional Oncology Therapy
Radiofrequency Ablation of Tumors

This minimally invasive technique is often used in the treatment of liver, lung, and bone tumors and results in a reduced hospital stay and complication rate. Under CT or ultrasound guidance, a radiofrequency ablation (RFA) needle is percutaneously inserted into the tumor. RFA involves the deposition of energy at 480 kHz causing coagulation necrosis by heating the tissue to 60°C at which temperature cell death occurs (Fig. 12.28). Percutaneous

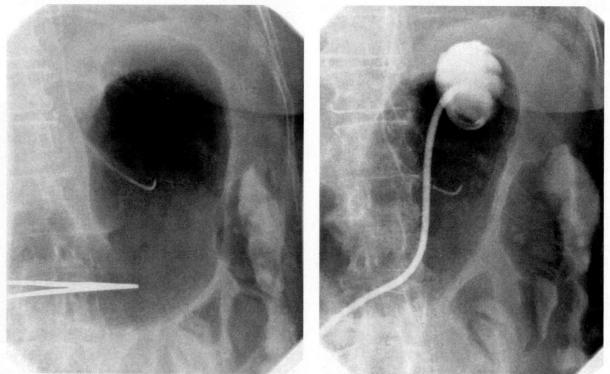

A   B

FIGURE 12.27. Fluoroscopic gastrostomy tube placement. **A:** The stomach is inflated and accessed percutaneously using a Seldinger technique. **B:** The tract is dilated over a guidewire and a 16F feeding tube placed.

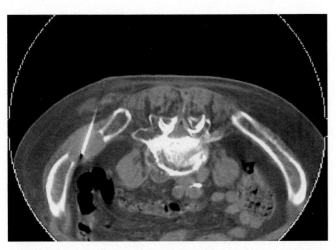

FIGURE 12.28. Radiofrequency ablation. CT pelvis shows a RFA needle in a bony metastasis in the right iliac bone, with the patient in the prone position. The heat generated locally will kill the pain fibers improving the patient's symptoms.

cryoablation which involves freezing, thawing, and refreezing a lesion is preferred for renal masses as there is less risk of urine leak.

Vertebroplasty

In the United States, there are more than 1.5 million osteoporosis-related fractures a year of which 700,000 are vertebral compression fractures. Vertebroplasty is the percutaneous injection of bone cement into a vertebral body fracture thereby stabilizing it and rendering it less painful. With the patient in the prone position and under fluoroscopic guidance an 11G or 13G needle is advanced percutaneously through each pedicle into the vertebral body, where 3 to 5 cc of liquid bone cement is then injected. The cement hardens and stabilizes the fracture, rendering it less painful (Fig. 12.29). A variant of this procedure is kyphoplasty where an attempt to augment the vertebral body height is made by temporarily inflating balloons. Following deflation and removal of the balloons, bone cement is then injected into the recently created cavity.

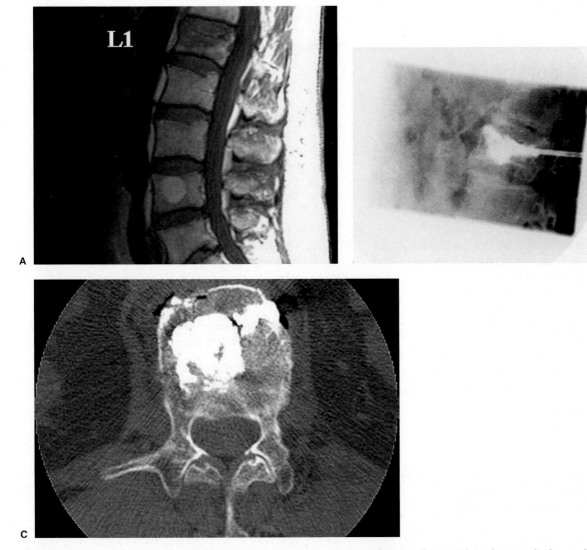

FIGURE 12.29. Vertebroplasty. **A:** MR of lumbar spine shows a compression fracture of L1. **B:** Bilateral transpedicular needle placement and injection of bone cement into the vertebral body. **C:** Postprocedure CT shows cement within the vertebral body.

Key Points

- IR is a specialty of medicine that provides patients diagnostic and therapeutic minimally invasive procedures using imaging guidance.
- Written informed consent is necessary for most angiographic and interventional procedures. The benefits, risks, and possible complications must be discussed with the patient.
- The Seldinger technique describes a method for gaining vascular or visceral access using a needle, a guidewire, and a catheter.
- Most arteriograms are performed via the common femoral artery, which should be punctured over the femoral head.
- Iodinated contrast is nephrotoxic, particularly in patients with diabetes and patients with preexisting renal impairment.

- CT has superseded pulmonary angiography and ventilation–perfusion scintigraphy in the diagnosis of PE. CT is also essential in the diagnostic workup of AAA and their follow-up postendograft placement.
- Some IVC filters are retrievable within 90 days of placement.
- A positive nuclear medicine scan is helpful in patients with GI bleeding because it not only confirms the diagnosis but also directs the angiographer to the site of bleeding.
- Arterial embolization is an important therapy for traumatic vascular injury, GI bleeding, uterine fibroids, and certain tumors.

FURTHER READINGS

Kandarpa K, Machan L. *Handbook of Interventional Radiologic Procedures.* 4th ed. Philadelphia, PA: Lippincott, 2010.

Kaufman J, Lee M. *Vascular and Interventional Radiology: The Requisites.* 1st ed. St. Louis, MO: Mosby, 2003.

QUESTIONS

1. Which of the following types of endoleak is the most common post endovascular repair (EVAR) of abdominal aortic aneurysms (AAA)?
   a. Type 1
   b. Type 2
   c. Type 3
   d. Type 4

2. The most common endoleak post AAA EVAR arises most commonly from which pair of arteries?
   a. Lumbar and inferior mesenteric
   b. Lumbar and superior mesenteric
   c. Inferior mesenteric and median sacral
   d. Inferior mesenteric and internal iliac

Questions 3 to 5: A patient is admitted with acute onset right upper extremity pain and swelling. Venography demonstrates axillosubclavian thrombosis with extensive collateral formation.

3. The most likely underlying cause for this is
   a. Pancoast tumor
   b. trauma
   c. external venous compression due to a rib or muscle at the level of the first rib
   d. external compression due to lymph nodes

4. The initial treatment should include
   a. anticoagulation alone
   b. catheter-directed thrombolysis
   c. surgical resection
   d. thrombectomy
   e. SVC filter placement

5. The preferred definitive treatment is
   a. surgical resection of the first rib
   b. balloon angioplasty of the RT subclavian vein
   c. stent placement in the RT subclavian vein
   d. creation of an arteriovenous fistula

Questions 6 to 9: A patient's chest film shows a peripheral 2-cm solitary lung nodule.

6. Initial workup includes
   a. review of previous imaging
   b. PET scan
   c. wedge resection
   d. transbronchial biopsy

7. Biopsy of this lesion is best accomplished using
   a. PET
   b. CT
   c. MR
   d. bronchoscopy

8. One hour after lung biopsy the patient complains of chest pain and dyspnea. A chest film is obtained and the most likely diagnosis is
   a. flail chest
   b. pneumothorax
   c. hydropneumothorax
   d. pneumopericardium

9. The patient's symptoms worsen and requires oxygen and IV analgesia. The next most appropriate treatment is
   a. more oxygen and analgesia
   b. a chest tube in the second intercostal space, midclavicular line
   c. a chest tube in the fifth intercostal space, midaxillary line
   d. bronchoscopy

10. A patient presents with back pain and weight loss. CT abdomen shows extensive retroperitoneal adenopathy. A biopsy is requested. This is best achieved
    a. by CT guided using a posterior approach
    b. by transjugular route
    c. by CT guided using an anterolateral approach
    d. endoscopically

11. A patient has end-stage renal disease and requires hemodialysis through a tunneled catheter which has recently started to malfunction. The following are likely causes for catheter malfunction except
    a. pericatheter fibrin sheath
    b. catheter thrombosis
    c. catheter malposition
    d. improving renal function

12. A patient is admitted with an upper GI bleed and abdominal distension. Endoscopy reveals esophageal varices which were sclerosed. A CT abdomen shows evidence of portal hypertension. The interventional radiologist refused to do a percutaneous liver biopsy because the patient had
    a. a prolonged prothrombin time
    b. a platelet count of less than 20,000
    c. ascites
    d. all of the above

13. A 35-year-old patient presents hypertension and hypokalemia. Serum aldosterone was elevated and serum renin was low, giving an elevated aldosterone to renin ratio. CT abdomen showed normal adrenal glands. The next appropriate radiology examination would be
    a. renal vein renin sampling
    b. adrenal vein sampling
    c. MRI abdomen with contrast
    d. iodine-131 MIBG scan

14. The following statements regarding the toxicity of Lidocaine are true except the following.
    a. It may present as hyperreflexia
    b. It may present as hyporeflexia
    c. May be treated with IV lipid emulsion
    d. It is not affected by hepatic function

15. Regarding iodinated contrast media, the following are true except
    a. Nonionic contrast media have lower osmolality and tend to have fewer side effects
    b. Allergic or anaphylactoid reactions to contrast are IgE mediated
    c. Pretreatment with steroids reduces the incidence of allergic reactions
    d. Cessation of metformin after contrast administration reduces the incidence of lactic acidosis

Answers

Answers to Chapter 1 Questions

1. c.
2. d.
3. c.
4. a.
5. a.
6. e.
7. b.
8. d.
9. c.
10. c.

Answers to Chapter 2 Questions

1. True.
2. False.
3. True.
4. True.
5. False.
6. False.

Answers to Chapter 3 Questions

1. d.
2. b.
3. d.
4. d.
5. c.
6. a.
7. b.
8. e.
9. b.
10. d.

Answers to Chapter 4 Questions

1a. False.
1b. True.
1c. True.
1d. False.
2a. True.
2b. True.
2c. True.
2d. False.
3a. True.
3b. True.
3c. False.
3d. False.
4a. False.
4b. False.
4c. True.
4d. True.
5a. True.
5b. False.
5c. False.
5d. True.
6a. False.
6b. True.
6c. True.
6d. True.

Answers to Chapter 5 Questions

1. d.
2. False.
3. a.
4. c.
5. False.
6. c.
7. b.
8. d.
9. False.
10. a.

Answers to Chapter 6 Questions

1. b.
2. d.
3. a.
4. c.
5. a.
6. b.
7. c.
8. d.
9. c.
10. b.

Answers to Chapter 7 Questions

1a. True.
1b. True.
1c. False.
1d. True.
2a. True.
2b. False.
2c. False.
2d. True.
3a. True.
3b. False.
3c. True.
3d. False.
4a. True.
4b. True.
4c. False.
4d. True.

Answers to Chapter 8 Questions

1. c.
2. b.
3. c.
4. c.
5. d.
6. a, b, c, d.

Answers to Chapter 9 Questions
1. c.
2. a.
3. c.
4. d.
5. b.
6. b.
7. a.
8. c.
9. d.
10. b.

Answers to Chapter 10 Questions
1. a.
2. b.
3. a.
4. a.
5. b.
6. d.
7. d.
8. c.
9. d.
10. b.
11. b.

Answers to Chapter 11 Questions
1. b.
2. d.
3. c.
4. d.
5. c.
6. c.
7. a.
8. c.
9. a.
10. d.

Answers to Chapter 12 Questions
1. b.
2. a.
3. c.
4. b.
5. a.
6. a.
7. b.
8. b.
9. b.
10. a.
11. d.
12. d.
13. b.
14. d.
15. b.

Index

Note: Page numbers followed by f denote figure; page numbers followed by t denote table.